Handbook of Diagnostic Endocrinology

Contemporary Endocrinology

P. Michael Conn, Series Editor

Androgens in Health and Disease, edited by Carrie Bagatell and William J. Bremner, 2003
Endocrine Replacement Therapy in Clinical Practice, edited by A. Wayne Meikle, 2003
Early Diagnosis and Treatment of Endocrine Disorders, edited by Robert S. Bar, 2003
Type I Diabetes: Etiology and Treatment, edited by Mark A. Sperling, 2003
Handbook of Diagnostic Endocrinology, edited by Janet E. Hall and Lynnette K. Nieman, 2003
Pediatric Endocrinology: A Practical Clinical Guide, edited by Sally Radovick and Margaret H. MacGillivray, 2003
Diseases of the Thyroid, 2nd ed., edited by Lewis E. Braverman, 2003
Developmental Endocrinology: From Research to Clinical Practice, edited by Erica A. Eugster and Ora Hirsch Pescovitz, 2002
Osteoporosis: Pathophysiology and Clinical Management, edited by Eric S. Orwoll and Michael Bliziotes, 2002
Challenging Cases in Endocrinology, edited by Mark E. Molitch, 2002
Selective Estrogen Receptor Modulators: Research and Clinical Applications, edited by Andrea Manni and Michael F. Verderame, 2002
Transgenics in Endocrinology, edited by Martin Matzuk, Chester W. Brown, and T. Rajendra Kumar, 2001
Assisted Fertilization and Nuclear Transfer in Mammals, edited by Don P. Wolf and Mary Zelinski-Wooten, 2001
Adrenal Disorders, edited by Andrew N. Margioris and George P. Chrousos, 2001
Endocrine Oncology, edited by Stephen P. Ethier, 2000
Endocrinology of the Lung: Development and Surfactant Synthesis, edited by Carole R. Mendelson, 2000
Sports Endocrinology, edited by Michelle P. Warren and Naama W. Constantini, 2000
Gene Engineering in Endocrinology, edited by Margaret A. Shupnik, 2000
Endocrinology of Aging, edited by John E. Morley and Lucretia van den Berg, 2000
Human Growth Hormone: Research and Clinical Practice, edited by Roy G. Smith and Michael O. Thorner, 2000
Hormones and the Heart in Health and Disease, edited by Leonard Share, 1999
Menopause: Endocrinology and Management, edited by David B. Seifer and Elizabeth A. Kennard, 1999
The IGF System: Molecular Biology, Physiology, and Clinical Applications, edited by Ron G. Rosenfeld and Charles T. Roberts, Jr., 1999
Neurosteroids: A New Regulatory Function in the Nervous System, edited by Etienne-Emile Baulieu, Paul Robel, and Michael Schumacher, 1999
Autoimmune Endocrinopathies, edited by Robert Volpé, 1999
Hormone Resistance Syndromes, edited by J. Larry Jameson, 1999
Hormone Replacement Therapy, edited by A. Wayne Meikle, 1999
Insulin Resistance: The Metabolic Syndrome X, edited by Gerald M. Reaven and Ami Laws, 1999
Endocrinology of Breast Cancer, edited by Andrea Manni, 1999
Molecular and Cellular Pediatric Endocrinology, edited by Stuart Handwerger, 1999
Gastrointestinal Endocrinology, edited by George H. Greeley, Jr., 1999

Handbook of Diagnostic Endocrinology

Edited by

Janet E. Hall, MD

Massachusetts General Hospital, Boston, MA

and

Lynnette K. Nieman, MD

National Institute of Child Health and Human Development, National Institutes of Health, Bethesda, MD

SPRINGER SCIENCE+BUSINESS MEDIA, LLC

Originally published by Humana Press Inc. in 2003
Softcover reprint of the hardcover 1st edition 2003

This publication is printed on acid-free paper. ∞
ANSI Z39.48-1984 (American National Standards Institute)
Permanence of Paper for Printed Library Materials.

Production Editor: Robin B. Weisberg
Cover Design: Patricia Cleary

10 9 8 7 6 5 4 3 2 1

Handbook of diagnostic endocrinology /edited by Janet E. Hall and Lynnette K. Nieman.
p. ; cm.—(Contemporary endocrinology)
Includes bibliographical references and index.
ISBN 978-1-61737-172-1 ISBN 978-1-59259-293-7 (eBook)
DOI 10.1007/978-1-59259-293-7
1. Endocrine glands—Diseases—Diagnosis—Handbooks, manuals, etc. I. Hall, Janet E.
II. Nieman, Lynnette, K. III. Contemporary endocrinology (Totowa, NJ).
[DNLM: 1. Endocrine Diseases—diagnosis. 2. Diagnostic Techniques, Endocrine. WK 140 H236 2003]
RC649 .H298 2003
616.4'075—dc21 2002032870

Preface

The aim of the *Handbook of Diagnostic Endocrinology* is to provide a comprehensive overview of current approaches to the diagnosis of endocrine disorders. Our ability to diagnose patients with diseases of the endocrine systems is expanding exponentially with the development of new and more reliable assay methods and the incorporation of both molecular and genetic approaches into our understanding of the pathophysiology of these diseases. Although the primary focus of this volume is on the diagnosis of endocrine disease, the vast majority of endocrine diseases require long-term management; therefore, many of the chapters also discuss approaches to follow-up in these patients.

The *Handbook of Diagnostic Endocrinology* comprises 16 chapters. Immunoassays have long been the cornerstones of endocrine diagnoses. As an important background, Sabrina Gill, Frances Hayes, and Patrick Sluss discuss the many methodological advances that have expanded our repertoire of diagnostic tests. With the increased number of tests available for endocrine evaluation, it is incumbent that we understand the factors that affect assay performance and their impact on our ability to use these tools to aid in clinical diagnosis. Joseph Verbalis reviews the regulatory mechanisms underlying water and sodium metabolism and presents a comprehensive approach to disorders of body fluids, which are among the most commonly encountered problems in clinical medicine. Mary Lee Vance outlines the diagnosis and long-term followup of patients presenting with pituitary tumors, and Lynnette Nieman provides an approach to the diagnosis and differential diagnosis of Cushing's syndrome that includes a critical appraisal of available tests. Although endocrine causes of hypertension occur in only 10% of hypertensive subjects, this small fraction represents a large number of patients. Jennifer Lawrence and Robert Dluhy present a thoughtful and efficient approach to the diagnosis of these disorders. Anastassios Pittas and Stephanie Lee then update the approach to the diagnosis of thyroid disease, including an important discussion of currently available assays. Regina Castro and Hossein Gharib present a cost-effective approach to evaluation of the common problem of thyroid nodules and discuss the preoperative evaluation and postoperative followup of patients with thyroid cancer. Allison Goldfine provides an overview of the diagnosis of the various forms of diabetes and a comprehensive discussion of long-term monitoring of the primary disease and its complications. Robert Ratner reviews the important area of gestational diabetes, both its diagnosis and consequences, and John Service presents a clear approach to the diagnosis of hypoglycemia. William Donahoo, Elizabeth Stephens, and

Robert Eckel provide a thorough discussion of the modalities that are currently available for the assessment of dyslipidemia and obesity. Benjamin Leder and Joel Finkelstein then review calcium metabolism and present a logical approach to the diagnosis of hyper- and hypocalcemia. Patrick Doran and Sundeep Khosla discuss the spectrum of osteoporosis and an approach to diagnosis and long-term followup based on the currently available tools. Margaret Wierman reviews the normal physiology of the hypothalamic–pituitary–testicular axis and the physiology of erection, both of which are critical to the approach to evaluation of hypogonadism and erectile dysfunction. Drew Tortoriello and Janet Hall then discuss the physiology of normal menstrual function as a backdrop to their approach to the evaluation and long-term followup of women with disorders of menstrual function. Ricardo Azziz completes this volume with a practical and focused discussion of the evaluation of androgen excess in women.

In *Handbook of Diagnostic Endocrinology* we provide the reader with a concise approach to the diagnosis of endocrine disorders that is based on an understanding of their pathophysiology and includes both clinical manifestations and the most current laboratory tests available. This work will serve as a reference for students and fellows in training as well as an update for practicing endocrinologists and internists.

We thank the contributors to this volume, without whose expertise and efforts this work would not be possible.

***Janet E. Hall,* MD**
***Lynnette K. Nieman,* MD**

Contents

Contributors

Ricardo Azziz, md, mph, mba, *Department of Obstetrics and Gynecology, Cedars-Sinai Medical Center, Los Angeles, CA*

M. Regina Castro, md, *Department of Medicine and Endocrinology, Albany Medical College, Stratton VA Medical Center, Albany, NY*

Robert G. Dluhy, md, *Division of Endocrinology-Hypertension, Brigham and Women's Hospital, Boston, MA*

William T. Donahoo, md, *Division of Endocrinology, Metabolism and Diabetes, University of Colorado Health Sciences Center, Denver, CO*

Patrick M. Doran, md, *Division of Endocrinology, McGill University Health Center, Montreal, Canada*

Robert H. Eckel, md, *Division of Endocrinology, Metabolism and Diabetes, University of Colorado Health Sciences Center, Denver, CO*

Joel S. Finkelstein, md, *Division of Endocrinology, Massachusetts General Hospital, Boston, MA*

Hossein Gharib, md, face, *Division of Endocrinology and Metabolism, Mayo Clinic and Mayo Foundation, Rochester, MN*

Sabrina Gill, md, *Division of Endocrinology and Metabolism, St. Paul's Hospital, Vancouver BC, Canada*

Allison B. Goldfine, md, *Research Division, Joslin Diabetes Center, Boston, MA*

Janet E. Hall, md, *Reproductive Endocrine Unit, Division of Endocrinology, Massachusetts General Hospital, Boston, MA*

Frances J. Hayes, md, *Reproductive Endocrine Unit, Division of Endocrinology, Massachusetts General Hospital, Boston, MA*

Sundeep Khosla, md, *Division of Endocrinology and Metabolism, Mayo Clinic, Rochester, MN*

Jennifer E. Lawrence, md, *Valdosta Specialty Clinic, Valdosta, GA*

Benjamin Z. Leder, md, *Division of Endocrinology, Massachusetts General Hospital, Boston, MA*

Stephanie L. Lee, md, *Division of Endocrinology, Diabetes and Metabolism, Boston Medical Center, Boston, MA*

Lynnette K. Nieman, md, *Pediatric and Reproductive Endocrinology Branch, National Institute of Child Health and Human Development, National Institutes of Health, Bethesda, MD*

Anastassios G. Pittas, md, *Division of Endocrinology, Diabetes, Metabolism and Molecular Medicine, New England Medical Center, Boston, MA*

Robert E. Ratner, MD, *MedStar Research Institute, Washington, DC*
F. John Service, MD, PhD, *Division of Endocrinology and Internal Medicine, Mayo Clinic, Rochester, MN*
Patrick M. Sluss, PhD, *Reproductive Endocrine Unit, Division of Endocrinology, Massachusetts General Hospital, Boston, MA*
Elizabeth Stephens, MD, *Division of Endocrinology, Diabetes, and Clinical Nutrition, Oregon Health and Science University, Portland, OR*
Drew V. Tortoriello, MD, *Department of Obstetrics and Gynecology, Columbia Presbyterian Medical Center, New York, NY*
Mary Lee Vance, MD, *Division of Endocrinology, University of Virginia Health Services Center, Charlottesville, VA*
Joseph G. Verbalis, MD, *Division of Endocrinology and Metabolism, Georgetown University School of Medicine, Washington, DC*
Margaret E. Wierman, MD, *Division of Endocrinology, Veterans Affairs Medical Center, University of Colorado School of Medicine, Denver, CO*

1 Issues in Endocrine Immunoassay

Sabrina Gill, MD, *Frances J. Hayes*, MD,
and *Patrick M. Sluss*, PhD

Contents

INTRODUCTION

Over the past 30 years, immunoassays have become a valuable and widely available tool among the repertoire of clinical methods to assess hormonal function *(1,2)*. The majority of hormonal proteins and steroids are bioactive at extremely low concentrations in the peripheral circulation, and hormone metabolites often play a significant physiological role at target tissue sites. Therefore, evaluation of a patient's endocrine status with a given immunoassay is dependent upon both the sensitivity and specificity of that assay. Hormone levels outside a given reference range can indicate a pathologic disease process. When clinical decisions regarding a patient's hormonal status or their response to a therapeutic intervention are based on hormone testing, it is important that due consideration be given to issues relating to the validity and utility of the assay.

In practice, the performance of an immunoassay can be influenced by a variety of physiological, pre-analytical and analytical factors, which may result in deviation from the "true" value, i.e., that which reflects the actual physiological status of the patient. Indeed, it is important to bear in mind that the clinical definition of a "true" value for many hormones is relative only to the reference ranges established for the individual assay methods. Furthermore, these issues often vitiate the ability to compare values generated by different laboratories.

From: *Contemporary Endocrinology: Handbook of Diagnostic Endocrinology*
Edited by: J. E. Hall and L. K. Nieman © Humana Press Inc., Totowa, NJ

The intent of this chapter is to provide the reader with an appreciation of how an endocrine immunoassay can be an effective tool provided that the methods are carefully chosen, monitored, and applied in the appropriate clinical setting.

CURRENT IMMUNOASSAY METHODS

Principles

Immunoassays were originally developed as competitive binding assays that utilized immunoglobulins as the binding protein. The first clinically important immunoassay developed for hormones was the radioimmunoassay (RIA). RIA is designed to utilize the competition, between hormone tagged with radioisotopes (the antigen) and unlabeled hormone in the patient specimen, for binding to a limited number of antibodies generated against that hormone *(3,4)*. After incubating the unlabeled specimens and standards (samples of known concentration of a hormone) with assay reagents (antibody, radiolabeled hormone, buffer, and stabilizers), the amount of radiolabeled hormone bound to the antibody is measured. The more unlabeled hormone present in the mixture, the less radiolabeled hormone will be bound to the antibody. The standards provide a calibration for the amount of bound radiolabeled hormone across a range of known hormone concentrations, thereby allowing for interpretation of the assay results in terms of clinically relevant hormone levels *(5,6)*.

The accuracy of the RIA depends on the ability to separate antibody-bound from unbound reagents, particularly the radiolabeled antigen being measured. A variety of methods can be used to separate bound from unbound hormone after the competitive binding has occurred. Historically, methods were used to precipitate the bound antibody and separate the unbound reagents by centrifugation *(7)*. With the development of automated immunoassay systems, the antibody is attached to solid materials, such as glass or latex beads, paramagnetic particles, or plastic surfaces of tubes or small reagent cups *(8–10)*. The antibody can be immobilized to a solid material either directly, attaching to the surface during the binding reaction, or indirectly, after the binding reaction has been completed. While the principle of the assay is the same in either case, there are significant design differences in these two approaches attributable to the kinetic relationships between the reagents *(11,12)*. Assays using indirect immobilization of the antibody to a solid surface (for example, biotinylated antibody to avidin-coated surfaces) are analogous to RIAs, differing only in the method of separation. In contrast, in assays in which the antibody binds to the solid material during the binding reaction, significant differences are observed in the kinetic properties of the antibody in solution vs attached to the solid material. These assays are designed to present an excess amount of antibody in order to maximize hormone binding both in solution and when immobilized to a solid surface. Such systems are referred to as immunoradiometric assays (IRMA), rather than RIA, to emphasize the differences between the design of these two approaches. In both cases, the amount of hormone present in a patient specimen is determined by comparing the amount of radioactive hormone bound to antibody in the specimen and in the standards. In addition to the standards and patient specimens, assays also include quality control specimens, which are standardized concentrations of hormone that are tested in every assay to confirm its accuracy and precision.

While RIA is still considered a "gold standard" in reference laboratories, it has now been largely replaced by more rapid, nonisotopic methods, primarily enzyme-linked immunosorbent assays (ELISAs). There are many different design strategies used for ELISAs *(2,13,14)*. Early forms utilized competition between hormone tagged with enzyme and unlabeled hormone. This design is analogous to RIA but substitutes enzyme activity for radioactivity for hormone detection. Enzyme activity is detected by washing away unbound reactants and then incubating the antibody–hormone complex with a substrate that produces a light-absorbing product. More recently, substrates that produce chemiluminescence upon enzymatic digestion have also been used effectively *(15)*. Enzyme turnover is then measured in a spectrophotometer or luminometer and is directly proportional to the amount of enzyme-linked hormone that is bound. As in RIA, the amount of labeled hormone is inversely proportional to the unlabeled hormone in the standards and unknown specimens.

Immunometric immunoassays have now found widespread clinical utility, primarily for measurement of protein hormones. These assays utilize multiple antibody systems based on noncompetitive, e.g., "immunometric" designs *(12)*. In these systems, it is not necessary for the hormone to be chemically manipulated by labeling with radioactivity or enzyme. Instead, endogenous hormone is captured with one antibody and quantitatively detected with another, which is chemically labeled with radioisotope (IRMA), enzyme, or luminescent chemicals, such as acrydinium esters. The amount of detection antibody bound is directly proportional to the amount of antigen captured and can be used to generate dose–response curves for assay standards. As with all immunoassays, the concentration of hormone in patient specimens is determined by comparing patient results to the dose–response curves developed from the assay standards.

Selected Survey of Current Methods

Commercially available systems with different methodologies in endocrine immumodiagnostics are widely used in clinical laboratories today (Table 1). The trend over the past decade has been toward automated nonisotopic systems. Automated systems not only decrease the turn-around time for laboratory results, but also support larger testing volumes and test menus. In addition, the overall cost of testing is reduced, as reportable results can be obtained efficiently with

Table 1
Overview of Selected Current Methods for Hormone Immunoassay

Instrument	*Manufacturer*	*Operation*	*Design* *Separation Method*[a]	*Design* *Detection Method*[b]
Reagent Kits				
	DPC	Manual	CT	R
	DSL	Manual	P, CT, CW	R, C
	Linco	Manual	P, CW	R, C
	Serotec	Manual	CW	C
Automated Systems				
Architect	Abbott	Continuous Access	MP	EL
AxSYM	Abbott	Continuous Access	PF	EL
IMx	Abbott	Batch	PF	EL
ACS180	Bayer	Continuous Access	MP	L
Centaur	Bayer	Continuous Access	MP	L
Immuno 1	Bayer	Continuous Access	MP	L
Access	Beckman	Continuous Access	MP	C
Immulite	DPC	Batch	CB	EL
Immulite 2000	DPC	Continuous Access	CB	EL
Advantage	Nichols	Continuous Access	MP	L. EL
Viros Eci	Ortho	Continuous Access	CW	EL
Elecsys	Roche	Continuous Access	MP	L

[a]*Codes:* CB, coated-bead; CT, coated-tube; CW, coated-well; MP, magnetic particle; P, precipitation; PF, particle-filtration.

[b]*Codes:* C, colorometric enzyme-linked immunoassay; EL, enzyme-chemiluminescent immunoassay, L, chemiluminescent immunoassay; R, radioimmunoassay.

less technical expertise. Reagent kits still, however, play a key role where highly specific tests for closely related proteins are required or when highly sensitive immunoassays are needed for analytical characterization of relatively small numbers of specimens in specialist chemistry laboratories.

IMMUNOASSAY ISSUES RELATED TO PHYSIOLOGICAL VARIATION

Overview

Perhaps the greatest challenge associated with use of immunoassays to assess endocrine status is the dynamic change in peripheral hormone concentrations. Hormone regulation involves an interplay of feed-forward and feedback interactions at different levels of the hypothalamic-pituitary-target organ axes. Interpretation of immunoassay measurements thus requires an appreciation of the dynamic nature of hormonal secretion and must be based upon appropriate reference ranges. In addition, immunoassays may vary based on differences in the nature of protein biosynthesis and hormone metabolism, dictating that only method-specific comparisons be made.

Biosynthesis of Protein Hormones

The biosynthesis, secretion, and clearance of hormones all contribute to the physiologic variation in their serum concentration across time and between normal individuals. Gonadotropin hormones provide a clear, albeit extreme, example. Gonadotropins are dimeric glycoprotein hormones composed of an α- and β-subunit. The gene for the α-subunit is expressed in both thyrotrope and gonadotrope cells and directs the synthesis of an α-subunit protein, which can be secreted free (free α-subunit) or complexed with one of three β-subunits. Gonadotropes express genes for the β-subunits of both luteinizing hormone (LH) and follicle-stimulating hormone (FSH), while thyrotropes express a gene for the synthesis of the thyroid-stimulating hormone (TSH) β-subunit. The bioactivity of glycoprotein hormones is determined by the β-subunit. Thus, a dimer composed of α-subunit complexed with a FSH β-subunit has FSH bioactivity, while the same α-subunit complexed with the TSH β-subunit has TSH bioactivity.

The α-subunit gene is also expressed in the placenta, where it can be secreted as either the free α-subunit or as the dimeric protein hormone human chorionic gonadotropin (hCG), in which it complexes with the hCG β-subunit. The β-subunits of hCG and LH closely resemble each other sharing 97 of 121 amino acids. Indeed, hCG expresses many LH-like activities at target tissues.

α- and β-subunit proteins are subject to posttranslational processing by glycosylation and proteolysis, both of which are well known to influence immunoassay measurements. Both subunits are glycosylated, resulting in a multitude of isoforms of each hormone, which differ in both the number and type of sugar moieties attached. Proteolytic enzymatic activity, either prior to or after secretion into the peripheral blood, can result in additional isoforms of these hormones, which can be either nicked (broken but still complexed into a dimeric protein) or truncated (protein sequence missing).

These aspects of the biosynthesis and posttranslational processing of gonadotropins are associated with differences in the specificity and accuracy of all current immunoassays. The presence of a shared α-subunit among gonadotropins, TSH, and hCG results in significant cross-reactivity in immunoassays, which depend on the specificity of the antibody for the α-subunit. Many of the early RIAs utilized polyclonal antibodies, which primarily recognized the α-subunit. Almost all current automated immunoanalyzers utilize at least one monoclonal or polyclonal antibody directed at the α-subunit, often resulting in inconsistent or conflicting results. Similarly, the high degree of structural homology between

Table 2
FSH Levels Measured in the Same Specimen by Different Laboratories Using Various Commercial Immunoassay Systems

Hormone	*Instrument*	*Manufacturer*	*No. Labs*	*Low*	*High*	*Mean*	*SD*	*CV*
FSH	Architect	Abbott	32	28.5	35.9	33.05	1.69	5.1%
	AxSYM	Abbott	561	26.9	38.9	32.63	2.09	6.4%
	Imx	Abbott	28	30.4	35.8	32.82	1.57	4.8%
	ACS180	Bayer	219	38.2	52.5	45.81	2.66	5.8%
	Centaur	Bayer	123	37.6	51.0	44.46	2.31	5.2%
	Immuno 1	Bayer	98	33.4	39.4	36.18	1.30	3.6%
	Access	Beckman	102	32.0	43.1	38.02	2.19	5.8%
	Immulite	DPC	106	33.4	44.4	38.51	2.23	5.8%
	Immulite 2000	DPC	37	31.3	41.3	36.39	2.39	6.6%
	IRMA (CAC)	DPC	14	33.9	39.8	36.12	1.70	4.7%
	Elecsys	Roche	49	32.8	47.0	38.91	3.60	9.3%
	Eci	Vitros	45	23.8	28.7	25.69	1.22	4.7%
	DELFIA	Wallac	5	26.5	31.2	—	—	

the LH and hCG β-subunits can lead to the inability to distinguish these two proteins in assays, which utilize nonspecific β-directed antibodies *(16)*. In addition, posttranslational processing, by either glycosylation or proteolysis, can alter antigenic epitopes and thus contribute to differences among immunoassays utilizing different, although specific antibodies. Finally, the effects of proteolysis on hCG are notorious for confounding differences among hCG immunoassays *(17)*.

Inaccuracies between methods, attributable at least in part to specificity issues, can be quite substantial *(18)*. For example, results of FSH measurements of an identical specimen (*Ligand–Special Series; August, 2000*) distributed in aliquots to different laboratories by the College of American Pathologists, revealed levels varying by almost 2-fold due to method-based differences in gonadotropin immunoassays of proven clinical utility (Table 2).

Regulated Secretion of Protein and Steroid Hormones

Physiological variation in serum hormone concentrations can significantly impact immunoassay utility. Use of hormonal measurements to assess a patient's physiological status relies upon the reference ranges established for each immunoassay. For many hormones, including growth hormone (GH), adrenocorticotrophic hormone (ACTH), cortisol, and gonadotropins, establishing reference ranges is confounded by their dynamic secretion, such that there is considerable variability from minute-to-minute, day-to-day, and over the lifetime of an individual.

Pulsatility

Neuroendocrine regulation of hormones involves a complex integrated network of feedback mechanisms between the hypothalamus, pituitary, and target organs. In the reproductive axis, gonadotropin-releasing hormone (GnRH) is secreted in a pulsatile fashion by hypothalamic neurons, which in turn stimulates pulsatile secretion of LH and FSH by the gonadotrope cells of the anterior pituitary. In young healthy men, pulses of LH are secreted approx every 120 min, and given this pulsatile secretion, concentrations of LH can vary 3–4-fold *(19)*. In women, there are dynamic changes in the hypothalamic-pituitary-ovarian axis across the menstrual cycle *(20–22)*. LH pulses occur every 90 min in the early follicular phase, increasing to every 60 min in the mid-follicular phase and then, following the mid-cycle LH surge and ovulation, slow progressively to 1 pulse every 4 h in the late luteal phase. Although secretion of most gonadal steroids is apulsatile, progesterone concentrations have been shown to fluctuate rapidly in the luteal phase increasing from 2 to 40 ng/mL within minutes *(22,23)*. Other pituitary hormones, such as GH and TSH, are also secreted in a pulsatile manner, regulated by their respective hypothalamic releasing hormones, growth hormone-releasing hormone (GHRH) and thyrotropin-releasing hormone (TRH), respectively. Such variability in serum hormone levels makes it difficult to interpret a single blood test.

Diurnal and Cyclic Variation in Hormone Levels

The secretion of many hormones, including cortisol, TSH, GH, and prolactin, follows a circadian pattern. The nocturnal rise of TSH begins in the early evening, peaks near midnight, and reaches nadir levels by early morning. Conversely, cortisol levels peak in the morning and decline throughout the day, with lowest levels achieved in the late afternoon–early evening. GH and prolactin concentrations increase at night at the onset of sleep and decline by early morning. Glucose response to food also increases in the evening, which, along with a decline in insulin secretion, results in decreased glucose tolerance in the late evening. An increase in the counter-regulatory hormones at this time of day may contribute to this relative insulin resistance.

During puberty, there is a nocturnal rise in LH pulse frequency and amplitude. In adult men, mean gonadotropin levels remain relatively constant. However, LH pulse patterns may be quite variable in some individuals, resulting in a wide range of testosterone concentrations. In one study, where blood was sampled every 10 min for 24 h, 15% of young healthy men had serum testosterone levels as low as 100 ng/dL documented following long interpulse intervals of LH secretion *(19)*. Testosterone also has a diurnal pattern with levels falling by approx 30% in the late afternoon and peaking in the early morning *(19,24)*.

In women, there are dynamic changes in reproductive hormone levels across the ovulatory menstrual cycle, which typically lasts approx 28 d *(22,25–27)*. LH and FSH levels are relatively low in the follicular and luteal phases, but increase by as much as 10-fold at the time of the mid-cycle surge. Estradiol levels begin to increase in the mid-follicular phase, reaching a peak approx 1 d prior to ovulation. Progesterone, which is secreted by the corpus luteum, reaches a peak in the mid-luteal phase of the cycle approx 7 d prior to menses. The nonsteroidal gonadal peptides, inhibins A and B, are also differentially regulated across the menstrual cycle. Inhibin B levels peak in the early and mid-follicular phase, while inhibin A rises rapidly during the late follicular phase to peak in the luteal phase which is consistent with it being a secretory product of the ovulatory follicle and corpus luteum *(28,29)*. Thus, interpretation of reproductive hormone levels requires a knowledge of normal reproductive physiology and, for women, must be viewed in the context of the time in the menstrual cycle at which the blood was drawn.

Effect of Aging

Although hormone levels fluctuate during childhood and puberty, the pulsatility of many hormones, including GH, TSH, and cortisol, is attenuated with aging *(24)*. In older subjects, there is a decrease in TSH pulse frequency and amplitude with an earlier TSH rise in the afternoon. The nadir in cortisol levels is advanced by 1 to 2 h in older individuals.

Women experience significant fluctuations in their menstrual cycle patterns as they get older *(30)*. After menopause, there is a gradual slowing of GnRH pulse frequency, and mean gonadotropin concentrations in older postmenopausal women are approx 40% lower than younger postmenopausal subjects *(31)*. In addition, the half-lives of LH and FSH are prolonged in postmenopausal women, due to a shift to more acidic isoforms *(32)*. During the perimenopausal transition, peak FSH levels are achieved by d 3, as opposed to d 6 of the cycle, and mean levels are higher than those of younger controls. Follicular phase estradiol levels are also higher in older than younger women, whereas progesterone levels are lower *(33)*.

Unlike menopause, reproductive aging in the male is a gradual process. Serum total testosterone levels begin to decline at the age of 40 yr. Cross-sectional studies suggest an annual decline in total testosterone of 0.4% and in free testosterone of 1.2% *(34)*. The proportionately greater decline in free testosterone could be attributed to the increase in sex hormone-binding globulin (SHBG) that may occur with aging. Furthermore, the diurnal variation in testosterone secretion is attenuated in older men *(24)*.

Clearance and Metabolism of Protein and Steroid Hormones

Factors that alter the metabolism and clearance of hormones are another source of specific interassay and intra-assay variation, with respect to reference ranges. Hormones undergo structural and/or functional changes during metabolism,

Table 3
Estradiol Levels Measured in the Same Specimen by Different Laboratories Using Various Commercial Immunoassay Systems

Hormone	*Instrument*	*Manufacturer*	*No. Labs*	*Low*	*High*	*Mean*	*SD*	*CV*
E2	AxSYM	Abbott	263	318.0	906.0	628.10	138.00	22.0%
	Imx	Abbott	53	614.0	1390.0	885.90	183.90	20.8%
	ACS180	Bayer	66	345.0	499.0	408.40	31.10	7.6%
	Centaur	Bayer	78	340.0	495.0	419.90	30.70	7.3%
	Immuno 1	Bayer	63	701.0	981.0	844.30	50.50	6.0%
	Access	Beckman	46	744.0	994.0	897.10	54.60	6.1%
	Immulite	DPC	129	732.0	997.0	842.30	56.90	6.8%
	Immulite 2000	DPC	44	698.0	920.0	815.10	49.20	6.0%
	IRMA (CAC)	DPC	64	508.0	796.0	650.30	58.50	9.0%
	Elecsys	Roche	41	826.0	1127.0	972.60	77.20	7.9%
	Eci	Vitros	30	737.0	991.0	843.20	55.30	6.6%

which can generate forms that are less biologically active yet still capable of binding antibody. Therefore, different levels of hormone reflect differences in the secretion of the biologically active fraction only if the metabolism and clearance of the hormone remain constant.

Additional complications exist for hormones that circulate bound to binding globulins. These physiological carrier proteins, such as thyroxine-binding globulin (TBG), cortisol-binding globulin (CBG), and SHBG, influence the distribution and biological activity of thyroid hormone, cortisol, and sex steroids, respectively. Issues related to the amount and nature of binding proteins in individual specimens may contribute to methodological differences in immunoassays for these hormones *(35)*. For steroid assays, method to method differences can be quite significant, as illustrated for estradiol measurements in Table 3.

Factors Influencing Interpretation of Hormone Levels

Reference values are established based on multiple measurements of a hormone sampled from a physiologically normal population to determine the range of values above and below which would be deemed abnormal. Many factors, including stress and medications, can interfere with hormone physiology or assay methodology resulting in an inaccurate interpretation of a laboratory value. As these factors may not exist in the population sampled to establish the reference ranges, it is prudent to account for these factors when interpreting hormone levels based on established reference values.

Exercise, emotional stress, and food deprivation can significantly increase catecholamine and cortisol secretion. Stress is also a potent stimulator of prolactin secretion. GH secretion increases in response to exercise and fasting and is decreased in obesity. In women, extreme stress, caloric restriction, and intensive exercise can suppress endogenous GnRH secretion leading to hypothalamic amenorrhea.

Various drugs can interfere with hormone levels in the absence of any glandular dysfunction. Anticonvulsants stimulate the hepatic drug-metabolizing system augmenting the metabolism of hormones, such as cortisol and thyroid hormones. Alterations in the binding affinity or concentrations of binding globulins can alter total hormone concentrations. Estrogen-containing drugs, such as oral contraceptives, can increase TBG and thus total thyroxine levels, while androgens and glucocorticoids decrease TBG concentrations. Drugs, such as dopamine, dobutamine, and glucocorticoids can decrease TSH levels and confound the interpretation of TSH levels.

IMMUNOASSAY ISSUES RELATED TO PRE-ANALYTIC VARIATION

Artifacts associated with the collection, handling, or storage of blood may alter test results by producing changes in the specimen that do not reflect the physiologic state of the patient. Many hormones are very stable in blood or serum as illustrated in Fig. 1. In contrast, some hormones are extremely sensitive to proteolytic degradation, which results in a loss of recognition by antibodies and an underestimation of the true hormone level in blood. For example, insulin is particularly sensitive to degradation by enzymes released from hemolyzed red blood cells, and thus, insulin measurements in hemolyzed specimens are invalid (Fig. 2).

IMMUNOASSAY ISSUES RELATED TO ANALYTIC VARIATION

All immunoassay methods are based upon the ability of antibodies to discriminate among hormones and to bind specific hormones with high affinity. Competitive and immunometric immunoassays are variants of competitive binding assays in which hormone levels in unknown specimens are determined by extrapolating their response to those generated by the assay standards *(36–38)*. The goal is always to obtain a measurement of the hormone that is as close as possible to the true value and, thus, provide an accurate assessment of the patient's endocrine status. Achieving this goal depends on four complementary characteristics of all immunoassays: *(i)* sensitivity; *(ii)* specificity; *(iii)* precision; and *(iv)* accuracy (bias).

Sensitivity

The sensitivity of an immunoassay can be defined in a number of ways *(39)*. However, in all cases, the definition of sensitivity is intended to describe quantitatively either the minimum measurable difference in hormone concentrations

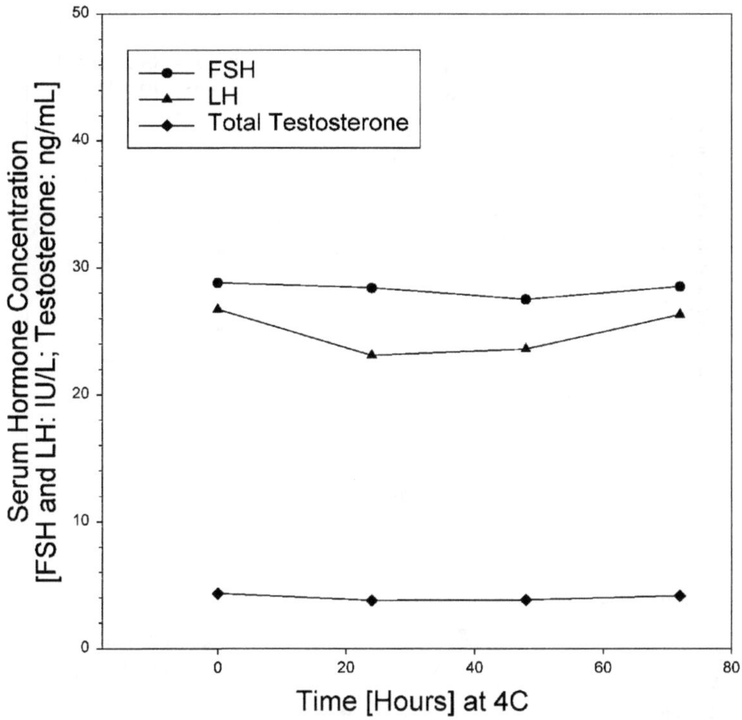

Fig. 1. Pre-analytical stability of hormones.

or the minimum hormone concentration that can be measured (limit of detection). The sensitivity of an immunoassay is system-dependent and a function of the antibody's affinity for the hormone as well as the error associated with repeated measurements (imprecision). As discussed below, the degree of measurement error is dependent not only on intrinsic factors such as the physical properties of liquid handling and detection equipment, but also on the concentration of hormone in the specimen. Classically, the sensitivity of an immunoassay or the relative ability to distinguish measurable concentrations of hormone is based upon the slope of the standard response curve and the precision characteristics of the assay. The clinically useful and more common definition of sensitivity is the minimum amount of hormone that can be measured.

The minimum amount of measurable hormone is generally defined in one of two ways. Analytical sensitivity is often referred to as the limit of detection (LOD), i.e., the lowest concentration that can be distinguished from no hormone. For immunometric assays with a positive dose–response curve, the LOD is the dose equivalent of the upper 95% confidence limit of replicate determinations (usually at least 10) of a "zero" dose standard (Fig. 3). For competitive immunoassays that

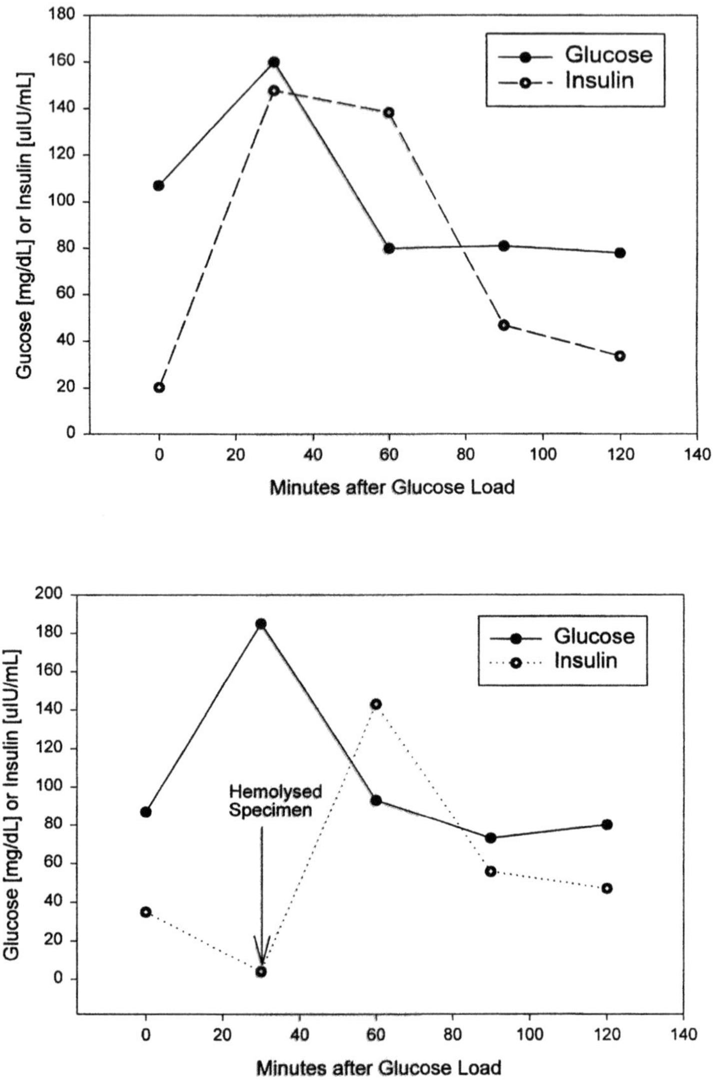

Fig. 2. Effect of pre-analytical hemolysis on insulin measurements.

have a negative dose–response curve, the lower 95% confidence limit is used. Alternatively, the minimum detectable concentration of hormone can be defined based upon the variance of repeated measurements of unknown specimens, referred to as the functional sensitivity or limit of quantitation (LOQ). The LOQ takes into account the fact that the variance of repeated measurements is related to the concentration of hormone being measured and is always nonuniform across the dose–

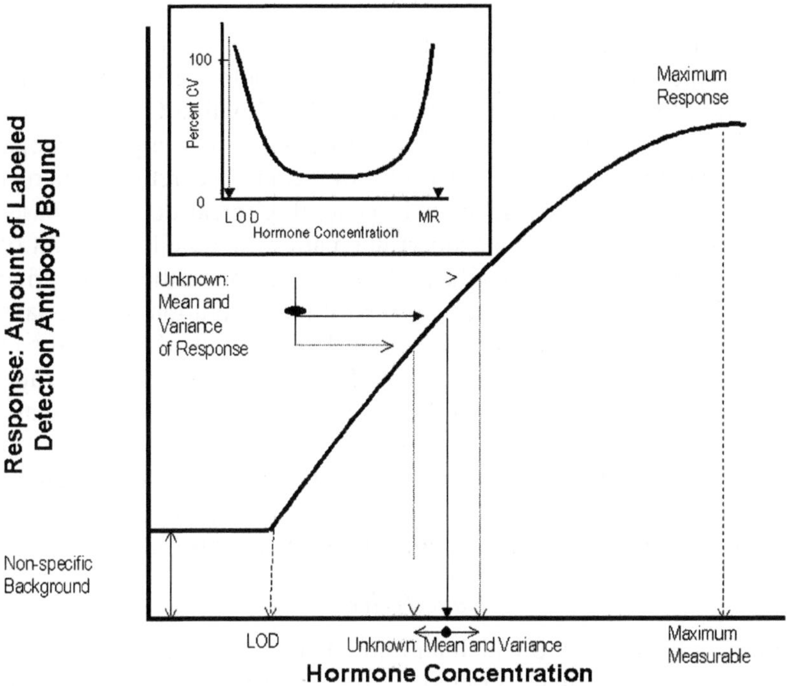

Fig. 3. Principles of immunoassay.

response curve of an immunoassay. Typically, the coefficient of variation (CV), defined as the standard deviation expressed as a percentage of the mean of replicated measurements, is used to represent variance. As shown in the insert of Fig. 3, the CV of repeated measurements is nonuniform across the dose–response curve of an assay. At very low or very high concentrations of hormone, there is no dose–respsonse relationship, and the CV approaches infinity. Thus, a functional sensitivity can be defined as the level associated with a minimally acceptable CV. In the absence of specific clinical requirements for greater precision, a CV of 20% is generally used to define functional sensitivity *(40,41)*.

The range of concentrations between the limit of detection (or functional sensitivity) and the maximum measurable concentration is called the reportable range of the assay. Generally, the maximum measurable concentration is defined based upon an acceptable between-assay variance (see discussion of precision below), and this concentration is chosen as the highest point on the standard curve.

Sensitivity is an important issue with respect to the clinical utility of immunoassays in assessing the endocrine status of an individual. It is important to appreciate that a standard definition of sensitivity does not exist; some assay results are reported based on LOD, while others use LOQ. Whenever measurements of a hormone at concentrations near the lower limits of the assay are required, it is important to know the reproducibility of the measurement. For example, in some estradiol assays, results reported below 40 pg/mL, although well above the LOD of 10 pg/mL, can be associated with a CV of up to 60%. Distinguishing between the upper limit for estradiol levels in postmenopausal women (20–40 pg/mL) from the lower limit of estradiol secretion from ovarian tumors (>50 pg/mL) is quite difficult. In general, clinical decisions based on lower than normal hormone levels are problematic when the lower limit of the normal reference range approaches the LOD or LOQ of the method. This principle is illustrated by the use of first, second, and third generation TSH assays for diagnosis of hyperthyroidism. First generation TSH assays had an LOD of 1 mU/L and were, therefore, useful in identifying hypothyroid patients, but failed to distinguish normal from suppressed TSH levels in mild to moderate cases of hyperthyroidism. In second generation assays, the LOD decreased to 0.1 mU/L, but this assay still fails to detect patients with mild hyperthyroidism. Only third generation assays, which have a detection limit of 0.01 mU/L, are effective in distinguishing mildly hyperthyroid from euthyroid patients *(42,43)*.

Specificity

Specificity is the degree to which an immunoassay measures only the target hormone. The specificity of an immunoassay is dependent not only on the ability of the antibodies to discriminate among antigens, but also on the extent to which measurements are free from interference by nonantigenic materials in the specimen. Artifacts associated with lack of antibody specificity are fairly intuitive and generally result in an overestimation of hormone levels, to the extent that the other compounds bind to the antibodies. However, it is also important to bear in mind that immunoassays, which utilize one or more highly specific monoclonal antibodies, can be too specific and measure only a subpopulation of biologically active hormone *(16,44,45)*. This point is best illustrated in the published case of a 31-yr-old women with a history of two previous pregnancies, whose LH levels were inappropriately low due to an immunological variant of LH that was poorly recognized or unrecognized by two monoclonal antibodies, but had normal bioactivity *(46)*.

Precision

Precision is a measure of the reproducibility of repeated measurements and varies tremendously among hormone immunoassays *(47,48)*. The typical approach to defining this parameter of immunoassay performance is based upon repeated measurements of stable aliquots of the same specimen. Intra-assay or within assay precision refers to repeated measurements in the same immunoassay, while interassay or "between assay" precision is the term used when the measurements are repeated in separate immunoassays. The precision associated with repeated measurements is meant to determine or monitor over time the error associated with immunoassay measurements.

It is important to recognize that the method of determining precision reflects the various sources of error associated with the method. Thus, the intra-assay precision reflects error associated with the dose–respsonse curve of the assay standard, specimen pipeting, and each of the procedural steps involved in performing the assay. Interassay precision reflects the additional errors associated with changes in reagents and equipment performance over time. Only by measuring multiple samples of the same individual in multiple assays under stable physiological conditions can biological sources of error be determined.

The variance associated with the dose–respsonse curve is most often the largest source of error in all approaches (intra-specimen, intra-assay, interspecimen, interassay) to determining precision, because at both extremes of the standard curve, the dose–respsonse relationship breaks down. For the purposes of defining and monitoring the performance of immunoassays, precision, or more precisely imprecision, is generally expressed as the %CV of repeated measurements. The %CV of an immunoassay is highly dependent on the concentration of hormone measured as illustrated in the insert of Fig. 3. At both the LOD and at the maximum response level, different concentrations of hormone give responses that are not statistically distinguishable, and the CV goes to infinity. Thus, assay variance is not uniform over the concentration range of the assay. Depending on the clinical uses of the immunoassay, the working range is usually defined as the concentration range of measurements associated with CVs below a maximum acceptable level, typically no more than 20% *(40,41)*.

In addition to their implications with respect to defining a meaningful lower limit of an immunoassay (see discussion of LOD vs functional sensitivity above), these principles imply that the precision of an assay should be monitored at concentrations spanning the working range of the immunoassay. Control specimens used for quality controls are designed to be as similar as possible to human serum, yet stable over long periods of time. Thus, not only can the performance of an individual assay be verified, but also trends (drift) in the accuracy of the method can be identified. Most clinical laboratories utilize carefully considered guidelines for determining when drift in the precision or accuracy of a method may impact on the validity of patient specimen measurements *(49)*.

Accuracy

Accuracy is the parameter that describes how closely the measurement obtained by an immunoassay agrees with the actual mass of hormone present in the specimen. The ideal immunoassay is completely accurate based upon the measurement of known masses of hormone added to patient specimens (spiked or analytical recovery) or by comparison to a method (gold standard) known to be accurate. Few, if any, current hormone immunoassays are completely accurate across their entire reportable range. Specificity is by far the most significant factor contributing to inaccuracy in hormone immunoassays. As discussed previously, hormone isoforms and metabolites can often contribute to a lack of specificity and thus inaccuracy. This issue is particularly acute in the case of gonadotropin hormones, which to this day are calibrated in terms of arbitrarily defined units rather than mass because of the heterogeneity of bioactive isoforms *(18)*. Furthermore, interference by serum components often limits accuracy either directly, by masking immunoreactivity of the hormone antigens, or indirectly, by reducing the affinity or availability of the antibodies upon which the assay depends. Interference by serum components can vary from patient to patient and is difficult to identify based upon single measurements. Generally, such interference is suggested by results that are disparate with other clinical parameters and can be confirmed by observing nonparallelism of patient dilutions relative to the standard response curve of the assay. In this regard, assay precision, which as noted above is not uniform across the reportable range of the assay, must also be considered. If the interassay precision is poor, then a majority of the replicate measurements may be inaccurate even though the mean of repeated measurements coincides with an accurate measurement.

Human anti-animal antibodies provide an illustrative example of serum factors that can vitiate the accuracy of an assay. Interference by human anti-animal antibodies is a special case of bridging protein interference where endogenous antibodies recognize the detection system antibody in two-site immunoassays *(50)*. For example, many immunoassays depend on mouse immunoglobulin G (IgGs) conjugated to an enzyme or chemiluminescent compound for detection of hormone bound to a solid-phase antibody, often a second monoclonal IgG. These assays are based upon measuring the amount of detection antibody as a direct index of the amount of hormone captured from the patient's serum specimen. While most individuals have very low levels of antibodies that recognize mouse proteins (human anti-mouse antibodies [HAMA]), patients exposed to therapeutic monoclonal mouse antibodies often develop high concentrations of antibodies against mouse IgG. Serum from such patients can interfere significantly with two-site mouse immunoassays. The bivalent HAMA in serum can form a bridge between the solid-phase and the detection system mouse IgGs in the immunoassay, resulting in the capture of detection antibody in the absence of hormone and an overestimation of the hormone concentration. Once the mechanism of interference is recognized, solutions to the interference are generally straightforward. To eliminate interference by HAMA, some manufacturers now add nonspecific mouse IgG to buffers to tie up the endogenous HAMA before detection antibody is added. In addition, assays are now being developed that rely on hybrid antibodies in which the antigenic portion of the detection antibody is human. The specific mechanisms underlying most cases of serum interference are still unknown.

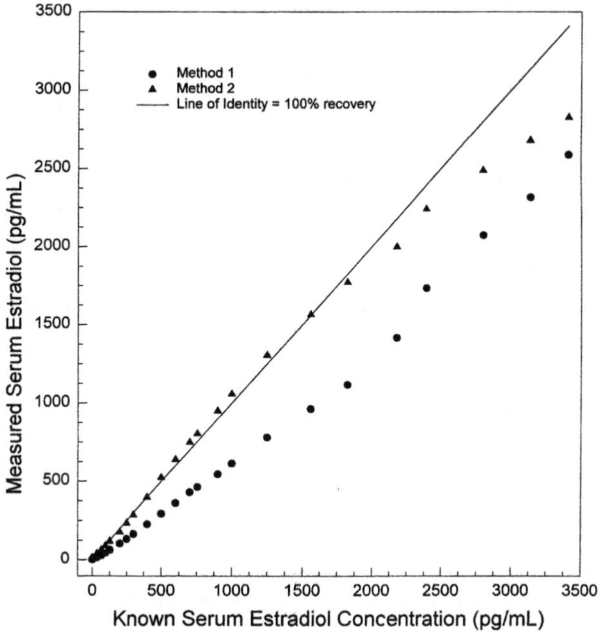

Fig. 4. Comparison of the analytical recovery of two estradiol immunoassays demonstrating nonuniformity of bias between assays.

The degree to which immunoassay measurements differ from the absolute amount of hormone is often referred to as the bias of the assay. Because the goal is to determine the physiological status of the patient, it is not essential that a clinical immunoassay be accurate to be useful. Indeed, it is arguable that a slightly biased assay with high precision is preferable to a more accurate assay with less precision. It is essential, however, to have an accurate reference range that is based on measurements of clinically characterized individuals. These reference ranges define expected values for physiological and pathological conditions *(51)*. Because there are currently few, if any, clinical immunoassays for hormones that qualify as gold standards, reference ranges must be determined for each method. Recognizing this principle, good laboratory practice requires that the reference ranges published for a given commercial method also be verified by each laboratory using that method.

Bias also refers to difference between methods, regardless of the accuracy of the methods. Indeed, it is bias rather than accuracy that is considered when applying for Food and Drug Administration (FDA) clearance for most hormone immunoassays for diagnostic purposes. It is important to emphasize that bias is seldom uniform across the reportable range of an assay as illustrated in Fig. 4, which shows analytical recovery data for two currently available commercial estradiol immunoassays. According to the manufacturers' package inserts, the reportable range for both assays was from less than 30 to 3000 pg/mL. Assay 1 is accurate at lower concentrations, but becomes increasingly inaccurate at concentrations greater than 1500 pg/mL. Assay 2, while uniformly biased at lower concentrations, becomes increasingly accurate at higher concentrations. Because of the nonuniformity of bias both between assays and relative to the known concentrations of estradiol, it is virtually impossible to compare measurements between these assays.

Finally, a special circumstance of inaccuracy in hormone immunoassays should be mentioned. This phenomenon, referred to as the hook effect *(52)*, can result in serious underestimations of hormone concentration in patient specimens. The mechanism of the hook effect in a single-step immunometric assay is illustrated in Fig. 5. Patient serum and labeled detection antibody are exposed simultaneously to the immobilized capture antibody. Initially, the capture and detection antibodies are in excess, so that the amount of hormone captured and therefore detected is directly proportional to the concentration of hormone in the specimen (Fig. 5A). At hormone concentrations exceeding the binding capacity of immobilized antibody, but under conditions when the detection antibody is still in excess, the dose-response relationship is lost (Fig. 5B). Because the response is higher than the reportable range of the assay, the operator knows to dilute the specimen in order to obtain an accurate measurement. The hook effect occurs at hormone concentrations above this point, where the binding capacity of the detection antibody becomes limiting, as hormone in excess of the capture antibody begins to tie up the detection antibody (Fig. 5C). Under these conditions, the response (i.e., the amount of detection antibody bound to captured hormone) is inversely proportional to the hormone concentration. Extrapolating the specimen response to the assay calibrators (e.g., the reportable range as illustrated in Fig. 5) results in a gross underestimation of hormone concentration in the specimen often with serious clinical implications *(53,54)*. Because the response is in the reportable range, the operator has no reason to dilute the specimen unless the clinician queries the laboratory, because the result is inconsistent with other clinical information. Once a problem is suspected, the hook effect is easily identified because a diluted specimen will contain more apparent hormone than the undiluted specimen. Error due to this type of hook effect can easily be corrected by using a two-step immunoassay in which the patient's serum is incubated with the immobilized antibody first, followed by the addition of the labeled antibody detection system after excess unbound hormone has been washed away.

CONCLUSION

Immunoassay of hormones can be an effective clinical tool only if the methods are carefully chosen, thoughtfully monitored, and applied in appropriate pathophysiological settings. The ease and precision of modern automated analyzers has made these powerful tools widely available. However, the methods

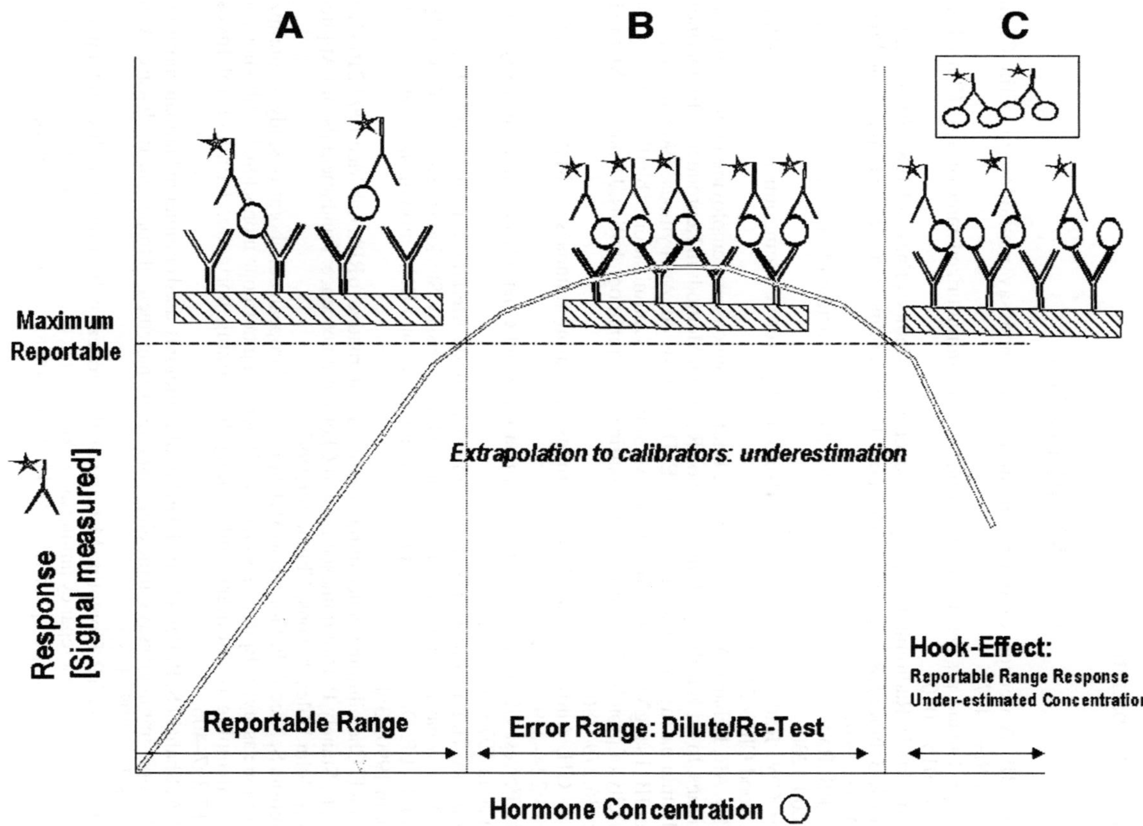

Fig. 5. Mechanism of the "hook effect" in a one-step immunometric assay.

remain highly complex, and it is essential to view immunoassay results within the whole clinical picture. Effective communication of disparate observations can lead to simple troubleshooting procedures in the laboratory, which greatly enhance the value of an immunoassay measurement in determining the endocrine status of a patient.

REFERENCES

1. Gosling JP. A decade of development in immunoassay methodology. Clin Chem 1990;36:1408–1427.
2. Ekins RP. Ligand assays: from electrophoresis to miniaturized microarrays. Clin Chem 1998;44:2015–2030.
3. Van Vunakis H. Radioimmunoassays: an overview. Methods Enzymol 1980;70:201–209.
4. Jaffe BM, Behram HR. Methods of Hormone Radioimmunoassay, 2nd ed. Academic Press, New York, 1978.
5. Yalow RS. Radioimmunoassay: a probe for the fine structure of biologic systems. Science 1978;200:1236.
6. Parker CW. Radioimmunoassay of Biologically Active Compounds. Prentice-Hall, Englewood Cliffs, NJ, 1976.
7. Midgley AR, Rebar RW, Niswender GD. Radioimmunoassays employing double antibody techniques. In 1st Karolinska Symposium on Research Methods in Reproductive Endocrinology: Immunoassay of gonadotropins. In: E. Diczfalusy, ed. Anonymous. 1969, p. 247.
8. Pilcher JB, Tsang VCW, Zhou W, Black CM, Sidman C. Optimization of binding capacity and specificity of protein G on various solid matrices for immunoglobulins. J Immunol Methods 1991;136:279–286,.
9. Parsons GH. Antibody-coated plastic tubes in radioimmunoassay. Methods Enzymol 1981;73:224–239.
10. Nye L, Forrest GC, Greenwood H. Solid-phase magnetic particle radioimmunoassay. Clin Chem Acta 1976;69:387–392.
11. Van Vunakis H, Langone JJ. Immunochemical Methods. Methods Enzymol 1980;70:1–525.
12. Price CP, Newman DJ. Principles and Practice of Immunoassay. Stockton Press, New York, 1991.
13. Diamandis EP. Detection techniques for immunoassay and DNA probing applications. Clin Biochem 1990;23:443.
14. Dudley RF. Chemiluminescence Immunoassay: an alternative to RIA. Lab Med 1990;216–222.
15. Kricka L, Stanely P. Bioluminescence and Chemiluminescence: Fundamentals and Applied Aspects. John Wiley & Sons, Chichester;1997.
16. Costagliola S, Niccoli P, Florentino M, Carayon P. European collaborative study of luteinizing hormone assay: 1. Epitope specificity of luteinizing hormone monoclonal antibodies and surface mapping of pituitary and urinary luteinizing hormone. J Endocrinol Invest 1994;17:397–406.
17. Cole LA, Shahabi S, Butler SA, et al. Utility of commonly used commercial human chorionic gonadotropin immunoassays in the diagnosis and management of trophoblastic diseases. Clin Chem 2001;47:308–315.
18. Costagliola S, Niccoli P, Florentino M, Carayon P. European collaborative study on luteinizing hormone assay: 2. Discrepancy among assay kits is related to variation both in standard curve calibration and epitope specificity of kit monoclonal antibodies. J Endocrinol Invest 1994;17:407–416.
19. Spratt DI, O'Dea LS, Schoenfeld DA, Butler J, Rao PN, Crowley WF Jr. Neuroendocrine-gonadol axis in men: frequent sampling of LH, FSH and testosterone. Am J Physiol 1988;254:E658–E666.
20. Santoro N, Butler JP, Filicori M, Crowley WF Jr. Alterations of the hypothalamic GnRH interpulse interval sequence over the normal menstrual cycle. Am J Physiol 1988;255:E696–701.

21. Veldhuis JD, Beitins IZ, Johnson ML, Serabian MA, Dufau ML. Biologically active luteinizing hormone is secreted in episodic pulsations that vary in relation to stage of the menstrual cycle. J Clin Endocrinol Metab 1984;58:1050–1058.
22. Filicori M, Butler JP, Crowley WF Jr. Hypothalamic control of goandotropin secretion in the human menstrual cycle. Proc Clin Biol Res 1986;225:55–74.
23. Filicori M, Butler JP, Crowley WF, Jr. Neuroendocrine regulation of the corpus luteum in the human. Evidence for pulsitile progesterone secretion. J Clin Invest 1984;73:1638–1647.
24. Bremner WJ, Vitiello MV, Prinz PN. Loss of circadian rhythmicity in blood testosterone levels with aging in normal men. J Clin Endocrinol Metab 1983;56:1278–1281.
25. Hall JE, Schoenfeld DA, Martin KA, Crowley WF Jr. Hypothalamic gonadotropin-releasing hormone secretion and follicle-stimulating hormone dynamics during the luteal-follicular transition. J Clin Endocrinol Metab 1992;74:600–607.
26. Ross GT, Cargille CM, Lipsett MB, et al. Pituitary and gonadal hormones during spontaneous and induced menstrual cycles. Recent Prog Horm Res 1970;26:1–62.
27. Sherman BM, Korenman SG. Hormonal characteristics of the human menstrual cycle throughout reproductive life. J Clin Invest 1975;55:699–706.
28. Groome NP, Illingworth PJ, O'Brien M, et al. Detection of dimeric inhibin throughout the human menstrual cycle by two-site enzyme immunoassay. Clin Endocr 1994;40:717–723.
29. Hall JE, Martin KA, Taylor AE, et al. Reciprocal changes in inhibin B and inhibin A during the normal menstrual cycle. Annual Meeting Endocrine Society. 1996.
30. Treloar AE, Boynton RE, Behn BG, Brown BW. Variation of the human menstrual cycle through reproductive life. Int J Fertil 1970;12:77–126.
31. Hall JE, Lavoie H, Marsh EE, Martin KA. Decrease in gonadotropin-releasing hormone pulse frequency with aging in postmenopausal women. J Clin Endocrinol Metab 2000;85:1794–1800.
32. Sharpless J, Supko JG, Martin, KA, Hall JE. Disappearance of endogenous luteinizing hormone is prolonged in postmenopausal women. J Clin Endocrinol Metab 1999;84:688–698.
33. Welt CK, McNicholl DJ, Taylor AE, Hall JE. Female reproductive aging is marked by decreased secretion of dimeric inhibin. J Clin Endocrinol Metab 1999;84:105–111.
34. Gray A, Feldman HA, McKinlay JB, Longcope C. Age, disease, and changing sex hormone levels in middle-aged men: result of the Massachusetts Male Aging Study. J Clin Endocrinol Metab 1999;73:1016–1025.
35. Masters AM, Hahnel R. Investigation of sex-hormone binding globulin interference in direct radioimmunoassays for testosterone and estradiol. Clin Chem 1989;35:979#-3984.
36. Rodbard D. Statistical quality control and routine data processing for radioimmunoassays and immunoradiometric assays. Clin Chem 1974;20:1255–1270.
37. Dudley RA. Guidelines for immunoassay data processing. Clin Chem 1985;31:1271.
38. Chan DW, Peristein MT. Immunoassay: A Practical Guide. Academic Press, New York, 1987.
39. Ekins RP, Edwards P. Point on the meaning of sensitivity. Clin Chem 1997;43:1824–1831.
40. Fraser CG, Petersen PH. Desirable standards for laboratory tests if they are to fulfill medical needs. Clinical Chemistry 39: 1447-1455, 1993.
41. Spencer CA, Takeuchi M, Kazarosyan M. Current status and performance goals for serum thyrotropin [TSH] assays. Clin Chem 1996;42:140–145.
42. De los Santos ET, Starich GH, Mazzaferri EL. Sensitivity, specificity, and cost-effectiveness of the sensitive thyrotropin assay in the diagnosis of thyroid disease in ambulatory patients. Arch Int Med 1989;149:526–532.
43. Squire CR, Fraser WD. Thyroid stimulating hormone measurement using a third generation immunometric assay. Ann Clin Biochem 1995;32:307–313.
44. Ferrand V, Niccoli P, Roux F, Carayon P. Accuracy of luteinizing hormone immunoassay is improved by changing epitope specificity of the labeled monoclonal antibody. Clin Chem 1995;41:953–955.
45. Pettersson K, Ding YQ, Huhtaniemi I. Monoclonal antibody-based discrepancies between two-site immunometric tests for lutropin. Clin Chem 1991;37:1745–1748.

46. Pettersson K, Ding YQ, Huhtaniemi I. An immunologically anomalous luteinizing hormone variant in a healthy woman. J Clin Endocrinol Metab 1992;74:164–171.
47. Westgard JO, Carey RN, Wold S. Criteria for judging precision and accuracty in method development and evaluation. Clin Chem 1974;20:825–833.
48. Westgard JO, Bawa N, Ross JW, Lawson NS. Laboratory precision performance: state of the art vs operating specifications that assure the analytical quality required by clinical laboratory improvement amendments proficiency testing. Arch Pathol Lab Med 1996;120:621–625.
49. Westgard JO, Falk H, Groth T. Influence of a between-run component of variation, choice of control limits, and shape of error distribution on the performance characteriztics of rules for internal quality control. Clin Chem 1979;25:394–400.
50. Kricka LJ, Schmerfeld-Pruss D, Senior M, Goodman DBP, Kaladas P. Interference by human anti-mouse antibody in two-site immunoassays. Clin Chem 1990;36:892–894.
51. Baxter RC. Methods of measuring confidence limits in radioimmunoassay. Methods Enzymol 1983;92:601–610.
52. Zweig MH. High-dose hook efffect in a two-site IRMA for measuring thyrotropin. Ann Clin Biochem 1990;27:495.
53. Levavi H, Neri A, Bar J, Nordenberg J, Ocadia J. "Hook effect" in complete hydatidiform molar pregnancy: a falsely low level of beta-hCG. Obstet Gynecol 1993;82:720–721.
54. Valdya HC, Wolf BA, Garrett N, Catalona WJ, Clayman RV, Nahm MH. Extremely high values of prostate-specific antigen in patients with adenocarcinoma of the prostate;demonstration of the "hook effect". Clin Chem 1988;34:2175–2177.

2 Disorders of Water Metabolism

Joseph G. Verbalis, MD

Contents

INTRODUCTION

Disorders of body fluids are among the most commonly encountered problems in the practice of clinical medicine. This is in large part because many different disease states can potentially disrupt the finely balanced mechanisms that control the intake and output of water and solute. Since body water is the primary determinant of the osmolality of the extracellular fluid (ECF), disorders of water metabolism can be broadly divided into hypoosmolar disorders, in which there is an excess of body water relative to body solute, and hyperosmolar disorders, in which there is a deficiency of body water relative to body solute. Because sodium is the main constituent of plasma osmolality (P_{osm}), these disorders are typically characterized by hyponatremia and hypernatremia, respectively. Before discussing these disorders, this chapter will first review the regulatory mechanisms underlying water and sodium metabolism, the two major determinants of body fluid homeostasis.

BODY FLUID COMPARTMENTS

Water constitutes approx 55–65% of body weight, varying somewhat with age, sex, and amount of body fat, and, therefore, constitutes the largest single constituent of the body. Total body water (TBW) is distributed between the intracellular fluid (ICF) and the ECF compartments. Estimates of the relative

From: *Contemporary Endocrinology: Handbook of Diagnostic Endocrinology*
Edited by: J. E. Hall and L. K. Nieman © Humana Press Inc., Totowa, NJ

sizes of these two important pools differ significantly depending on the tracer used to measure the ECF volume, but most studies in animals and man have suggested that 55–65% (or just under two-thirds) of TBW resides in the ICF, and 35–45% (or slightly more than one-third) is in the ECF *(1)*. Approximately three-fourths of the ECF compartment is interstitial fluid, and one-fourth is intravascular fluid (blood volume). Figure 1 summarizes the estimated body fluid spaces of an average weight adult. The solute composition of the ICF and ECF differ considerably, since membrane-bound Na^+/K^+ pumps maintain Na^+ in a primarily extracellular location and K^+ in a primarily intracellular location. Nonetheless, it is important to remember that the osmotic pressure, which is a function of the concentrations of all the solutes in a fluid compartment, must always be equivalent in the ICF and ECF, because most biological membranes are semipermeable (i.e., freely permeable to water, but not to aqueous solutes). Thus, water will flow across membranes into a compartment with a higher solute concentration until a steady state is reached, in which the osmotic pressures have equalized on both sides of the cell membrane. An important consequence of this thermodynamic law is that the volume of distribution of body Na^+ and K^+ is actually the TBW rather than just the ECF or ICF volume, respectively *(2)*. For example, any increase in ECF [Na^+] will cause water to shift from the ICF to the ECF until the ICF and ECF osmotic pressures are equal, thereby in effect distributing the Na^+ across both extracellular and intracellular water.

TOTAL AND EFFECTIVE OSMOLALITY

Osmolality is defined as the concentration of all of the solutes in a given weight of water. P_{osm} can be measured directly (via determination of freezing point depression or vapor pressure, since each of these are colligative properties of the number of free solute particles in a given volume of plasma) or estimated as:

$$P_{osm}\ (\text{mOsm/kg } H_2O) = 2 \times \text{plasma } [Na^+]\ (\text{mEq/L}) + \text{glucose (mg/dL)}/18 + \text{BUN (mg/dL)}/2.8$$

Both methods produce comparable results under most conditions, as will simply doubling the plasma sodium concentration ([Na^+]), since sodium and its accompanying anions are by far the predominant solutes present in plasma. However, the total osmolality of plasma is not always equivalent to the "effective" osmolality (sometimes referred to as the "tonicity" of the plasma), because the latter is a function of the relative solute permeability properties of the membranes separating the two compartments. Solutes that are impermeable to cell membranes (Na^+, mannitol) are restricted to the ECF compartment and are effective solutes, since they create osmotic pressure gradients across cell membranes, leading to osmotic movement of water from the ICF to the ECF compartments. Solutes that are permeable to cell membranes (urea, ethanol, methanol) are

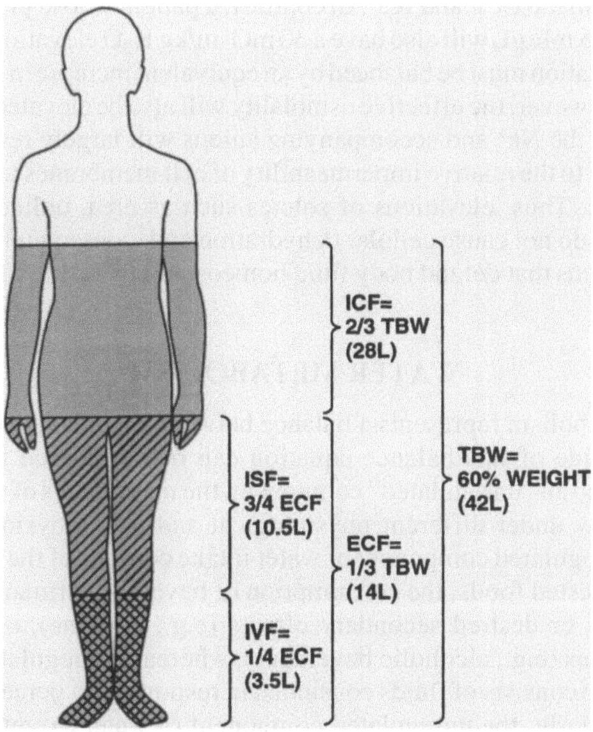

Fig. 1. Schematic representation of body fluid compartments in man. The shaded areas depict the approximate size of each compartment as a function of body weight. The figures indicate the relative sizes of the various fluid compartments and the approximate absolute volumes of the compartments (in L) in a 70-kg adult. Abbreviations: TBW, total body water; ICF, intracellular fluid; ECF, extracellular fluid; ISF, interstitial fluid; IVF, intravascular fluid.

ineffective solutes, since they do not create osmotic pressure gradients across cell membranes and, therefore, are not associated with such water shifts *(3)*. Glucose is a unique solute, since at normal physiologic plasma concentrations, it is taken up by cells via active transport mechanisms and, therefore, acts as an ineffective solute, but under conditions of impaired cellular uptake (e.g., insulin deficiency), it becomes an effective extracellular solute *(4)*.

The importance of this distinction between total and effective osmolality lies with the fact that only the effective solutes in plasma are determinants of whether clinically significant hyperosmolality or hypoosmolality is present. An example of this is uremia: a patient with a urea concentration that has increased by 30 mEq/L will have a corresponding 30 mOsm/kg H_2O elevation in P_{osm}, but the effective osmolality will remain normal, since the increased urea is proportionally distributed across both the ECF and ICF. In contrast, a patient whose plasma [Na^+] has increased by 15 mEq/L will also have a 30 mOsm/kg H_2O elevation of P_{osm}, since the increased cation must be balanced by an equivalent increase in plasma anions. In this case, however, the effective osmolality will also be elevated by 30 mOsm/kg H_2O, since the Na^+ and accompanying anions will largely remain restricted to the ECF due to the relative impermeability of cell membranes to Na^+ and other univalent ions. Thus, elevations of solutes such as urea, unlike elevations in plasma [Na^+], do not cause cellular dehydration and, consequently, do not activate mechanisms that defend body fluid homeostasis by acting to increase body water stores.

WATER METABOLISM

Water metabolism represents a balance between the intake and excretion of water. Each side of this balance equation can be considered to consist of a "regulated" and an "unregulated" component, the magnitudes of which can vary quite markedly under different physiological and pathophysiological conditions. The unregulated component of water intake consists of the intrinsic water content of ingested foods, the consumption of beverages primarily for reasons of palatability or desired secondary effects (e.g., caffeine), or for social or habitual reasons (e.g., alcoholic beverages), whereas the regulated component of water intake consists of fluids consumed in response to a perceived sensation of thirst. Similarly, the unregulated component of water excretion occurs via insensible water losses from a variety of sources (cutaneous losses from sweating, evaporative losses in exhaled air, gastrointestinal losses), as well as the obligate amount of water that the kidneys must excrete to eliminate solutes generated by body metabolism. The regulated component of water excretion is comprised of the renal excretion of free water in excess of the obligate amount necessary to excrete metabolic solutes *(5)*. In effect, the regulated components are those that act to maintain water balance by compensating for whatever perturbations result from unregulated water losses or gains. Within this framework, it is clear that the two major mechanisms responsible for regulating water metabolism are thirst and pituitary secretion of the hormone vasopressin.

Thirst

Thirst is the body's defense mechanism to increase water consumption in response to perceived deficits of body fluids. Thirst can be stimulated in animals and man either by intracellular dehydration, caused by increases in the effective osmolality of the ECF, or by intravascular hypovolemia, caused by losses of ECF. Substantial evidence to date has supported mediation of the former by osmoreceptors located in the anterior hypothalamus of the brain, whereas the latter appears to be stimulated primarily via activation of low- and/or high-pressure baroreceptors, with a likely contribution from circulating angiotensin II during more severe degrees of intravascular hypovolemia and hypotension *(6,7)*. Controlled studies in animals have consistently reported thresholds for osmotically induced drinking, ranging from 1–4% increases in P_{osm} above basal levels, and analogous studies in humans using quantitative estimates of subjective symptoms of thirst have confirmed that increases in P_{osm} of similar magnitudes are necessary to produce an unequivocal sensation described as thirst *(8,9)*.

Conversely, the threshold for producing hypovolemic, or extracellular, thirst is significantly greater in both animals and humans. Studies in several species have shown that sustained decreases in plasma volume or blood pressure of at least 4–8%, and in some species 10–15%, are necessary to consistently stimulate drinking. In humans, it has been difficult to demonstrate any effects of mild to moderate hypovolemia to stimulate thirst independently of osmotic changes occurring with dehydration. This blunted sensitivity to changes in ECF volume or blood pressure in humans probably represents an adaptation that occurred as a result of the erect posture of primates, which predisposes them to wider fluctuations in blood and atrial filling pressures as a result of orthostatic pooling of blood in the lower body; stimulation of thirst (and vasopressin secretion) by such transient postural changes in blood pressure might lead to overdrinking and inappropriate antidiuresis in situations where the ECF volume was actually normal but only transiently maldistributed. Consistent with a blunted response to baroreceptor activation, recent studies have also shown that systemic infusion of angiotensin II to pharmacological levels is a much less potent stimulus to thirst in humans than in animals *(10)*. Nonetheless, this response is not completely absent in humans, as demonstrated by rare cases of polydipsia in patients with pathological causes of hyperreninemia.

Although osmotic changes clearly are more effective stimulants of thirst than are volume changes in humans, it is not clear whether relatively small changes in P_{osm} are responsible for day-to-day fluid intakes. Most humans consume the majority of their ingested water as a result of the unregulated components of fluid intake discussed previously, and generally ingest volumes in excess of what can be considered to be actual “need” *(11)*. Consistent with this observation is the fact that, under most conditions, P_{osm}s in man remain within 1–2% of basal levels, and these relatively small changes in P_{osm} are generally below the threshold levels that have been found to stimulate thirst in most individuals. This suggests that despite the obvious vital importance of thirst during pathological situations of hyperosmolality and hypovolemia, under normal physiological conditions, water balance in man is accomplished more by regulated free water excretion than by regulated water intake *(5)*.

Arginine Vasopressin Secretion

The prime determinant of free water excretion in animals and man is the regulation of urinary flow by circulating levels of arginine vasopressin (AVP) in plasma. Before AVP was biochemically characterized, early studies of antidiuresis used the term "antidiuretic hormone" (ADH) to describe this substance. Now that its structure and function as the only naturally-occurring antidiuretic substance are known, it is more appropriate to refer to it by its real name. AVP is a 9-amino acid peptide that is synthesized in specialized (magnocellular) neural cells located in two discrete areas of the hypothalamus, the supraoptic (SON) and paraventricular (PVN) nuclei. The synthesized peptide is enzymatically cleaved from its prohormone and is transported to the posterior pituitary where it is stored within neurosecretory granules until specific stimuli cause secretion of AVP into the bloodstream *(12)*. Antidiuresis then occurs via interaction of the circulating hormone with AVP V_2 receptors in the kidney, which results in increased water permeability of the collecting duct through the insertion of a water channel called aquaporin-2 into the apical membranes of collecting tubule principal cells *(13)*. The importance of AVP for maintaining water balance is underscored by the fact that the normal pituitary stores of this hormone are very large, allowing more than a week's supply of hormone for maximal antidiuresis under conditions of sustained dehydration. Knowledge of the different conditions that stimulate pituitary AVP release in man is, therefore, essential for understanding water metabolism.

Osmotic Regulation

The primary renal response to AVP is an increase in water permeability of the kidney collecting tubules. Although an increase in solute reabsorption (primarily urea) occurs as well, the total solute reabsorption is proportionally much less than water. Consequently, a decrease in urine flow and an increase in U_{osm} occur as secondary responses to the increased net water reabsorption. With refinement of radioimmunoassays for AVP, the unique sensitivity of this hormone to small changes in osmolality, as well as the corresponding sensitivity of the kidney to small changes in plasma AVP levels, have become apparent *(14)*. Although some debate still exists with regard to the exact pattern of osmotically stimulated AVP secretion, most studies to date have supported the concept of a discrete osmotic threshold for AVP secretion above which a linear relationship between P_{osm} and AVP levels occurs (Fig. 2). The slope of the regression line relating AVP to P_{osm} can vary significantly across individual human subjects, in part because of genetic factors *(12)*. In general, each 1 mOsm/kg H_2O increase in P_{osm} causes an increase in plasma AVP level from 0.4 to 0.8 pg/mL. The renal response to circulating AVP is similarly linear, with urinary concentration that is directly proportional to AVP levels from 0.5 to 4–5 pg/mL, after which urinary osmolality (U_{osm}) is maximal and cannot increase further despite additional increases in AVP levels.

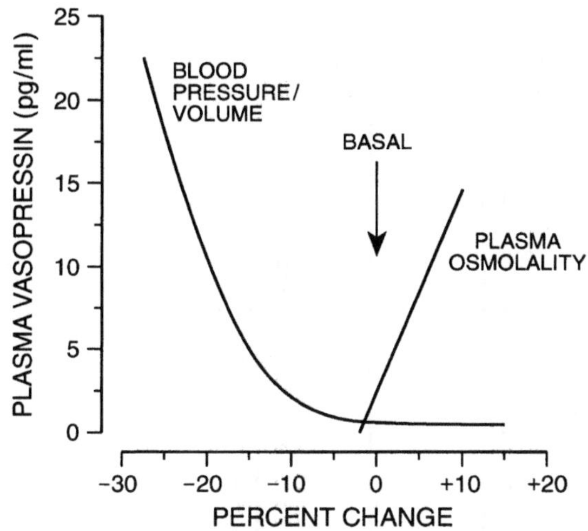

Fig. 2. Comparative sensitivity of AVP secretion in response to increases in P_{osm} vs decreases in blood volume or blood pressure in human subjects. The arrow indicates the low plasma AVP concentrations found at basal P_{osm} (modified with permission from ref. *12*).

Thus, changes of 1% or less in P_{osm} are sufficient to cause significant increases in plasma AVP levels with proportional increases in urine concentration, and maximal antidiuresis is achieved after increases in P_{osm} of only 5–10 mOsm/kg H_2O (2–4%) above the threshold for AVP secretion.

However, even this analysis underestimates the sensitivity of this system to regulate free water excretion for the following reason. U_{osm} is directly proportional to plasma AVP levels as a consequence of the fall in urine flow induced by the AVP, but urine volume is inversely related to U_{osm} (Fig. 3). Thus, an increase in plasma AVP concentration from 0.5–2 pg/mL has a much greater relative effect to decrease urine flow than does a subsequent increase in AVP concentration from 2–5 pg/mL, thereby further magnifying the physiological effects of small initial changes in plasma AVP levels *(15)*. The net result of these relations is a finely tuned regulatory system that adjusts the rate of free water excretion accurately to the ambient P_{osm} via changes in pituitary AVP secretion. Furthermore, the rapid response of pituitary AVP secretion to changes in P_{osm} coupled with the short half-life (10–20 minutes) of AVP in human plasma enables this regulatory system to adjust renal water excretion to changes in P_{osm} on a minute-to-minute basis.

Volemic Regulation

As in the case of thirst, hypovolemia also is a stimulus for AVP secretion in man; an appropriate physiological response to volume depletion should include urinary concentration and renal water conservation. But similar to thirst, AVP

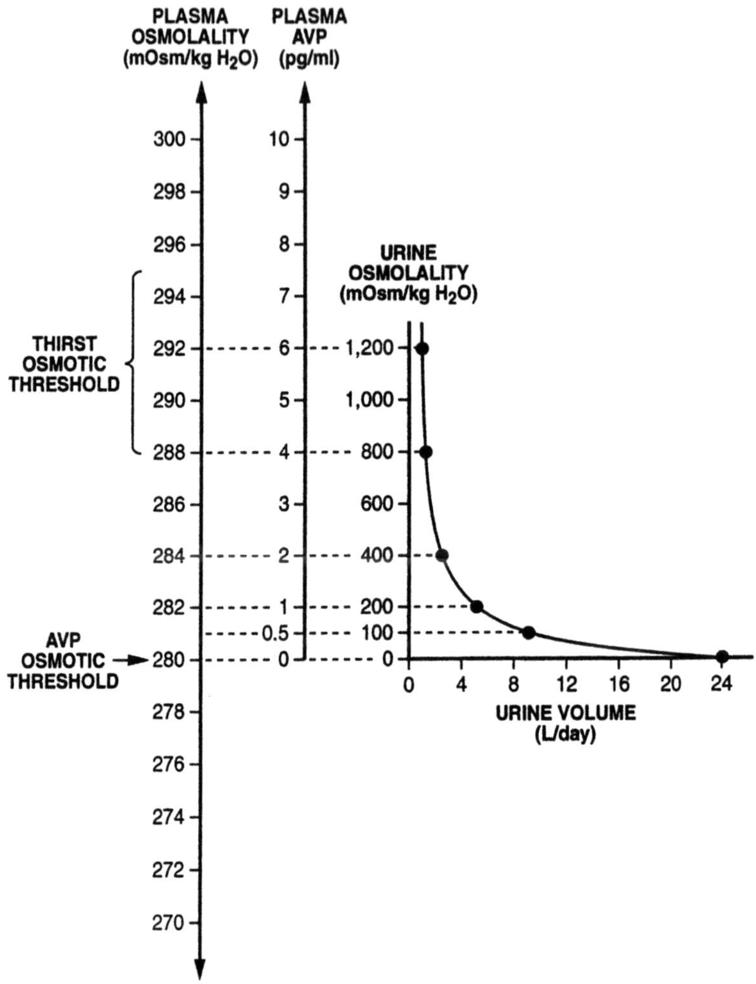

Fig. 3. Schematic representation of normal physiological relationships among P_{osm}, plasma AVP concentrations, U_{osm}, and urine volume in man. Note particularly the inverse nature of the relation between U_{osm} and urine volume, resulting in disproportionate effects of small changes in plasma AVP concentrations on urine volume at lower AVP levels (modified with permission from ref. *15*).

secretion is much less sensitive to small changes in blood volume and blood pressure than to changes in osmolality *(12)*; some have even suggested that the AVP response to decreases in blood volume is absent in man, though this most likely is simply a manifestation of the significantly higher threshold for AVP secretion to volemic stimuli. Such marked differences in AVP responses represent additional corroborative evidence that osmolality represents a more sensitive regulatory system for water balance than does blood or ECF volume.

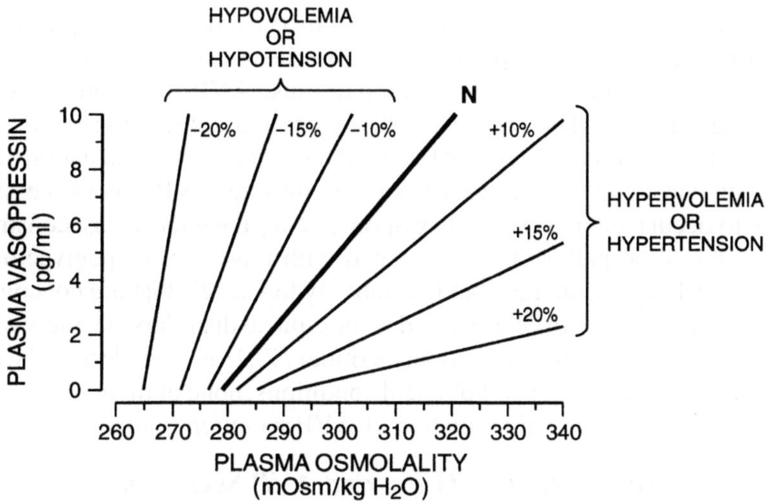

Fig. 4. Relation between plasma AVP concentrations and P_{osm} under conditions of varying blood volume and pressure. The line labeled "N" depicts the linear regression line associating these variables in euvolemic normotensive adult subjects. The lines to the left depict the changes in this regression line with progressive decreases in blood volume and/or pressure and the lines to the right depict the opposite changes with progressive increases in blood volume and/or pressure (in each case the numbers at the ends of the lines indicate the relative percent changes in blood volume and/or blood pressure associated with each regression line) (modified with permission from ref. *12*).

Nonetheless, modest changes in blood volume and pressure influence AVP secretion indirectly, even though they are weak stimuli by themselves. This occurs via shifting the sensitivity of AVP secretion to osmotic stimuli, so that a given increase in osmolality will cause a greater secretion of AVP during hypovolemic conditions than during euvolemic states (Fig. 4). Although this effect has been demonstrated in human as well as in animal studies, it has only been shown convincingly with substantial degrees of hypovolemia, and the magnitude of this effect during mild degrees of volume dumeepletion remains conjectural. Consequently, it is reasonable to conclude that the major effect of moderate degrees of hypovolemia on both AVP secretion and thirst is to modulate the gain of the osmoregulatory responses, with direct effects on thirst and AVP secretion occurring only during more severe degrees of hypovolemia (e.g., 10% reductions in blood volume).

Other Stimuli

Several other nonosmotic stimuli to AVP secretion have been described in man. Most prominent among these is nausea. The sensation of nausea, with or without vomiting, is by far the most potent stimulus to AVP secretion known in man. While 20% increases in osmolality will typically elevate plasma AVP levels to the range of 5–20 pg/mL, and 20% decreases in blood pressure to 10–100 pg/mL, nausea has been described to cause AVP elevations in excess of 200–400 pg/mL *(16)*. The reason for this profound stimulation is not known (although it has been speculated that the AVP response assists evacuation of stomach contents via contraction of gastric smooth muscle, AVP is not necessary for vomiting to occur), but it is probably responsible for the intense vasoconstriction, which produces the pallor often associated with this state. Hypoglycemia also stimulates AVP release in man, but to relatively low levels that are not consistent among individuals. As will be discussed in the clinical disorders, a variety of drugs also stimulate AVP secretion, including nicotine *(17)*. However, despite the importance of these stimuli during pathological conditions, none of them is a significant determinant of physiological regulation of AVP secretion in man.

Integration of Thirst and AVP Secretion

A synthesis of what is presently known about the regulation of thirst and AVP secretion in man leads to a relatively simple but elegant system to maintain water balance. Under normal physiological conditions, the sensitivity of the osmoregulatory system for AVP secretion accounts for maintenance of P_{osm} within narrow limits by adjusting renal water excretion to small changes in osmolality. Stimulated thirst does not represent a major regulatory mechanism under these conditions, and unregulated fluid ingestion supplies adequate water in excess of true need, which is then excreted in relation to osmoregulated pituitary AVP secretion. However, when unregulated water intake cannot adequately supply body needs in the presence of plasma AVP levels sufficient to produce maximal antidiuresis, then P_{osm} rises to levels that stimulate thirst and produce water intake proportional to the elevation of osmolality above this threshold. In such a system, thirst essentially represents a backup mechanism called into play when pituitary and renal mechanisms prove insufficient to maintain P_{osm} within a few percent of basal levels. This arrangement has the advantage of freeing man from frequent episodes of thirst that would require a diversion of activities toward behavior oriented to seeking water when water deficiency is sufficiently mild to be compensated for by renal water conservation, but would stimulate water ingestion once water deficiency reaches potentially harmful levels. Stimulation of AVP secretion at P_{osm}s below the threshold for subjective thirst acts to maintain an excess of body water sufficient to eliminate the need to drink whenever slight elevations in P_{osm} occur. This system of differential effective thresholds for thirst and AVP secretion nicely complements many studies that have demonstrated excess unregulated, or need-free, drinking in both man and animals *(6)*.

Therefore, in summary, during normal day-to-day conditions, body water homeostasis appears to be maintained primarily by *ad libitum*, or unregulated, fluid intake in association with AVP-regulated changes in urine flow, most of which occurs before the threshold is reached for osmotically stimulated, or regulated, thirst. But when these mechanisms become inadequate to maintain body fluid homeostasis, then thirst-induced regulated fluid intake becomes the predominant defense mechanism for the prevention of dehydration.

SODIUM METABOLISM

Maintenance of sodium homeostasis requires a simple balance between intake and excretion of Na^+. As in the case of water metabolism, it is possible to define regulated and unregulated components of both Na^+ intake and Na^+ excretion. Unlike water intake, however, there is little evidence in humans to support a significant role for regulated Na^+ intake, with the possible exception of some pathological conditions. Consequently, there is an even greater dependence on mechanisms for regulated renal excretion of sodium than is the case for excretion of water *(18)*. Whether for this reason or not, the mechanisms for renal excretion of sodium are more numerous and substantially more complex than the relatively simple, albeit quite efficient, system for AVP-regulated excretion of water.

Salt Appetite

The only solute for which any specific appetite has been clearly demonstrated in man is sodium (as with animals, this is generally expressed as an appetite for the chloride salt of sodium, so it is usually called NaCl, or salt, appetite). Because of the importance of Na^+ for ensuring maintenance of the ECF volume, which in turn directly supports blood volume and pressure, its uniqueness insofar as meriting a specific mechanism for regulated intake seems appropriate. However, despite abundant evidence in many different species demonstrating a salt appetite that is proportionately related to Na^+ losses *(19)*, there is only one pathological condition in which a specific stimulated sodium appetite has been unequivocally observed in humans, namely Addison's disease, which is caused by adrenal insufficiency. Almost since the initial discovery of this disorder, salt craving has remained one of the well-known manifestations of Addison's disease *(20)*. A robust salt appetite also occurs prominently in adrenalectomized animals, and appears to be related in part to the high plasma levels of adrenocorticotropin (ACTH) produced as a result of the loss of cortisol feedback on the pituitary. However, despite the presence of Na^+ deficiency in most patients with untreated Addison's disease, only 15–20% of such patients manifest salt-seeking behavior *(21)*.

Even more striking is the apparent absence of salt appetite during a variety of other disorders causing severe Na^+ and ECF volume depletion in humans (patients with hemorrhagic blood loss, diuretic-induced hypovolemia, or hypotension of any etiology become thirsty when intravascular deficits are marked, but almost never express a pronounced desire for salty foods or fluids). Yet, as with thirst, the possibility of subclinical activation of neural mechanisms stimulating salt intake without a conscious subjective sensation of salt "hunger" must be entertained. However, this possibility cannot be supported either, because many such patients actually become hyponatremic as a result of continued ingestion of only water or osmotically dilute fluids in response to their volume depletion *(18)*. It is also interesting to note that athletes must be instructed to ingest sodium as NaCl tablets or electrolyte solutions during periods of sodium losses from profuse sweating since they fail to develop a salt appetite, which would be protective under these circumstances. As a corollary to the infrequency of stimulated salt appetite in man, there is also no evidence to support inhibition of sodium intake under conditions of Na^+ and ECF excess, as demonstrated by the difficulty in maintaining even moderate degrees of sodium restriction in patients with edema-forming diseases such as congestive heart failure.

Renal Sodium Excretion

Although specific mechanisms exist for regulated renal excretion of all major electrolytes, none is as numerous or as complex as those controlling Na^+ excretion, which is not surprising in view of the fact that maintenance of ECF volume is crucial to normal health and function. The most important of these mechanisms are discussed briefly below, but given their complexity, the reader is referred to more complete reviews of this subject *(22,23)*.

Glomerular Filtration Rate

Glomerular filtration rate (GFR) is one of two classical mechanisms known to regulate renal Na^+ excretion. Multiple factors influence GFR, including the glomerular plasma flow, the glomerular capillary surface area, the hydrostatic pressure gradient between the glomerular capillaries and Bowman's capsule, and the oncotic pressure produced by the proteins in glomerular capillaries. Because the amount of Na^+ filtered through the kidney is huge (approx 25,000 mmol/d in healthy adults), relatively small changes in GFR can potentially have large effects on filtered Na^+. However, changes in filtered load of Na^+ are compensated for by concomitant changes in proximal tubular sodium reabsorption via a process known as tubuloglomerular feedback *(24)*. As the filtered Na^+ load increases, Na^+ absorption in the proximal tubule also increases, largely compensating for the increased filtered load. Although the mechanisms(s) responsible for tubuloglomerular feedback are not completely understood, one important factor appears to be changes in peritubular capillary forces, which is analogous to the Starling forces in systemic capillaries. An increase in filtered fluid at the glomerulus decreases the hydrostatic pressure and increases the oncotic pressure of the nonfiltered fluid delivered to the peritubular capillaries, thereby increasing the pressure gradient for reabsorbing the Na^+, which is actively transported from the proximal tubular epithelial cells into the extracellular fluid surrounding the proximal tubule. Although this mechanism dampens the effects of alterations in

GFR on renal Na^+, excretion and prevents large changes in urine Na^+ excretion in response to minor changes in GFR, nonetheless, many experimental results indicate that sustained alterations of GFR can significantly modulate renal Na^+ excretion.

Aldosterone

The second major factor long known to influence renal Na^+ excretion is adrenal aldosterone secretion, which increases Na^+ resorption in the distal nephron by inducing the synthesis and activity of ion channels that affect sodium reabsorption and sodium–potassium exchange in tubular epithelial cells, particularly the epithelial sodium channel (ENaC) *(25)*. The importance of this hormone for Na^+ homeostasis is best illustrated by the well-known renal Na^+ wasting of patients with primary adrenal insufficiency. Multiple factors stimulate adrenal mineralocorticoid secretion. Most prominent of these is angiotensin II, which is formed as the end result of renin secretion from the juxtaglomerular apparatus in response to renal hypoperfusion. High plasma K^+ concentrations also stimulate aldosterone secretion, thereby increasing urinary K^+ excretion at the expense of Na^+ retention. More recently two inhibitors of aldosterone secretion have been described: atrial natriuretic peptide (ANP) and hyperosmolality; both of these stimuli appear to be sufficiently potent to completely block stimulated aldosterone secretion *(26)*. Although aldosterone clearly plays an important role in sodium homeostasis, its effects to stimulate Na^+ resorption in the distal tubule can be overridden by other natriuretic factors. This is evident in the phenomenon of renal "escape" from mineralocorticoids, in which experimental animals and man reestablish sodium balance after an initial period of Na^+ retention and ECF volume expansion. Potential mechanisms responsible for this phenomenon are discussed below.

Intrarenal Hemodynamic and Peritubular Factors

Although GFR and aldosterone effects can account for much of the observed variation in renal Na^+ excretion, it has long been known that they cannot completely explain the natriuresis that occurs in the absence of measurable changes in GFR or aldosterone secretion during isotonic saline volume expansion. This led to the postulation of the existence of a "third factor" or factors regulating Na^+ excretion. Intrarenal hemodynamic factors are now known to be important in this regard, particularly changes in renal perfusion pressure. This is illustrated by aldosterone escape described above, which appears to be mediated primarily by increased renal perfusion pressure with subsequent increased fractional sodium excretion *(27)*. In effect, this represents a "safety-valve" mechanism; when renal artery pressure rises as a result of volume expansion, the increase in filtered load of Na^+ is sufficient to overwhelm the aldosterone-mediated distal sodium resorption. This phenomenon has been called a pressure diuresis and natriuresis. Note that the term escape is somewhat of a misnomer, since aldosterone effects are still present, but a new steady-state of volume expansion has been reached in which no additional sodium retention occurs due to activation of compensatory mechanisms for sodium excretion. Although sodium balance is reestablished, a substantial degree of volume expansion persists nonetheless, thus confirming the presence of continued systemic mineralocorticoid effects.

Other Factors

Several factors in addition to those discussed above have also been found to influence renal sodium excretion. These include angiotensin II, arginine vasopressin, atrial natriuretic peptide, dopamine, renal sympathetic nerve activity, and renal prostaglandins. However, none of these have yet been clearly demonstrated to play a major role in regulating renal sodium excretion in man.

HYPEROSMOLALITY AND HYPERNATREMIA

Pathogenesis

Hyperosmolality indicates a deficiency of water relative to solute in the ECF. Because water moves freely between the ICF and ECF, this also indicates a deficiency of TBW relative to total body solute. Although hypernatremia can be caused by an excess of body sodium, the vast majority of cases are due to losses of body water in excess of body solutes, caused by either insufficient water intake or excessive water excretion. Consequently, most of the disorders causing hyperosmolality are those associated with inadequate water intake and/or deficient AVP secretion (Table 1). The best known of these is diabetes insipidus (DI), in which AVP secretion, or its renal effects, is impaired without an abnormality of thirst. Much less common are disorders of osmoreceptor function, resulting in abnormalities of both AVP secretion and thirst. Although hyperosmolality from inadequate water intake is seen frequently in clinical practice, this is usually not due to an underlying defect in thirst, but rather results from a generalized incapacity to obtain and/or ingest fluids, often stemming from a depressed sensorium. An example is hyperosmolar coma caused by renal water losses from hyperglycemia-induced diuresis in elderly patients who eventually are unable to drink enough fluid to keep up with their unrelenting osmotic diuresis.

Differential Diagnosis

Evaluation of hyperosmolar patients should include a careful history, clinical assessment of ECF volume, a thorough neurological evaluation, serum electrolytes, glucose, blood urea nitrogen (BUN), and creatinine, calculated and/or directly measured P_{osm}, simultaneous urine electrolytes and osmolality, and urine glucose *(28)*. Hypernatremia is always synonymous with hyperosmolality, since Na^+ is the main constituent of P_{osm}, but hyperosmolality can exist without

Table 1
Pathogenesis of Hyperosmolar Disorders

Water depletion (decreases in total body water in excess of body solute):

1. Insufficient water intake
   - Unavailability of water.
   - Hypodipsia (osmoreceptor dysfunction, age).
   - Neurological deficits (cognitive dysfunction, motor impairments).
2. Hypnotic fluid loss[a]
   - A. Renal: Diabetes Insipidus
     - Insufficient AVP secretion (central DI, osmoreceptor dysfunction).
     - Insufficient AVP effect (nephrogenic DI).
   - B. Renal: Other Fluid Loss
     - Osmotic diuresis (hyperglycemia, mannitol).
     - Diuretic drugs (furosemide, ethacrynic acid, thiazides).
     - Postobstructive diuresis
     - Diuretic phase of acute tubular necrosis.
   - C. Nonrenal fluid loss
     - Gastrointestinal (vomiting, diarrhea, nasogastric suction).
     - Cutaneous (sweating, burns).
     - Pulmonary (hyperventilation).
     - Peritoneal dialysis.

Solute excess (increases in total body solute in excess of body water):

1. Sodium
   - Excess Na^+ administration (NaCl, $NaHCO_3$).
   - Sea water drowning.
2. Other
   - Hyperalimentation (intravenous, parenteral).

[a]Most hypotonic fluid losses will not produce hyperosmolality unless insufficient free water is ingested or infused to replace the ongoing losses, so these disorders also usually involve some component of insufficient water intake.

hypernatremia when there is an excess of non-sodium solute. This occurs most often with marked elevations of plasma glucose, as in patients with nonketotic hyperglycemic hyperosmolar coma. As for cases of artifactual hyponatremia caused by elevated plasma lipids or protein, misdiagnosis can be avoided by direct measurement of P_{osm}, or by correcting the serum [Na^+] by 1.6 mEq/L for each 100 mg/dL increase in plasma glucose concentration above 100 mg/dL *(29)*, though more recent studies have indicated a more complex relation between hyperglycemia and serum [Na^+] and suggested that a more accurate correction factor is closer to 2.4 mEq/L *(30)*. Evaluation of the patient's ECF volume status is important as a guide to fluid replacement therapy, but is not as useful for differential diagnosis, since most hyperosmolar patients will manifest some degree of hypovolemia. Rather, assessment of urinary concentrating ability provides the most useful data with regard to the type of disorder present. Using this approach, disorders of hyperosmolality can be categorized as those in which renal water conservation mechanisms are intact, but are unable to compensate for inadequately replaced losses of hypotonic fluids from other sources, or those in which renal concentrating defects are a contributing factor to the deficiency of body water.

An appropriately concentrated urine in a hyperosmolar patient usually eliminates the possibility of a primary renal cause of the disorder in most cases. Maximum urine concentrating ability varies between individuals and decreases with age, but in general U_{osm}s above 800 mOsm/kg H_2O are considered sufficient to verify normal AVP secretion and renal response. In such cases, potential causes of nonrenal fluid losses should be investigated, particularly gastrointestinal and cutaneous losses (although subsequent ingestion of free water can produce hypoosmolality in such patients as a result of AVP-induced water retention). In the absence of disorders causing fluid losses, primary disorders of thirst should be considered, especially in the elderly who have a decreased sensation of thirst and ingest lesser amounts of fluids in response to induced dehydration *(31)*. One situation in which a normally concentrated urine may not completely eliminate the possibility of an underlying renal concentrating defect is in patients with mild partial central DI, who can sometimes achieve maximally concentrated urine during extreme dehydration through a combination of severely limited GFR and stimulated AVP secretion at high P_{osm}s, as will be discussed below. However, as P_{osm} is corrected, these patients will demonstrate inappropriate dilution of their urine before reaching normal levels of P_{osm}.

An inappropriately low U_{osm} (e.g., less than 800 mOsm/kg H_2O in a hyperosmolar patient) signifies the presence of a renal concentrating defect. The urine should always be checked for glucose, since a solute diuresis will limit urine concentrating ability and U_{osm} can approach isotonicity at high rates of urine excretion. In the absence of glucosuria or any other cause of osmotic diuresis, inadequate urine concentration in a hyperosmolar patient generally indicates the presence of DI and further testing is then indicated to ascertain the etiology.

Diabetes Insipidus

DI can result from either inadequate AVP secretion (central or neurogenic DI) or inadequate renal response to AVP (nephrogenic DI) (Table 2). Central DI is caused by a variety of acquired or congenital anatomic lesions that disrupt the hypothalamic-posterior pituitary axis, including pituitary surgery, tumors, trauma, hemorrhage, thrombosis, infarction, or granulomatous disease *(12)*. Severe nephrogenic DI is most commonly congenital, due to defects in the gene

Table 2
Common Etiologies of Polydipsia and Hypotonic Polyuria

Central (neurogenic) diabetes insipidus
Congenital (congenital malformations; autosomal dominant: AVP-neurophysin gene mutations).
Drug/toxin-induced (ethanol, diphenylhydantoin, snake venom).
Granulomatous (histiocytosis, sarcoidosis).
Neoplastic (craniopharyngioma, meningioma, germinoma, pituitary tumor, or metastases).
Infectious (meningitis, encephalitis).
Inflammatory/autoimmune (lymphocytic infundibuloneurohypophysitis).
Trauma (neurosurgery, deceleration injury).
Vascular (cerebral hemorrhage or infarction).
Nephrogenic diabetes insipidus
Congenital (X-linked recessive: AVP V_2 receptor gene mutations; autosomal recessive: aquaporin-2 water channel gene mutations).
Drug-induced (demeclocycline, lithium, cisplatin, methoxyflurane).
Hypercalcemia.
Hypokalemia.
Infiltrating lesions (sarcoidosis, amyloidosis).
Vascular (sickle cell anemia).
Osmoreceptor dysfunction
Granulomatous (histiocytosis, sarcoidosis).
Neoplastic (craniopharyngioma, pinealoma, meningioma, metastases).
Vascular (anterior communicating artery aneurysm/ligation, intrahypothalamic hemorrhage).
Other (hydrocephalus, ventricular/suprasellar cyst, trauma, degenerative diseases, idiopathic).
Increased AVP metabolism
Pregnancy
Primary polydipsia
Psychogenic (schizophrenia).
Dipsogenic (downward resetting of thirst threshold: similar lesions as central DI).

for the AVP V_2 receptor (X-linked recessive pattern of inheritance) or in the gene for the aquaporin-2 water channel (autosomal recessive pattern of inheritance) *(32)*, but relief of chronic urinary obstruction or therapy with drugs, such as lithium, can cause an acquired form sufficient to warrant treatment. Short-lived nephrogenic DI can result from hypokalemia or hypercalcemia, but the mild concentrating defect generally does not by itself cause hypertonicity and responds to correction of the underlying disorder. Regardless of the etiology of the DI, the end result is a free water diuresis due to an inability to concentrate urine appropriately. Because renal mechanisms for sodium conservation are unimpaired, there is no accompanying sodium deficiency. Although untreated DI can lead to both hyperosmolality and volume depletion, until the water losses become severe, volume depletion is minimized by osmotic shifts of water from the ICF to the more osmotically concentrated ECF. This phenomenon is not as evident following increases in ECF [Na^+], since such osmotic shifts result in a slower increase in the serum [Na^+] than would otherwise occur. However, when nonsodium solutes such as mannitol are infused, this effect is more obvious due to the progressive dilutional decrease in serum [Na^+] caused by translocation of intracellular water to the ECF compartment.

Because patients with DI do not have impaired urine Na^+ conservation, the ECF volume is generally not markedly decreased, and regulatory mechanisms for maintenance of osmotic homeostasis are primarily activated: stimulation of thirst and AVP secretion (to whatever degree the neurohypophysis is still able to secrete AVP). In cases where AVP secretion is totally absent (complete DI), patients are dependent entirely on water intake for maintenance of water balance. However, in cases where some residual capacity to secrete AVP remains (partial DI), P_{osm} can eventually reach levels that allow moderate degrees of urinary concentration (recall from Fig. 3 that even small concentrations of AVP can have substantial effects to limit urine volume). As the P_{osm} increases, some patients with partial DI can secrete enough AVP to achieve near maximal U_{osm}s (Fig. 5). However, this should not cause confusion about the diagnosis of DI, since in such patients the U_{osm} will still be inappropriately low at P_{osm}s within normal ranges, and they will respond to exogenous AVP administration with a further rise in U_{osm}.

Distinguishing between central and nephrogenic DI in a patient who is already hyperosmolar is straightforward and consists simply of evaluating the response to administered AVP (5 U subcutaneously [sc]) or, preferably, the AVP V_2 receptor agonist desmopressin (1-deamino-8-D-arginine vasopressin [dDAVP]; 1 μg sc or intravenously [IV]). A significant increase in U_{osm} within 1 to 2 h after injection indicates insufficient endogenous AVP secretion and, therefore, central DI, whereas an absent response indicates renal resistance to AVP effects and, therefore, nephrogenic DI (NDI) *(15)*. Although conceptually simple, interpretational difficulties often arise because the water diuresis produced by AVP deficiency produces a "wash-out" of the renal medullary concentrating gradient, so that increases in U_{osm} in response to administered AVP or dDAVP are not as great as would be expected (more recent experimental results suggest that down-regulation of collecting tubule aquaporin-2 water channels as a result of

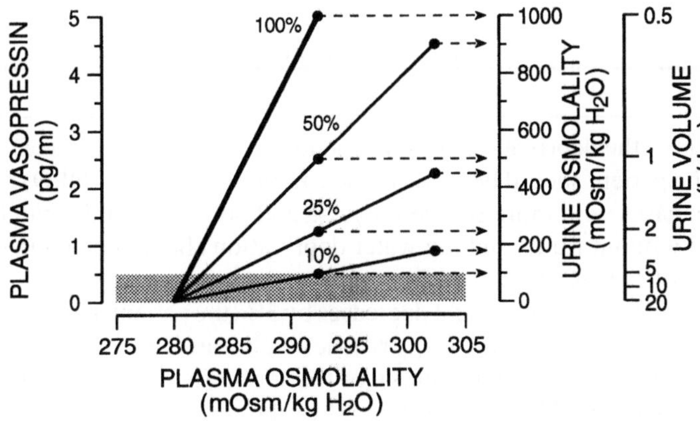

Fig. 5. Relation between plasma AVP levels, U_{osm}, and P_{osm} in subjects with normal posterior pituitary function (100%) compared to patients with graded reductions in AVP-secreting neurons (to 50, 25, and 10% of normal). Note that the patient with a 50% secretory capacity can only achieve half the plasma AVP level and half the U_{osm} of normal subjects at a P_{osm} of 293 mOsm/kg H_2O, but with increasing P_{osm} this patient can nonetheless eventually stimulate sufficient AVP secretion to reach a near maximal U_{osm}. In contrast, patients with more severe degrees of AVP-secreting neuron deficits are unable to reach maximal U_{osm}s at any levels of P_{osm} (modified with permission from ref. *12*).

AVP deficiency also contributes to the blunted response to subsequent acute AVP or dDAVP administration *[33]*). Generally, increases of U_{osm} of 50% reliably indicate central DI, and responses of 10% indicate nephrogenic DI, but responses between 10–50% are less certain *(34)*. For this reason, plasma AVP levels should be measured to aid in this distinction: hyperosmolar patients with nephrogenic DI will have clearly elevated AVP levels, while those with central DI will have absent (complete) or blunted (partial) AVP responses relative to their P_{osm}. Since it will not be known beforehand which patients will have diagnostic vs indeterminate responses to AVP or dDAVP, a plasma AVP level should be drawn prior to AVP or dDAVP administration in all patients *(35)*. One drawback to using the AVP levels for diagnosis is the relatively long turnaround time (4–10 d in most laboratories) for results. An alternative in such cases is to continue dDAVP treatment for 1 to 2 d as a clinical trial; if central DI is present, the medullary tonicity will gradually reestablish itself, and as it does, more pronounced responses to successive administered dDAVP doses will occur, thereby confirming the diagnosis.

Since patients with DI have intact thirst mechanisms, most often they do not present with hyperosmolality, but rather with a normal P_{osm} and [Na^+] and symptoms of polyuria and polydipsia. In these cases it is most appropriate to perform a water deprivation test (Table 3). This entails following the patient's serum [Na^+], urine volume, and U_{osm} in the absence of fluid intake until the serum [Na^+]

Table 3
Water Deprivation Test

Procedure

1. Initiation of the deprivation period depends on the severity of the DI; in routine cases, the patient should be made to have nothing by mouth (NPO) after dinner, while in cases with more severe polyuria and polydipsia, this may be too long a period without fluids and the water deprivation should be begun early in the morning of the test (e.g., 6 AM).
2. Stop the test when body weight decreases by 3%, the patient develops orthostatic blood pressure changes, the U_{osm} reaches a plateau (i.e., less than 10% change over 3 consecutive measurements), or the serum [Na^+] is >145 mmol/L.
3. Obtain a plasma AVP level at the end of the test when the P_{osm} is elevated, preferably above 300 mOsm/kg H_2O.
4. If the serum [Na^+] is <146 mmol/L or the P_{osm} is <300 mOsm/kg H_2O, then consider infusion of hypertonic saline (3% NaCl at a rate of 0.1 mL/kg/min for 1 to 2 h) to reach these endpoints.
5. Administer AVP (5 U) or dDAVP (1 μg) sc and continue following U_{osm} and volume for an additional 2 h.

Interpretation

1. An unequivocal urine concentration after AVP/dDAVP (>50% increase) indicates neurogenic DI and an unequivocal absence of urine concentration (<10%) strongly suggests NDI or primary polydipsia (PP).
2. Differentiating between NDI and PP, as well as for cases in which the increase in U_{osm} after AVP administration is more equivocal (e.g., 10–50%) is best done using the plasma AVP levels obtained at the end of the dehydration period and/or hypertonic saline infusion and the relation between pAVP levels and U_{osm} under basal conditions.

is 146 mEq/L or the U_{osm} reaches a plateau (generally defined as 3 successive urines with less than 10% differences in osmolality from the preceding sample) and the patient has lost at least 2% of body weight. At this point, a plasma AVP level is drawn and the patient is given AVP or dDAVP (as discussed above for hyperosmolar patients). The same criteria are used to evaluate the etiology of the DI following this test, but one additional entity, primary polydipsia, must be considered in the differential diagnosis of normonatremic polyuria and polydipsia (Table 2). Primary polydipsia is usually a result of psychiatric disease. Such patients ingest large amounts of fluids for a variety of reasons, but generally not because of physiological sensations of thirst; this is referred to as psychogenic polydipsia. A smaller subset of patients with primary polydipsia have a true disorder of thirst regulation, usually manifested by a downward resetting of the osmotic threshold for stimulated thirst; this is sometimes called dipsogenic diabetes insipidus *(36)*. Regardless of the cause of the excessive fluid intake, because the ensuing water diuresis can wash out the medullary concentration gradient and down-regulate kidney aquaporin-2 water channels, such patients may concentrate their urine subnormally in response to water deprivation and therefore, resemble partial central DI. In contrast to central DI, however, patients with primary polydipsia will generally concentrate their urine <10% in response to administered AVP or dDAVP and will have plasma AVP levels appropriate to their P_{osm}. With use of the water deprivation test combined with plasma AVP determinations, greater than 95% of all cases of polyuria and polydipsia can be diagnosed appropriately; diagnoses in the remaining patients will generally become evident over time based on their responses to therapeutic clinical trials.

Osmoreceptor Dysfunction

There is an extensive literature in animals indicating that the primary osmoreceptors that control AVP secretion and thirst are located in the anterior hypothalamus. Lesions of this region in animals cause hyperosmolality through a combination of impaired thirst and osmotically stimulated AVP secretion *(37,38)*. Initial reports in humans described this syndrome as "essential hypernatremia," and subsequent studies used the term "adipsic hypernatremia" in recognition of the profound thirst deficits found in most of the patients. Rather than focus on semantic issues, it makes more sense to group all of these syndromes as disorders of osmoreceptor function. Four major patterns of osmoreceptor dysfunction have been described as characterized by defects in thirst and/or AVP secretory responses: *(i)* upward resetting of the osmostat for both thirst and AVP secretion (normal AVP and thirst responses but at an abnormally high P_{osm}); *(ii)* partial osmoreceptor destruction (blunted AVP and thirst responses at all P_{osm}s); *(iii)* total osmoreceptor destruction (absent AVP secretion and thirst regardless of P_{osm}); and *(iv)* selective dysfunction of thirst osmoregulation with intact AVP secretion *(39)*. Most of the cases reported to date have represented various degrees of osmoreceptor destruction associated with different brain lesions. As opposed to lesions causing central DI, these lesions usually occur more anteriorly in the hypothalamus, consistent with the anterior hypothalamic location of the primary osmoreceptor cells *(12)*. Whether some of these patients also have an inability to suppress as well as stimulate AVP secretion, thereby leading to hypoosmolality in some situations, remains an interesting but incompletely evaluated possibility. For all cases of osmoreceptor dysfunction, it is important to remember that afferent pathways from the brainstem to the hypothalamus remain intact; therefore, these patients will usually have normal AVP and renal concentrating responses to baroreceptor-mediated stimuli, such as hypovolemia and hypotension *(39)*. This often causes confusion, since at some times these patients appear to have DI, and yet at other times they can concentrate their urine quite normally.

Clinical Manifestations

The clinical manifestations of any disease entity are important aids to the differential diagnosis, and therefore, it is essential that the clinician be aware of the clinical manifestations of hyperosmolar patients. These can be divided into the signs and symptoms produced by dehydration, which are largely cardiovascular, those caused by the hyperosmolality itself, which are largely neurological and reflect brain dehydration as a result of osmotic water shifts out of the central nervous system, and those that are secondary to excessive renal water losses in patients with DI. Cardiovascular manifestations of hypertonic dehydration include hypotension, azotemia, acute tubular necrosis secondary to renal hypoperfusion or rhabdomyolysis, and shock. Neurological manifestations range from nonspecific symptoms, such as irritability and decreased sensorium, to more severe manifestations, such as chorea, seizures, coma, focal neurological deficits, and cerebral infarction. The severity of symptoms can be roughly correlated with the degree of hyperosmolality, but individual variability is marked and for any single patient, the level of serum [Na^+] at which symptoms will appear cannot be predicted. Similar to hypoosmolar syndromes, the length of time over which hyperosmolality develops can markedly affect clinical symptomatology. Rapid development of severe hyperosmolality is frequently associated with marked neurologic symptoms, whereas gradual development over several days or weeks generally causes milder symptoms. In this case, the brain counteracts osmotic shrinkage by increasing intracellular content of solutes. These include electrolytes such as potassium and a variety of organic osmolytes which previously had been called "idiogenic osmoles" (for the most part these are the same organic osmolytes that are lost from the brain during adaptation to hypoosmolality) *(40)*. The net effect of this process is to protect the brain against excessive shrinkage during sustained hypertonicity. However, once the brain has adapted by increasing its solute content, rapid correction of the hyperosmolality can cause brain edema, since it takes a finite time (24–48 h in animal studies) to dissipate the accumulated solutes, and until this process has been completed, the brain will accumulate excess water as P_{osm} is normalized. This effect is most often seen in dehydrated pediatric patients, who can develop seizures with rapid rehydration, but has been described only rarely in adults, including the most severely hyperosmolar patients with nonketotic hyperglycemic hyperosmolar coma.

The characteristic symptoms of DI are the polyuria and polydipsia that result from the underlying impairment of urinary concentrating mechanisms. Interestingly, patients with DI typically describe a craving for cold water, which seems to quench their thirst better. Patients with central DI also typically describe a precipitous onset of their polyuria and polydipsia, which simply reflects the fact that urinary concentration can be maintained fairly well until the number of

AVP-producing neurons in the hypothalamus decreases to 10–15% of normal, after which plasma AVP levels decrease to the range where urine output increases dramatically (see Fig. 3) *(15)*.

HYPOOSMOLALITY AND HYPONATREMIA

Pathogenesis

Hypoosmolality indicates excess water relative to solute in the ECF; because water moves freely between ECF and ICF, this also indicates an excess of TBW relative to total body solute. Imbalances between body water and solute can be generated either by depletion of body solute more than body water, or by dilution of body solute from increases in body water more than body solute (Table 4) *(3)*. This represents an oversimplification, because most hypoosmolar states include components of both solute depletion and water retention (e.g., isotonic solute losses, as occurs during an acute hemorrhage, do not produce hypoosmolality until subsequent retention of ingested or infused hypotonic fluids causes a secondary dilution of the remaining ECF solute). Nonetheless, this concept has proven to be useful because it provides a simple framework for understanding the diagnosis and therapy of hypoosmolar disorders.

Differential Diagnosis

Evaluation of hypoosmolar patients should include a careful history (especially concerning medications), clinical assessment of ECF volume, thorough neurological evaluation, serum electrolytes, glucose, uric acid, BUN, and creatinine, calculated and/or directly measured P_{osm}, and simultaneous urine electrolytes and osmolality *(28)*. Hyponatremia and hypoosmolality are usually synonymous, with two exceptions. First, pseudohyponatremia can be produced by marked elevation of serum lipids and/or proteins; although the [Na^+]/L plasma water is unchanged, the [Na^+]/L plasma is decreased because of the increased nonaqueous portion of the plasma occupied by lipid or protein. However, the directly measured P_{osm} is not affected by increased lipids or proteins. Second, high concentrations of effective solutes other than Na^+, e.g., glucose, cause relative decreases in serum [Na^+] despite an unchanged P_{osm}. Misdiagnosis can be avoided again by direct measurement of P_{osm}, or in the case of hyperglycemia by correcting the serum [Na^+] by 1.6 mEq/L for each 100 mg/dL increase in the plasma glucose concentration above 100 mg/dL, which provides an estimate of the contribution of the glucose to the P_{osm}. Definitive identification of the etiology of the hypoosmolality is not always possible at the time of presentation, but categorization according to the patient's ECF volume status will allow determination of an appropriate initial therapy in the majority of cases (Fig. 6).

Table 4
Pathogenesis of Hypoosmolar Disorders

Solute depletion
(primary decreases in total body solute plus secondary water retention[a])

1. Renal solute loss
   - Diuretic use.
   - Solute diuresis (glucose, mannitol).
   - Salt wasting nephropathy.
   - Mineralocorticoid deficiency.
2. Nonrenal solute loss
   - Gastrointestinal (diarrhea, vomiting, pancreatitis, bowel obstruction).
   - Cutaneous (sweating, burns).
   - Blood loss.

Solute dilution
(primary increases in total body water ± secondary solute depletion[a])

1. Impaired renal free water excretion
   - A. Increased proximal nephron reabsorption
     - Congestive heart failure.
     - Cirrhosis.
     - Nephrotic syndrome.
     - Hypothyroidism.
   - B. Impaired distal nephron dilution
     - SIADH.
     - Glucocorticoid deficiency.
2. Excess water intake
   - Primary polydipsia.

[a]Virtually all disorders of solute depletion are accompanied by some degree of secondary retention of water by the kidneys in response to the resulting intravascular hypovolemia; this mechanism can lead to hypoosmolality even when the solute depletion occurs via hypotonic or isotonic body fluid losses. Disorders of water retention can cause hypoosmolality in the absence of any solute losses, but often some secondary solute losses occur in response to the resulting intravascular hypervolemia, and this can then further aggravate the dilutional hypoosmolality.

Decreased ECF Volume

Clinically detectable hypovolemia indicates some degree of solute depletion. Elevation of BUN is a useful laboratory correlate of decreased ECF volume. Even isotonic or hypotonic fluid losses can cause hypoosmolality if water or hypotonic fluids are subsequently ingested or infused. A low urine [Na^+] (U_{Na}) suggests a nonrenal cause of solute depletion, whereas a high U_{Na} suggests renal causes of solute depletion (Table 4). Diuretic use is the most common cause of hypovolemic hypoosmolality; thiazides are more commonly associated with severe hyponatremia than are loop diuretics such as furosemide *(41)*. Although

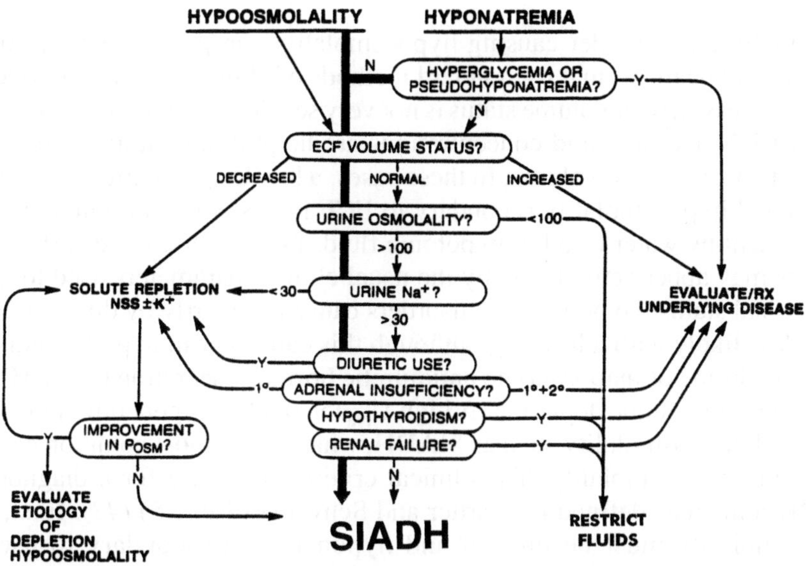

Fig. 6. Schematic summary of the evaluation of hypoosmolar patients. The dark arrow in the center emphasizes that the presence of CNS dysfunction due to hyponatremia should always be assessed immediately, so that appropriate therapy can be started as soon as possible in symptomatic patients while the outlined diagnostic evaluation is proceeding. Abbreviations: N, no; Y, yes; ECF, extracellular fluid volume; NSS, normal (isotonic) saline; Rx, treat; 1°, primary; 2°, secondary; P_{osm}, P_{osm}; d/c, discontinue; SIADH, syndrome of inappropriate antidiuretic hormone secretion; numbers referring to osmolality are in mOsm/kg H_2O, numbers referring to [Na^+] are in mEq/L (modified with permission from ref. *28*).

this seemingly is a simple example of solute depletion, the pathophysiological mechanisms underlying the hypoosmolality are complex and include multiple components. Many such patients do not present with clinical evidence of hypovolemia, in part because ingested water has been retained in response to nonosmotically stimulated vasopressin (AVP) secretion, which occurs in all disorders of solute depletion as an attempt to maintain volume homeostasis. In addition, U_{Na} may be high or low depending on when the last diuretic dose was taken. Consequently, any suspicion of diuretic use mandates careful consideration of this diagnosis regardless of clinical or laboratory findings. Most other etiologies of solute losses causing hypovolemic hypoosmolality will be clinically apparent, although some salt-wasting nephropathies (chronic interstitial nephropathy, polycystic kidney disease, obstructive uropathy, or Bartter's syndrome) or mineralocorticoid deficiency (Addison's disease) may be challenging to diagnose during early phases of these diseases.

Normal ECF Volume

Virtually any disorder causing hypoosmolality can present with a volume status that appears normal by standard methods of clinical evaluation. Because clinical assessment of volume status is not very sensitive, the presence of normal or low BUN and uric acid concentrations are helpful laboratory correlates of relatively normal ECF volume. In these cases, a low U_{Na} (<30 mEq/L) suggests depletional hypoosmolality secondary to ECF losses with subsequent volume replacement by water or other hypotonic fluids *(42)*; as discussed earlier, such patients may appear euvolemic by the usual clinical parameters used to assess hydrational status. Hypoosmolar disorders caused primarily by dilution (Table 4) are less likely with a low U_{Na}, although this can occur in hypothyroidism or in the syndrome of inappropriate antidiuretic hormone secretion (SIADH) with superimposed volume depletion. A high U_{Na} (>30 mEq/L) generally indicates a dilutional hypoosmolality such as SIADH, which is the most common cause of euvolemic hypoosmolality. The clinical criteria necessary for a diagnosis of SIADH remain as defined by Bartter and Schwartz (Table 5) *(43)*. First, ECF hypoosmolality must be present and hyponatremia secondary to pseudohyponatremia or hyperglycemia excluded. Second, U_{osm} must be inappropriate for plasma hypoosmolality; this simply requires that the urine be less than maximally dilute (i.e., Uosm >100 mOsm/kg H_2O). Furthermore, U_{osm} need not be inappropriately elevated at all levels of P_{osm}, but simply at some level below 275 mOsm/kg H_2O. In patients with a reset osmostat, AVP secretion is suppressed at some lower level of P_{osm}, resulting in maximal urinary dilution and free water excretion at P_{osm}s below this level. Third, clinical euvolemia must be present; this does not mean that patients with SIADH cannot become hypovolemic for other reasons, but in such cases, it is impossible to make a diagnosis of SIADH until the patient is made euvolemic. The fourth criterion, an elevated U_{Na}, has caused much confusion; its importance lies in differentiating hypoosmolality caused by decreased relative intravascular volume, in which renal Na^+ conservation occurs, from dilutional disorders, in which urinary Na^+ excretion is normal or increased due to ECF volume expansion. The continued excretion of ingested Na^+ by such patients reflects the importance of mechanisms for volume homeostasis, which in this case override osmotic homeostatic mechanisms that would favor Na^+ conservation. However, U_{Na} can also be high in renal causes of solute depletion, such as diuretic use or Addison's disease, and conversely, patients with SIADH can have a low urinary Na^+ excretion if they subsequently become hypovolemic or solute depleted. Consequently, although elevated urinary Na^+ excretion is the rule in most patients with SIADH, its presence does not confirm this diagnosis nor does its absence rule it out. Finally, SIADH is a diagnosis of exclusion, and other potential causes of hypoosmolality must always be excluded (Fig. 6). Glucocorticoid deficiency and SIADH can be especially difficult to distinguish,

Table 5
Criteria for the Diagnosis of SIADH

Essential

1. Decreased effective osmolality of the ECF (P_{osm} <275 mOsm/kg H_2O).
2. Inappropriate urinary concentration (U_{osm} > 100 mOsm/kg H_2O with normal renal function) at some level of hypoosmolality.
3. Clinical euvolemia, as defined by the absence of signs of hypovolemia (orthostasis, tachycardia, decreased skin turgor, dry mucous membranes) or hypervolemia (subcutaneous edema, ascites).
4. Elevated urinary sodium excretion while on a normal salt and water intake.
5. Absence of other potential causes of euvolemic hypoosmolality: hypothyroidism, hypocortisolism (Addison's disease or pituitary ACTH insufficiency) and diuretic use.

Supplemental

6. Abnormal water load test (inability to excrete at least 80% of a 20 mL/kg water load in 4 h and/or failure to dilute Uosm to <100 mOsm/kg H_2O).
7. Plasma AVP level inappropriately elevated relative to P_{osm}.
8. No significant correction of serum [Na^+] with volume expansion but improvement after fluid restriction.

since hypocortisolism can cause elevated plasma AVP levels and impair maximal urinary dilution *(44)*; no patient should be diagnosed as having SIADH without an evaluation of adrenal function, preferably via a rapid ACTH stimulation test. Although additional testing is generally not necessary to establish a diagnosis of SIADH, abnormal excretion (<80%) of a standard water load (20 mL/kg body weight) within 4 h can be helpful in confirming the diagnosis in difficult cases *(45)*. However, water loading should be avoided in patients with more severe hypoosmolality (serum [Na^+] <125 mEq/L), since abnormal retention of the ingested water can cause a significant (4–6 mEq/L) further decrease in plasma [Na^+]. Many different disorders have been associated with SIADH; these can be divided into four major etiologic groups: tumors, central nervous system (CNS) disorders, drug effects, and pulmonary diseases (Table 6).

Increased ECF Volume

Clinically detectable hypervolemia indicates whole body sodium excess, and hypoosmolality in these patients suggests a relatively decreased intravascular volume and/or pressure leading to water retention as a result of elevated plasma AVP levels and decreased distal delivery of glomerular filtrate *(46,47)*. Such patients usually have a low U_{Na} because of secondary hyperaldosteronism, but under certain conditions, the U_{Na} may be elevated (e.g., diuretic therapy).

Table 6
Common Etiologies of SIADH

Tumors
Pulmonary/mediastinal (bronchogenic carcinoma, mesothelioma, thymoma).
Nonchest (duodenal carcinoma, pancreatic carcinoma, ureteral/prostate carcinoma, uterine carcinoma, nasopharyngeal carcinoma, leukemia).
CNS disorders
Mass lesions (tumors, brain abscesses, subdural hematoma).
Inflammatory diseases (encephalitis, meningitis, systemic lupus).
Degenerative/demyelinative diseases (Guillan-Barré, spinal cord lesions).
Miscellaneous (subarachnoid hemorrhage, head trauma, acute psychosis, delirium tremens, pituitary stalk section).
Drug induced
Stimulated AVP release (nicotine, phenothiazines, tricyclics).
Direct renal effects and/or potentiation of AVP effects (dDAVP, oxytocin, prostaglandin synthesis inhibitors).
Mixed or uncertain actions (chlorpropamide, clofibrate; carbamazepine, cyclo phosphamide, vincristine).
Pulmonary diseases
Infections (tuberculosis, aspergillosis, pneumonia, empyema).
Mechanical/ventilatory (acute respiratory failure, chronic obstructive pulmonary disease [COPD], positive pressure ventilation).

Hyponatremia generally does not occur until advanced stages of congestive heart failure, cirrhosis, or nephrotic syndrome, so diagnosis is usually not difficult. Renal failure can also cause retention of both sodium and water, but in this case, the factor limiting excretion of excess body fluid is not decreased effective circulating volume but rather decreased glomerular filtration. Although primary polydipsia can sometimes cause hypoosmolality, especially if renal free water excretion is impaired, these patients rarely, if ever, manifest signs of hypervolemia, since water retention alone without sodium excess does not cause significant volume expansion.

Clinical Manifestations

The clinical manifestations of hyponatremia are largely neurological, and primarily reflect brain edema resulting from osmotic water shifts into the brain *(3,48)*. These range from nonspecific symptoms, such as headache and confusion, to more severe manifestations, such as decreased sensorium, coma, seizures, and death. Significant CNS symptoms generally do not occur until serum [Na^+] falls below 125 mEq/L, and the severity of symptoms can be roughly correlated with the degree of hypoosmolality *(49)*. Individual variability is marked, and for any patient the level of serum [Na^+] at which symptoms will appear cannot be predicted. Several factors other than the severity of the hypoosmolality also affect the degree of neurological dysfunction. The most important is the time-course over which hypoosmolality develops. Rapid development of severe hypoosmolality frequently causes marked neurologic symptoms, whereas gradual development over several days or weeks is often associated with relatively mild symptomatology despite profound degrees of hypoosmolality. This is because the brain counteracts osmotic swelling by extruding extracellular and intracellular solutes (including potassium and organic osmolytes) *(50)*. Since this is a time-dependent process, rapid development of hypoosmolality can result in brain edema before this adaptation occurs, but with slower development of the same degree of hypoosmolality brain cells can lose solute sufficiently rapidly to prevent cell swelling, brain edema, and neurological dysfunction *(3)*. Underlying neurological disease also affects the level of hypoosmolality at which CNS symptoms appear; moderate hypoosmolality is of little concern in an otherwise healthy patient, but can cause morbidity in a patient with an underlying seizure disorder. Non-neurological metabolic disorders (hypoxia, hypercapnia, acidosis, hypercalcemia, etc.) can similarly affect the level of P_{osm} at which CNS symptoms occur *(51)*. Recent clinical studies have suggested that menstruating females and young children may be particularly susceptible to the development of neurological morbidity and mortality during hyponatremia, especially in the acute postoperative setting *(52,53)*. The true clinical incidence, as well as the underlying mechanisms responsible for these sometimes catastrophic cases, remains to be determined.

REFERENCES

1. Fanestil DD. Compartmentation of body water. In: Narins RG, ed. Clinical Disorders of Fluid and Electrolyte Metabolism. McGraw-Hill, New York, 1994, 3–20.
2. Rose BD. New approach to disturbances in the plasma sodium concentration. Am J Med 1986; 81:1033–1040.
3. Verbalis JG. The syndrome of inappropriate antidiuretic hormone secretion and other hypoosmolar disorders. In: Schrier RW, ed. Diseases of the Kidney and Urinary Tract. Lippincott Williams & Wilkins, Philadelphia, 2001, 2511–2548.
4. Vokes TP, Aycinena PR, Robertson GL. Effect of insulin on osmoregulation of vasopressin. Am J Physiol 1987; 252:E538–E548.
5. Verbalis JG. Body water and osmolality. In: Jamison RL, Wilkinson R, eds. Nephrology. Chapman & Hall Medical, London. 1997, 89–94.
6. Fitzsimons JT. Physiology and pathophysiology of thirst and sodium appetite. In: Seldin DW, Giebisch G, eds. The Kidney, Physiology and Pathophysiology. Raven Press, New York, 1992, 1615–1648.
7. Stricker EM, Verbalis JG. Water intake and body fluids. In: Zigmond MJ, Bloom FE, Landis SC, Roberts JL, Squire LR, eds. Fundamental Neuroscience. Academic Press, San Diego, 1999, 1111–1126.

8. Robertson GL. Thirst and vasopressin function in normal and disordered states of water balance. J Lab Clin Med 1983; 101:351–371.
9. Thompson CJ, Bland J, Burd J, Baylis PH. The osmotic thresholds for thirst and vasopressin release are similar in healthy man. Clin Sci (Colch) 1986; 71:651–656.
10. Phillips PA, Rolls BJ, Ledingham JG, Morton JJ, Forsling ML. Angiotensin II-induced thirst and vasopressin release in man. Clin Sci (Colch) 1985; 68:669–674.
11. de Castro J. A microregulatory analysis of spontaneous fluid intake in humans: evidence that the amount of liquid ingested and its timing is mainly governed by feeding. Physiol Behav 1988; 3:705–714.
12. Robertson GL. Posterior pituitary. In: Felig P, Baxter J, Frohman L, eds. Endocrinology and Metabolism. McGraw-Hill, New York, 1995, 385–432.
13. Knepper MA. Molecular physiology of urinary concentrating mechanism: regulation of aquaporin water channels by vasopressin. Am J Physiol 1997; 272:F3–F12.
14. Robertson GL. The regulation of vasopressin function in health and disease. Recent Prog Horm Res 1976; 33:333–385.
15. Robinson AG. Disorders of antidiuretic hormone secretion. Clin Endocrinol Metab 1985; 14:55–88.
16. Rowe JW, Shelton RL, Helderman JH, Vestal RE, Robertson GL. Influence of the emetic reflex on vasopressin release in man. Kidney Int 1979; 16:729–735.
17. Robertson GL, Aycinena P, Zerbe RL. Neurogenic disorders of osmoregulation. Am J Med 1982; 72:339–353.
18. Verbalis JG. Body sodium and extracellular fluid volume. In: Jamison R, Wilkinson R, eds. Nephrology. Chapman & Hall Medical, London, 1997, 95–101.
19. Denton D. The Hunger for Salt: An Anthropological, Physiological and Medical Analysis. Springer-Verlag, Berlin. 1982.
20. Wilkins L, Richter CP. A great craving for salt by a child with cortico-adrenal insufficiency. JAMA 1940; 114:866–868.
21. Orth DN, Kovacs WJ. The adrenal cortex. In: Wilson JD, Foster DW, Kronenberg HM, Larsen PR, eds. Williams Textbook of Endocrinology. W.B. Saunders, Philadelphia. 1998, 517–664.
22. Kirchner KA Stein JH. Sodium metabolism. In: Narins RG ed. Clinical Disorders of Fluid and Electrolyte Metabolism. McGraw-Hill, New York, 1994, 45–80.
23. Reeves WB and Andreoli TE. Tubular sodium transport. In: Schrier RW, editor. Diseases of the Kidney and Urinary Tract. Lippincott Williams & Wilkins, Philadelphia. 2001, 135–175.
24. Baylis C, Lemley KV. Glomerular filtration. In: Jamison RL, Wilkinson R, eds. Nephrology. Chapman & Hall, London, 1997, 25–33.
25. Masilamani S, Kim GH, Mitchell C, Wade JB, Knepper MA. Aldosterone-mediated regulation of ENaC alpha, beta, and gamma subunit proteins in rat kidney. J Clin Invest 1999; 104:R19–R23.
26. Schneider EG, Radke KJ, Ulderich DA, Taylor R.E., Jr. Effect of osmolality on aldosterone secretion. Endocrinology 1985; 116:1621–1626.
27. Hall JE, Granger JP, Smith MJ Jr, Premen AJ. Role of renal hemodynamics and arterial pressure in aldosterone "escape". Hypertension 1984; 6:I183–I192.
28. Verbalis JG. Hyponatremia and hypoosmolar disrders. In: Greenberg A, ed. Primer on Kidney Diseases. Academic Press, San Diego. 2001, 57–63.
29. Katz MA. Hyperglycemia-induced hyponatremia—calculation of expected serum sodium depression. N Eng J Med 1973; 289:843–844.
30. Hillier TA, Abbott RD, Barrett EJ. Hyponatremia: evaluating the correction factor for hyperglycemia. Am J Med 1999; 106:399–403.
31. Phillips PA, Rolls BJ, Ledingham JG, et al. Reduced thirst after water deprivation in healthy elderly men. N Engl J Med 1984; 311:753–759.

32. Fujiwara TM, Morgan K, Bichet DG. Molecular biology of diabetes insipidus. Annu Rev Med 1995; 46:331–343.
33. Knepper MA, Verbalis JG, Nielsen S. Role of aquaporins in water balance disorders. Curr Opin Nephrol Hypertens 1997; 6:367–371.
34. Zerbe RL, Robertson GL. A comparison of plasma vasopressin measurements with a standard indirect test in the differential diagnosis of polyuria. N Eng J Med 1981; 305:1539–1546.
35. Robertson GL. Diabetes insipidus. Endocrinol Metab Clin North Am 1995; 24:549–572.
36. Robertson GL. Dipsogenic diabetes insipidus: a newly recognized syndrome caused by a selective defect in the osmoregulation of thirst. Trans Assoc Am Physicians 1995; 100:241–249.
37. Thrasher TN, Keil LC, Ramsay DJ. Lesions of the organum vasculosum of the lamina terminalis (OVLT) attenuate osmotically-induced drinking and vasopressin secretion in the dog. Endocrinology 1982; 110:1837–1839.
38. Johnson AK, Buggy J. Periventricular preoptic-hypothalamus is vital for thirst and normal water economy. Am J Physiol 1978; 234:R122–R129.
39. Baylis PH, Thompson CJ. Diabetes insipidus and hyperosmolar syndromes. In: Becker KL, ed. Principles and Practice of Endocrinology and Metabolism. Lippincott Williams & Wilkins, Philadelphia. 2001, 285-293.
40. Gullans SR, Verbalis JG. Control of brain volume during hyperosmolar and hypoosmolar conditions. Annu Rev Med 1993; 44:289–301.
41. Spital A. Diuretic-induced hyponatremia. Am J Nephrol 1999; 19:447–452.
42. Chung HM, Kluge R, Schrier RW, Anderson RJ. Clinical assessment of extracellular fluid volume in hyponatremia. Am J Med 1987; 83:905–908.
43. Bartter FC, Schwartz WB. The syndrome of inappropriate secretion of antidiuretic hormone. Am J Med 1987; 42:790–806.
44. OelkersW. Hyponatremia and inappropriate secretion of vasopressin (antidiuretic hormone) in patients with hypopituitarism. N Eng J Med 1989; 321:492–496.
45. Carroll PB, McHenry L, Verbalis JG. Isolated adrenocorticotrophic hormone deficiency presenting as chronic hyponatremia. NY State J Med 1990; 90:210–213.
46. Schrier RW. Pathogenesis of sodium and water retention in high-output and low-output cardiac failure, nephrotic syndrome, cirrhosis, and pregnancy (1). N Eng J Med 1988; 319:1065–1072.
47. Schrier RW. Pathogenesis of sodium and water retention in high-output and low-output cardiac failure, nephrotic syndrome, cirrhosis, and pregnancy (2). N Eng J Med 1988; 319:1127–1134.
48. Adrogue HJ, Madias NE. Hyponatremia. N Engl J Med 2000; 342:1581–1589.
49. Arieff AI, Llach F, Massry SG. Neurological manifestations and morbidity of hyponatremia: correlation with brain water and electrolytes. Medicine 1976; 55:121–129.
50. Verbalis JG, Gullans SR. Hyponatremia causes large sustained reductions in brain content of multiple organic osmolytes in rats. Brain Res 1991; 567:274–282.
51. Vexler ZS, Ayus JC, Roberts TP, Fraser CL, Kucharczyk J, Arieff AI. Hypoxic and ischemic hypoxia exacerbate brain injury associated with metabolic encephalopathy in laboratory animals. J Clin Invest 1994; 93:256–3264.
52. Ayus JC, Wheeler JM, Arieff AI. Postoperative hyponatremic encephalopathy in menstruant women. Ann Intern Med 1992; 117:891–897.
53. Arieff Al, Ayus J C, Fraser CL. Hyponatraemia and death or permanent brain damage in healthy children. Br Med J 1992; 304:1218–31222.

3 Pituitary Tumors

Prolactinomas, Acromegaly, Gonadotropin-Producing, Nonfunctioning

Mary Lee Vance, MD

CONTENTS

INTRODUCTION

Pituitary tumors are not uncommon and are diagnosed because of hormone disturbance, mass effect, or as an incidental finding when an imaging study is obtained because of head trauma or headache. The exact prevalence of pituitary tumors is not known, but autopsy studies of patients without suspected endocrine disease demonstrated an adenoma of the pituitary in up to 26% of specimens, and 40% of these produced prolactin with immunocytochemical staining *(1)*. With more clinical awareness, improved hormone assays, and modern imaging (computed tomography[CT], magnetic resonance imaging [MRI]), diagnosis of a pituitary tumor is relatively straightforward. The presenting features of a pituitary tumor depend upon the type and size of tumor. Headache is a common feature and occurs with a microadenoma (<10 mm) or a macroadenoma (>10 mm). Unfortunately, many patients are mistakenly assumed to have a migraine syndrome resulting in a delay in diagnosis. A fairly consistent occurrence in premenopausal women and men is gonadal dysfunction, such as amenorrhea, oligomenorrhea, or infertility in women and decreased libido and erectile dysfunction in men. In postmenopausal women, the most common presentation is that

From: *Contemporary Endocrinology: Handbook of Diagnostic Endocrinology*
Edited by: J. E. Hall and L. K. Nieman © Humana Press Inc., Totowa, NJ

of a mass—headache and/or visual loss. If the tumor compromises normal pituitary function, the patient may have secondary adrenal insufficiency, secondary hypothyroidism, secondary hypogonadism, and growth hormone deficiency; one or more pituitary deficiencies may occur. The occurrence of adrenal insufficiency or hypothyroidism, requires immediate replacement. Diabetes insipidus is uncommon in a patient with a pituitary adenoma. Diabetes insipidus as an initial feature is more suggestive of metastatic disease, sarcoidosis, a craniopharyngioma, or a Rathke's cleft cyst. The challenge is to determine the type of pituitary adenoma, the need for hormone replacement, and the appropriate therapy or therapies.

HYPOPITUITARISM

A patient with a large pituitary tumor is at risk for secondary adrenal insufficiency, secondary hypothyroidism, secondary hypogonadism, and growth hormone (GH) deficiency. The immediate need is to determine if glucocorticoid and/or thyroid hormone replacement is necessary. This can be accomplished by measuring a morning serum cortisol and a serum thyroxine or free thyroxine level (thyroid-stimulating hormone [TSH] is of no value and may be misleading in secondary hypothyroidism). If the morning serum cortisol level is below normal, the patient requires glucocorticoid replacement. If the morning serum cortisol is normal, this does not guarantee that the patient will have a normal response to stress. In this situation, an insulin hypoglycemia test is the most accurate to determine the need for replacement. An adrenocorticotrophic hormone (ACTH) stimulation test may be misleading if adrenal insufficiency is of recent onset—the adrenal glands may respond normally (peak serum cortisol 18 μg/dL or greater) despite impaired ACTH reserve. Serum sodium and potassium concentrations are usually normal, since aldosterone secretion remains normal, because it is independent of ACTH control. If there is doubt about ACTH reserve, it is prudent to administer glucocorticoid replacement and test the patient at a later time. A caveat is that replacement of thyroid hormone in the setting of compromised ACTH secretion may precipitate an adrenal insufficiency crisis, emphasizing the importance of determining the need for glucocorticoid replacement before beginning thyroid hormone therapy. The most common deficiencies are the gonadotropins and growth hormone, which do not require immediate replacement. Depending on the tumor type and treatment, it is prudent to assess these hormones after treatment to determine continuing need for replacement.

PROLACTINOMA

The most common type of secretory pituitary tumor produces prolactin and hyperprolactinemia, which most commonly causes gonadal dysfunction in premenopausal women and in men. Serum prolactin may range from mildly elevated (30–60 ng/mL) to several thousand. Because prolactin, is a stress hormone and affected by venipuncture and nipple stimulation, it is advisable to obtain more than one serum prolactin when the first value is less than 60 ng/mL, to make sure this is a consistent finding.

Men and postmenopausal women usually have a macroadenoma at the time of diagnosis, while a microadenoma is more common in premenopausal women. Gonadal dysfunction in premenopausal women may include amenorrhea, oligomenorrhea, or regular menses with infertility. Galactorrhea may be an indicator of increased prolactin; however, approx 50% of women with galactorrhea do not have hyperprolactinemia. One caveat about evaluating young women is that they may harbor a tumor that secretes both prolactin and growth hormone without the classical clinical features of acromegaly. Similarly, men with hyperprolactinemia may not have obvious features of excessive GH secretion. Thus, every patient with hyperprolactinemia should be screened with a serum insulin-like growth factor-1 (IGF-1) measurement to exclude acromegaly, since the disease may be of recent onset and the patient has not yet developed the classical features of acromegaly. Postmenopausal women do not have menses to indicate a problem; thus, these women usually present with symptoms or signs of a mass—headache, visual loss, and cranial nerve dysfunction. Men are most commonly diagnosed because of a mass effect, headache, or visual loss. On careful questioning, decreased libido and erectile dysfunction are common but usually attributed to stress or getting older.

In Table 1 is listed causes of an elevated serum prolactin. These etiologies should be considered before assuming the patient has a pituitary tumor. Medications are a common cause of hyperprolactinemia; discontinuation of the medication may result in a normal serum prolactin. Primary hypothyroidism is a common cause of increased prolactin, thus a TSH and serum thyroxine or free thyroxine level should be obtained. Once other causes of hyperprolactinemia have been excluded, the pituitary and hyopthalamus should be imaged with an MRI scan, the best method of visualizing these structures. The anatomy must be correlated with the serum prolactin concentration in order to select appropriate therapy. An elevated prolactin does not always indicate a true prolactinoma. In a patient with a macroadenoma, >10 mm, a prolactin level of >200 ng/mL is chacteristic of a true prolactinoma. Any type of macroadenoma may cause an elevation in prolactin by interfering with dopamine transport through the pituitary stalk; serum prolactin is usually <200 ng/mL in this situation *(2,3)*. In the situation of no visible tumor on MRI and no other cause of hyperprolactinemia, the patient may harbor a small adenoma, which cannot be visualized, or possibly lactotrope hyperplasia. In general, the serum prolactin in a patient with a microadenoma (<10 mm) is less than 200 ng/mL and occasionally may be higher.

The correct diagnosis cannot be overemphasized, since the treatment decision is based on this assessment. In the situation of hyperprolactinemia, less than 200 ng/mL, and a macroadenoma, treatment with a dopamine-agonist drug will

Table 1
Causes of Hyperprolactinemia

Pituitary adenoma	
	Prolactinoma
	Acromegaly
	Macroadenoma (secondary hyperprolactinemia)
Pituitary lesion	
	Craniopharyngioma
	Rathke's cleft cyst
	Meningioma
	Chordoma
	Hemangiopericytoma
	Germinoma
Pituitary radiation	
Primary hypothyroidism	
Infiltrative disease (hypothalamic, pituitary)	
	Sarcoidosis
	Giant cell granuloma
	Lymphocytic hypophysitis
	Hystiocytosis X
	Tuberculosis
Chronic renal failure	
Cirrhosis	
Medications	
	Metoclopramide, Domperidone
	Resperidol, Haldol, Stelazine, Chlorpromazine
	Amoxapine
	Verapamil
	Morphine
	Estrogen
Chest wall stimulation	
	Nipple stimulation
	Spinal cord injury
	Breast implants
Stress	
	Physical
	Psychological
Idiopathic	

reduce the serum prolactin concentration, but shrinkage of the tumor does not usually occur. Medical treatment of a true prolactinoma results in reduction in prolactin and in tumor size in more than 90% of patients *(4)*. There are three dopamine-agonist drugs available in the United States, bromocriptine, pergolide and cabergoline. Pergolide, is not Food and Drug Administration (FDA) approved for treatment of hyperprolactinemia, but is less expensive than the other two preparations.

ACROMEGALY

Acromegaly is a multisystem disease resulting from excessive GH. The classical features of enlargement of hands, feet, and face (prognathism, dental malocclusion, frontal bossing, thickening of nose and lips) may take many years to become evident. Prior to the recognition of these classical characteristics, patients develop carpal tunnel syndrome, hyperhidrosis, oily skin, skin tags, cystic acne, joint pain (large joints: shoulders, hips, back, knees), hypertension, glucose intolerance or diabetes, sleep apnea, nodular goiter, and less commonly, congestive cardiomyopathy. An unfortunate reality is that most patients have the disease for 7 yr or more before correct diagnosis is made. Another unfortunate fact is that acromegaly is associated with premature mortality, approx 10 yr earlier than the normal population. The most common cause of death is cardiovascular disease; additionally, there is a 13.7-fold increased risk of colorectal cancer. Lowering of GH and IGF-1 to normal age-adjusted levels reverses the risk of premature mortality *(5,6)*.

Although the most common features of acromegaly are hyperhidrosis and enlargement of hands, feet, and face, other manifestations include other common medical conditions that may not raise the question of acromegaly. For example, at the time of diagnosis, 25% of patients have diabetes and over 50% have glucose intolerance, 82% of patients have sleep apnea, and more than one-third have hypertension. The precise incidence of carpal tunnel syndrome is unknown, but it is quite common, with many patients having previously undergone surgery. Patients rarely report excessive sweating or enlargement of hands and feet, often attributing these to aging, weight gain, or just a natural occurrence.

The diagnosis of acromegaly is usually straightforward. The best screening test is a serum IGF-1 concentration. IGF-1 is an indicator of overall growth hormone secretion and is the primary mediator of GH action. The IGF-1 assay is important, since some commercial laboratories do not provide a suitable range of normal values according to age and sex. GH production declines with age, and women produce more GH than men; thus, IGF-1 also varies with age and gender. A single serum GH measurement is of little value, since GH is released in a pulsatile fashion. Additionally, patients with acromegaly may have a "normal" random GH level, but the pattern of GH release is abnormal, with failure of GH levels to decline to undetectable or very low values. The pattern of GH secretion is more important than a single value; when GH is measured every 5 min over 24 h, the secretory profile is quite different from that of normal subjects (Fig. 1). The definitive test for diagnosis acromegaly is an oral glucose tolerance test with administration of 75 or 100 g glucose and measurement of serum glucose and GH concentrations every 30 min for 2 h. With the refinement of GH assays, the definition of a normal response has changed. Using sensitive radio immunoassay (RIA) or immunoradiometric

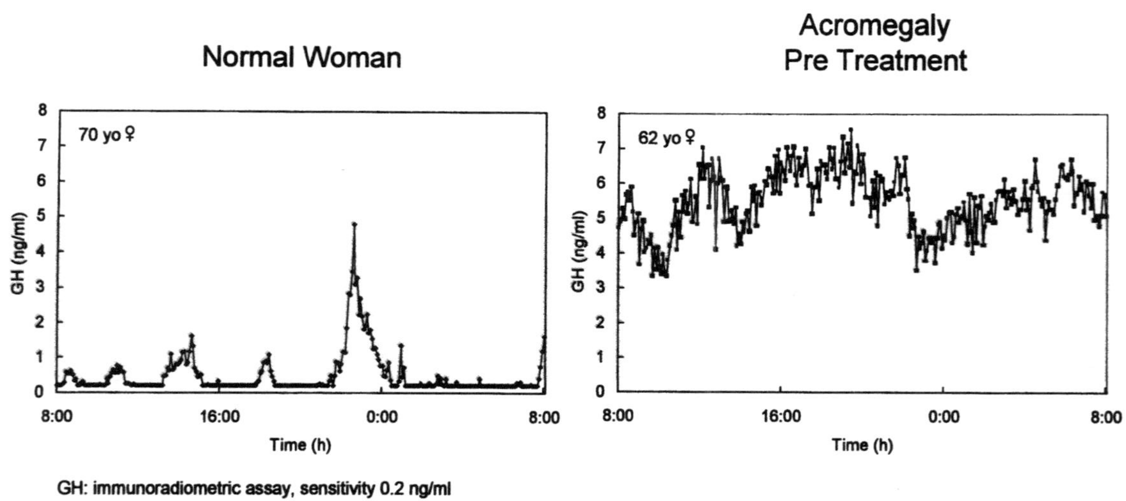

Fig. 1. Serum growth hormone levels measured every 5 min for 24 h in a normal woman and a woman with acromegaly.

assays (IRMA) methods, the normal GH response to oral glucose is <1 μg/L *(7)*. Using a more sensitive chemiluminescence assay, the nadir GH was 0.029 ± 0.014 μg/L in men and 0.25 ± 0.23 μg/L in women; this assay is not currently in widespread use *(8)*. A random GH level is not adequate to diagnose acromegaly unless the level is very elevated, e.g., >40 ng/mL.

If a patient has an elevated serum IGF-1 level and an abnormal GH response to oral glucose, an MRI is indicated. Approx 75% of patients with acromegaly have a macroadenoma at the time of diagnosis. This is consequential, since successful surgery for acromegaly is 50–60% when surgery is performed by an experienced pituitary surgeon. Thus, additional treatment or treatments (medical treatment and pituitary radiation) are often required to lower GH and IGF-1 to normal. The importance of lowering GH and IGF-1 levels to normal cannot be overemphasized, since elevated GH levels are associated with in premature mortality, and this is reversible with successful therapy *(5)*.

Medical treatment with a somatostatin analog (octreotide, Sandostatin LAR, lanreotide) reduces serum IGF-1 to normal in 50–60% of patients *(9–20)*. A substantial number of patients will not have reduction in GH and IGF-1 to normal, and medical therapy does not cure, but controls, the disease. Thus, pituitary radiation offers the prospect of reducing GH secretion permanently. The drawback to pituitary radiation, conventional or stereotactic, is that it is not effective immediately. Conventional fractionated radiation may not be effective for 10–20 yr; stereotactic (γ Knife) radiation is effective earlier in some patients, but again, may take several years to reduce IGF-1 to normal. A combination of medical therapy with a somatostatin analog and pituitary radiation offers the possibility of control of GH secretion while awaiting the effect of pituitary radiation. Patients who have undergone radiation therapy should be withdrawn from medical therapy at regular intervals (e.g., every 6 mo) and reevaluated to determine if radiation has become effective. Dopamine agonist treatment may reduce serum IGF-1 to normal, but this occurs in less than 10% of patients. Acromegaly often requires more than one treatment and involves a combination of surgical, medical, and radiotherapy treatments to effect reduction in excessive GH secretion.

GONADOTROPIN-PRODUCING ADENOMA

A gonadotropin-producing adenoma may secrete excessive amounts of lutenizing hormone (LH), follicle stimulating hormone (FSH), α-subunit, singly or in combination *(21,22)*. Additionally, this tumor type may secrete only the β-subunit of LH or FSH. Detection of these secretory products requires a specific assay, which is not readily available commercially. The precise prevalence of gonadotropin-producing adenomas is variable, from 45–90% of clinically nonfunctioning tumors are positive by immunostaining for LH, FSH, α-subunit, FSH β and LH β *(23–25)*. Most commonly, these secretory tumors cause hypogonadism, probably because of abnormal pulsatile gonadotropin secretion, with failure to stimulate ovarian and testicular function. A few cases of increased testosterone associated with an LH-secreting adenoma have been reported, as have several cases of ovarian hyperstimulation, associated with an FSH-secreting adenoma. Identifying a gonadotropin-secreting adenoma prior to treatment is useful to assess success of treatment (most commonly surgery) by having a serum tumor marker to follow.

The diagnosis of a gonadotroph adenoma is dependent on the presence of an excessive serum concentration of the particular hormone (LH, FSH, α-subunit). Administration of gonadotropin-releasing hormone (GnRH) with measurement of LH, FSH, and α-subunit responses has been proposed as a method of diagnosis. However, this has not proven to be of clinical utility. In general, a nonsecretory pituitary macroadenoma is associated with "normal" or suppressed levels of LH, FSH, and α-subunit. These tumors are found in men with secondary hypogonadism and in postmenopausal women. Thus, a slightly increased LH, FSH, or α-subunit may indicate a secretory gonadotropin tumor. The importance of identifying a gonadotrope adenoma is the use of a serum tumor marker to assess the effect of therapy.

Initial therapy is surgical removal with postoperative serum measurement of the hormone produced in excess, as well as an MRI study to assess anatomy (optimally 3 mo after surgery). At the postoperative evaluation (usually 6 wk after surgery), gonadotropin and α-subunit concentrations should be measured to determine the response to surgery. Serial hormone measurement of the elevated hormone or hormones every 6–12 mo allows for detection of tumor recurrence and for early intervention. There are no consistently effective medical therapies for this type of tumor *(24)*, thus emphasizing the need for lifelong follow up for recurrence, including hormone measurements and at least a yearly imaging study (MRI). Tumor recurrence may be treated with surgery and/or pituitary radiation, the choice depending on the size of the tumor, clinical features (headache, visual abnormality), and patient preference. In general once a tumor has recurred, it can be presumed to be "aggressive", which usually warrants a combination of a second surgical removal and postoperative pituitary radiation (conventional or stereotactic).

NONFUNCTIONING ADENOMA

Nonfunctioning pituitary adenomas are so designated, because they do not secrete an excess of a pituitary hormone into the circulation. However, the majority of these tumors synthesize a hormone or hormones when examined by immunostaining. The most common type are immunopositive for LH, FSH, and α-subunit, either singly or in combination. Uncommonly, a tumor may be positive on immunostaining for TSH, which is biologically inactive. Electron microscopic examination of these tumors confirms that they are gonadotrope in origin.

Clinically, these are nonfunctioning, since excess LH, FSH, or α-subunit is not detected in the serum. Explanations for this observation are that the hormone is either not released into the circulation or that posttranslational processing or glycosylation is altered and the antibody does not recognize the product. Other types of nonsecretory adenomas include "silent" ACTH, "silent" GH, "silent" subtype 3, and null cell adenomas. Patients with a silent ACTH or silent GH adenoma do not have clinical features of Cushing's syndrome or acromegaly, and biochemical measures (24-h urine free cortisol, serum ACTH, serum IGF-1, GH response to oral glucose) do not indicate ACTH or GH hypersecretion. Null cell adenomas do not have positive immunostaining for any hormone while silent ACTH and GH tumors are immunopositive for ACTH and GH, respectively. The "silent" ACTH, GH, and subtype 3 tumors are clinically important, since they have been described as being more "aggressive" regarding growth and risk of recurrence compared with other nonfunctioning adenomas.

The diagnosis of a nonfunctioning adenoma resides solely with the examination of the surgical specimen. Immunostaining for all of the pituitary hormones and electron microscopy are the most precise methods to chacterize the tumor type.

Treatment for a nonfunctioning adenoma is surgical removal with close monitoring for recurrence. The reported recurrence rate for nonsecretory adenomas is 16% within 10 yr, with a symptomatic recurrence rate of 10% within 10 yr *(26–28)*. Since there is no method to predict which patient will have a recurrence, all patients should be followed lifelong, with a yearly MRI study. Pituitary adenomas have been known to recur 20 yr after initial treatment. The use of adjunctive pituitary radiation is indicated in some patients, and the criteria for treatment are identical to those of gonadotrope adenomas. Although the goal of pituitary radiation is to prevent recurrence, a tumor may recur after such treatment, again emphasizing the need for lifelong monitoring.

SUMMARY

Pituitary tumors are more common than is generally recognized. Once a patient is diagnosed with a pituitary mass, it is necessary to characterize the type of tumor, the presence of hypopituitarism, begin essential hormone replacement, and recommend appropriate therapy. Dopamine agonist is the preferred therapy for a prolactinoma, and surgical resection by an experienced pituitary surgeon is recommended for all other tumor types. Regardless of the tumor type and the treatment or treatments, a patient with a pituitary tumor requires lifelong follow-up.

REFERENCES

1. Burrow GN, Wortzman G, Rewcastle NB, Holgate RC, Kovacs K. Microadenomas of the pituitary and abnormal sellar tomograms in an unselected autopsy series. N Engl J Med 1981;304:156–158.

2. Balagura S, Frantz AG, Houspain EM, et al. The specificity of serum prolactin as a diagnostic indicator of pituitary adenoma. J Neurosurg 1979;51:42–46.
3. Antunes JL, Houspain EM, Frantz AG. Proalctin-secreting pituitary tumors. Ann Neurol 1977;2:148–153.
4. Vance ML, Evans WS, Thorner MO. Drugs five years later: bromocriptine. Ann Intern Med 1984;100:78–91.
5. Bates AS, Van't Hoff W, Jones JM, Clayton RN. 1993 An audit of outcome of treatment in acromegaly. Q J Med 1993;86:293–299.
6. Orme SM, McNally RJ, Cartwright RA, Belchetz PE. Mortality and cancer incidence in acromegaly: a retrospective cohort study. United Kingdom Acromegaly Study Group. J Clin Endocrinol Metab 1998;83:2730–2734.
7. Stoffel-Wagner B, Springer W, Bidlingmaier F, Klingmüller. A comparison of different methods for diagnosing acromegaly. Clin Endocrinol 1997;46:531–537.
8. Chapman IM, Hartman ML, Straume M, Johnson ML, Veldhuis JD, Thorner MO. Enhanced sensitivity growth hormone (GH) chemiluminescence assay reveals lower post glucose nadir GH concentration in men and women. J Clin Endocrinol Metab 1994;78:1312–1319.
9. Quabbe HJ, Plockinger U. Dose-response study and long-term effects of the somatostatin analog octreotide in patients with therapy-resistant acromegaly. J Clin Endocrinol Metab 1989;68:873#-3881.
10. McKnight JA, McCance DR, Sheridan B, et al. A long-term dose-response study of somatostatin analogue (SMS 201-995, octreotide) in resistant acromegaly. Clin Endocrinol 1991;34:119–125
11. Vance ML, Harris AG. Long term treatment of 189 acromegalic patients with the somatostatin analog octreotide. Arch Intern Med 1991;151:1573–1578.
12. Ezzat S, Snyder PJ, Young WF, et al. Octreotide treatment of acromegaly: a randomized multicenter trial. Ann Intern Med 1992;117:711–718.
13. Newman CB, Melmed S, Snyder PJ, et al. Safety and efficacy of long-term octreotide therapy of acromegaly: results of a multicenter trial in 103 patients. J Clin Endocrinol Metab 1995;80:2768–2775.
14. Lucas-Morante T, Garcia-Urda J, Estada J, et al. Treatment of invasive growth hormone pituitary adenomas with long-acting somatostatin analog SMS 201-995 before transsphenoidal surgery. J Neurosurg 1994;81:10–14.
15. Stewart PM, Kane KF, Stewart SE, Lancranjan I, Sheppard MC. Depot long-acting somatostatin analog (Sandostatin-LAR) is an effective treatment for acromegaly. J Clin Endocrinol Metab 1995;80:3267–3272.
16. Flogstad AK, Halse J, Bakke S, et al. Sandostatin LAR in acromegalic patients: long term treatment. J Clin Endocrinol Metab 1997;82:23#-328.
17. Morange I, DeBoisvilliers F, Chanson P, et al. Slow release lanreotide treatment in acromegalic patients previously normalized by octreotide. J Clin Endocrinol Metab 1994;79:145–151.
18. Giusti M, Gussoni G, Cuttica CM, et al. Effectiveness and tolerability of slow release lanreotide treatment in active acromegaly: six-month report on an Italian Multicenter Study. J Clin Endocrinol Metab 1996;81:2089–2097
19. Al-Maskari M, Gebbie J, Kendall-Taylor P. The effect of a new slow-release, long-acting somatostatin analogue, lanreotide, in acromegaly. Clin Endocrinol 1996;45:415–421
20. Caron P, Morange-Ramos I, Cogne M, Jaquet P. Three year follow-up of acromegalic patients treated with intramuscular slow-release lanreotide. J Clin Endocrinol Metab 1996;82:18–22.
21. Vance ML, Ridgway EC, Thorner MO. Follicle-stimulating hormone- and α-subunit-secreting pituitary treated with bromocriptine. J Clin Endocrinol Metab 1985;61:580–584.
22. Borges JLC, Ridgway EC, Kovacs K, Rogol AD, Thorner MO. Follicle-stimulating hormone-secreting pituitary tumor with concomitant elevation of serum α-subunit levels. J Clin Endocrinol Metab 1984;58:937–941.

23. Katznelson, L, Alexander JM, Klibanski A. Clinical review 45 clinically nonfunctioning pituitary adenomas. J Clin Endocrinol Metab 1993;76:1089–1094.
24. Daneshdoost L, Gennarelli TA, Bashey HM, et al. Recognition of gonadotroph adenomas in women. N Engl J Med 1991;324:589–627.
25. Black PM, Hsu DW, Klibanski A, et al. Hormone production in clinically non-functioning pituitary adenomas. J Neurosurg 1987;66:244–250.
26. Ebersold MJ, Quast LM, Laws ER, Scheithauer B, Randall RV. Long-term results in transsphenoidal removal of nonfunctioning pituitary adenomas. J Neurosurg 1986;64:713–719.
27. Ciric I, Mikhael M, Stafford T, Lawson L, Garces R. Transsphenoidal microsurgery of pituitary macroadenomas with long-term follow-up results. J. Neurosurg 1983;59:395–401.
28. Vlahovitch B, Reynaud C., Rhiati J, Mansour H, Hammond F. Treatment and recurrences in 135 pituitary adenomas. Acta Neurochirurgica 1988;42(Suppl):120–123.

4 Cushing's Syndrome

Lynnette K. Nieman, MD

Contents

CLINICAL FEATURES OF CUSHING'S SYNDROME

Cushing's syndrome is a symptom complex that reflects excessive tissue exposure to cortisol. The diagnosis cannot be made without both clinical features and biochemical abnormalities. Thus, clinical features consistent with the syndrome will provoke laboratory testing.

Clinical features of Cushing's syndrome (Table 1) reflect the amount and duration of exposure to excess cortisol *(1–6)* . Not all patients have all features, and patients with mild or intermittent cortisol excess usually have fewer features than those with very high glucocorticoid production. Thus, while the full-blown Cushingoid phenotype is unmistakable (Fig. 1), it may be difficult to make a clinical diagnosis in patients with a less typical presentation.

While Cushing's syndrome is rare, many of its clinical features are common in the general population and raise the dilemma of who should be screened. The signs that are most indicative of glucocorticoid excess are shown in Table 2. These patients have the greatest likelihood of having Cushing's syndrome.

In the patient who does not have clinical features with a high positive likelihood ratio for Cushing's syndrome, it is helpful to look for additional signs of hypercortisolism and to look for clinical indicators of progression. For example, changes in mood and cognition may be recognized as signs of hypercortisolism in retrospect, especially if these represent a change from the patient's baseline status. These complaints include increased fatigue, irritability, crying and restlessness, depressed mood, decreased libido, insomnia, anxiety, decreased concentration, impaired memory (especially for recent events), and changes in

From: *Contemporary Endocrinology: Handbook of Diagnostic Endocrinology*
Edited by: J. E. Hall and L. K. Nieman © Humana Press Inc., Totowa, NJ

Table 1
The Sensitivity, Specificity, and Likelihood Ratio of Clinical Signs and Symptoms of Cushing's Syndrome[a]

			Likelihood ratio	
Sign/symptom	*Sensitivity (%)*	*Specificity (%)*	*Positive result*	*Negative result*
Increased fatigue	100			
Decreased libido	33–100			
Weight gain	79–97			
Irritability; emotional lability	40–86			
Insomnia	69			
Decreased concentration	66			
Impaired short-term memory	83			
Changes in appetite	54			
Lethargy, depression	40–67			
Menstrual changes	35–86	49	.68–1.68	1.3–0.29
Osteopenia or fracture	48–83	94	8–13.8	0.55–0.18
Headache	47–58	63	1.27–1.57	0.67–0.84
Backache	39–83			
Recurrent infections	14–25			
Generalized obesity or weight gain	51–90	71	1.75–3.10	0.14–0.69
Truncal obesity	3–97	38	0.05–1.56	0.08–2.6
Plethora	78–94	69	2.51–3.03	0.09–0.32
Round face	88–92			
Hirsutism	64–84	61	2.21–2.90	0.26–0.59
Hypertension	74–90	83	4.35–5.29	0.12–0.31
Eccymoses	60–68	94	10–11.3	0.34–0.43
Striae wider than 1 cm and purple color	50–64	78	2.72–2.91	0.46–0.64
Weakness, especially of proximal muscles	56–90	93	8–12.6	0.11–0.69
Abnormal fat distribution: centripetal, dorsocervical, supraclavicular, and temporal	34–67			
Edema	48–66	83	2.82–3.88	0.41–0.63
Thinness and fragility of skin	84			
Abdominal pain	21			
Acne	21–82	76	0.88–3.42	0.24–1.01
Female balding	13–51			

[a]Abstracted from refs. *1–6*

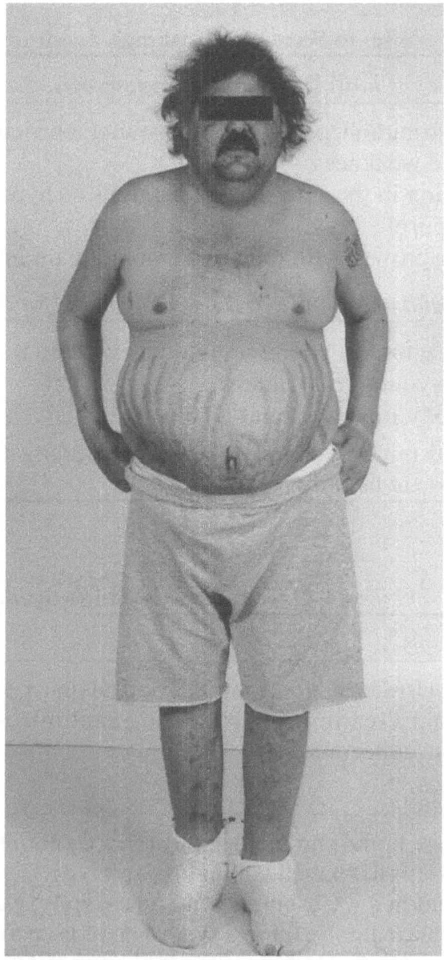

Fig. 1. Clinical features of Cushing's syndrome apparent in this patient include central obesity, plethora, edema, striae and supraclavicular fat.

appetite. Irritability, expressed as a decreased threshold for uncontrollable verbal outbursts, is often an early symptom. Serial 7 subtractions and recall of three cities (or three objects) can be used by the clinician to quantify this symptom complex *(5)*. Inspection of old photographs may also assist in recognition of physical changes over time.

When the physical features are not convincing, one option is to observe the patient over time. However, many endocrinologists will decide to perform one of the screening tests described below, usually with the expectation of excluding any abnormality.

Table 2
Who to Screen for Cushing's Syndrome

Screen patients with signs most suggestive of hypercortisolism:

1. Abnormal fat distribution, particularly in the supraclavicular and temporal fossae.
2. Proximal muscle weakness.
3. Excessive bruising in the setting of other signs of hypercortisolism.
4. Wide (>1 cm), purple striae.
5. Failure of linear growth with continued weight gain in a child.

Also screen patients with unexplained or unusual features for their age group, such as:

1. Nontraumatic fracture in young individuals with no risk for osteopenia.
2. Hypertension in young individuals.
3. Cutaneous atrophy in young individuals.

Screen any patient with multiple clinical features, particularly if there is progression over time (old photographs are helpful).

Table 3
UFC for the Diagnosis of Cushing's Syndrome

How

Collect all urine for 24 h (discard first morning void on first d, and keep it on the second). Measure UFC (and creatinine if collecting multiple specimens, to evaluate completeness of the collection).

Interpretation

Note that high-pressure liquid chromatography (HPLC) normal range is about half that of radioimmunoassay (RIA) methodology.
> 4× Upper limit of normal = Cushing's syndrome (rarely, glucocorticoid resistance).
1–4× Upper limit of normal = Cushing's syndrome or pseudo-Cushing's syndrome.
Within the normal range = no Cushing's syndrome (up to 5% false negative rate).

Caveats

UFC is not reliable when creatinine clearance <20 cc/min.

DIAGNOSTIC EVALUATION OF CUSHING'S SYNDROME

Overproduction of cortisol and reduced sensitivity to feedback inhibition by glucocorticoids are the hallmark laboratory findings in endogenous Cushing's syndrome *(7,8)*. The tests used to make the diagnosis of Cushing's syndrome take advantage of these physiologic abnormalities.

Table 4
Midnight Plasma Cortisol for the Diagnosis of Cushing's Syndrome

How

Insert an indwelling line by 11 PM. Ensure that the patient rests and fasts. Measure plasma cortisol at midnight.

Interpretation

Cortisol 7.5 μg/dL = not Cushing's syndrome.
Higher values = Cushing's syndrome.

Caveats

Patients who do not normally sleep at night and those travelling from other time zones may have false positive results.
5% False negative rate (usually intermittent or mild Cushing's syndrome).

Laboratory Screening Tests

Urine Free Cortisol

Urine free cortisol (UFC) (Table 3) is the gold standard test for the diagnosis of Cushing's syndrome *(7,8)*. If patients with Cushing's syndrome are compared to normal or obese individuals, and values exceed the upper limit of normal, the sensitivity and specificity of the test are greater than 94% *(9)*. However, the specificity decreases dramatically, to 23%, when the responses of patients with pseudo-Cushing states are evaluated *(10)*. Pseudo-Cushing states, characterized by mild overactivation of the hypothalamic–pituitary–adrenal axis without true Cushing's syndrome, include certain psychiatric disorders (depression, anxiety disorder, obsessive–compulsive disorder), morbid obesity, poorly controlled diabetes mellitus, and alcoholism. Mildly elevated UFC also may be seen without any associated condition *(11,12)*. In one small study, patients with pseudo-Cushing states all had urine cortisol excretion of less than 388 μg/d, about 4-fold the upper limit of normal in the radioimmunoassay used in the study *(13)*. Thus, if the criterion for the diagnosis of Cushing's syndrome is increased to this level, pseudo-Cushing states can be excluded, at the expense of a decreased sensitivity (45%) for Cushing's syndrome.

UFC may be falsely negative if the patient has cyclic or intermittent Cushing's syndrome and collects urine during an inactive time.

Measurement of Plasma Cortisol at Midnight

Midnight plasma cortisol values (Table 4) can distinguish pseudo-Cushing states from Cushing's syndrome, with 95% diagnostic accuracy using a cutpoint of 7.5 μg/dL *(10)*. Although measurement of midnight plasma cortisol has a high diagnostic accuracy, inconvenience and/or cost limit its use. Recent research at the National Institutes of Health (NIH) and in Milwaukee indicates that measurement of salivary cortisol at bedtime or midnight works as well as the midnight plasma cortisol. However, the cutpoints used in the two studies are different, due to differences in the assays for salivary cortisol. Because of this, salivary cortisol assays may need local validation before they are used for this purpose *(14)*.

Stimulation and Suppression Tests for the Diagnosis of Cushing's Syndrome

The 1-mg Overnight Dexamethasone Suppression Test (DST)

The 1-mg DST is a simple screening test *(11,12)* that takes advantage of the blunted sensitivity to glucocorticoid feedback in patients with Cushing's syndrome (Table 5). Recently, a number of authors have advocated increasingly conservative cutpoints for interpretation of the test. Traditionally, a serum cortisol value of more than 5 μg/dL was considered to indicate Cushing's syndrome. This cutpoint yields a diagnostic sensitivity of 98% and a specificity of 89% *(8)*. However, a number of patients with Cushing's syndrome suppress cortisol to <5 μg/dL, so that cutpoints of 1.16–3.62 μg/dL have been proposed *(15,16)*. The ability of the test to exclude Cushing's syndrome in those without the condition decreases when a lower cutpoint is used. Thus, these new cutpoints increase the sensitivity to 100%, but decrease the specificity to 41–89%. This trade-off may result in a need for further testing in patients with an abnormal response to dexamethasone.

The 2-mg 2-Day DST

Compared to the 1-mg overnight test, the 2-mg 2-d DST (low dose DST) has an improved specificity (97–100%), with a slightly diminished sensitivity (>90 %) if a plasma cortisol of 1.4–2.2 μg/dL is used as a cutpoint (Table 6) *(13,17)*. However, the disadvantage of this test is the requirement for strict attention to administration of the medication every 6 h. When used with urinary endpoints, the 2-mg 2-d test has an unacceptably high false-positive rate *(11,13)*.

The Dexamethasone–Corticotropin-Releasing Hormone Stimulation Test

This test (Table 7) distinguishes patients with pseudo-Cushing's syndrome from those with Cushing's syndrome *(13)*. The disadvantages of the test are that it requires strict compliance with the timing of dexamethasone and corticotropin-releasing hormone (CRH) administration, and it is costly in comparison to the DSTs or urine cortisol measurement.

CRH is available commercially (ACTHREL™, Ferring Corp., Tarrytown, NY) with Food and Drug Administration (FDA)-approved labeling for the differential diagnosis of Cushing's syndrome. Use of the agent in the dexamethasone–CRH test represents an off-label use. Only about 100 patients have been reported using this test *(13)*.

Table 5
Overnight 1-mg DST for the Diagnosis of Cushing's Syndrome

How
Give 1 mg dexamethasone orally between 11 PM and midnight. Measure plasma cortisol between 8 and 9 AM the following morning.
Interpretation
Cortisol <5 μg/dL (or 1.16–3.6 μg/dL) = not Cushing's syndrome.
Higher values = Cushing's syndrome or pseudo-Cushing's syndrome or other diseases or normal.
Caveats
2% False negative rate.
Up to 30% false positive rate in chronic illness, obesity, psychiatric disorders, and even normal individuals *(11)*.
Dexamethasone clearance can be increased or decreased by medications, giving false results.

Table 6
2-Day 2-mg DST for the Diagnosis of Cushing's Syndrome

How
Give 0.5 mg dexamethasone orally every 6 h for eight doses beginning at 9 AM. At 48 h, exactly 6 h after the final dose of dexamethasone, measure cortisol.
Interpretation
Cortisol <1.8 μg/dL = pseudo-Cushing's syndrome or normal (2% false negative rate).
Higher values = Cushing's syndrome.
Caveats
Dexamethasone clearance can be increased or decreased by medications, giving false results.

Caveats Regarding the Diagnostic Evaluation of Cushing's Syndrome

Any dexamethasone test may give either false positive or false negative results in conditions that alter the metabolic clearance of the agent. Alcohol, rifampin, phenytoin, and phenobarbital induce the cytochrome P450-related enzymes and enhance dexamethasone clearance, while renal or hepatic failure retard dexamethasone clearance *(18)*. It is advisable to stop these medications if possible, or to measure plasma dexamethasone levels to determine if its clearance has been altered.

Table 7
Dexamethasone–CRH Stimulation Test for the Diagnosis of Cushing's Syndrome

How

Give 0.5 mg dexamethasone orally every 6 h for eight doses beginning at noon, and give CRH, 1 μg/kg body weight (BW), intravenously 2 h after the last dose. Measure cortisol 15 min later. (Measure dexamethasone just before CRH is given to verify normal metabolism.)

Interpretation

Cortisol 1.4 μg/dL = pseudo-Cushing's syndrome or normal (2% false negative rate).
Higher values = Cushing's syndrome (2% false positive rate).

Caveats

Dexamethasone clearance can be increased or decreased by medications, giving false results.

Patients with intermittent Cushing's syndrome may have normal results and may require additional testing over time to establish the diagnosis.

APPROACHES TO THE DIFFERENTIAL DIAGNOSIS OF CUSHING'S SYNDROME

The etiologies of Cushing's syndrome can be divided into adrenocorticotrophic hormone (ACTH)-dependent and ACTH-independent disorders. The ACTH-dependent group is characterized by excessive ACTH production from a pituitary corticotrope tumor (Cushing's disease) or from a non-pituitary ectopic source. Rarely, ACTH overproduction is stimulated by ectopic CRH production from a tumor. ACTH-independent causes of Cushing's syndrome, apart from exogenous administration of glucocorticoids, represent autonomous adrenal activation. This enlarging group includes unilateral tumors and bilateral disease.

Measurement of ACTH

ACTH-independent causes of Cushing's syndrome are characterized by autonomous cortisol production, which inhibits the CRH neuron and the corticotrope and so decreases basal ACTH secretion (Table 8). Thus, this group can be differentiated biochemically from ACTH-dependent conditions by measurement of plasma ACTH *(11)*. Modern ACTH assays include a polyclonal ACTH radioimmunoassay with a detection limit of about 5 pg/mL and 2-site immunoradiometric assay (IRMA) and immunochemiluminometric assay (ICMA) assays with a lower sensitivity. ACTH levels are low or undetectable in the primary adrenal causes of Cushing's syndrome. A normal or increased value identifies patients with ACTH-dependent Cushing's syndrome.

Table 8
Plasma ACTH for the Differential Diagnosis of Cushing's Syndrome

How

Measure plasma ACTH using an assay with a detection limit 6 pg/mL

Interpretation

ACTH undetectable = ACTH-independent Cushing's syndrome (if hypercortisolemic).
ACTH measurable but <10 pg/mL = probably ACTH-independent cause of Cushing's syndrome; occasional cases of ACTH-dependent Cushing's with values 5–10 pg/mL.
ACTH 10– 15 pg/mL = probably ACTH-dependent cause; occasionally ACTH-independent.
ACTH >15 pg/mL = almost always ACTH-dependent (unless intermittent).

Caveats

ACTH must be drawn into prechilled tube, put on ice, and spun quickly, otherwise plasma proteases will degrade it, giving a spuriously low value.

A low ACTH level also identifies exogenous causes of Cushing's syndrome, which include iatrogenic Cushing's syndrome caused by prescribed glucocorticoids (oral, intramuscular, or inhaled) or ACTH. Patients with factitious Cushing's syndrome often have had multiple surgical procedures and do not reveal that they are self-administering steroids. Demonstration of a suppressed dehydroepiandrosterone sulfate (DHEAS) value may help confirm the ACTH-independent nature of the process, as low DHEAS values reflect diminished ACTH secretion.

Imaging studies are the next testing strategy once a low or suppressed ACTH value is obtained.

Stimulation and Suppression Tests for the Differential Diagnosis of ACTH-Dependent Cushing's Syndrome

These biochemical tests distinguish between the ACTH-dependent causes of Cushing's syndrome. Cushing's disease, secondary to an ACTH-secreting pituitary adenoma, is the most common cause of Cushing's syndrome. These tumors tend to retain the normal corticotrope responsiveness to metyrapone and dexamethasone (though they are more resistant), as well as to CRH. Cushing's disease is more common in women than men (6:1), with a mean age of onset in the fourth decade. In some patients, tonic ACTH secretion leads to adrenal nodularity, which may be unilateral or bilateral *(19)*. Ectopic ACTH secretion from a non-pituitary source accounts for about 20% of ACTH-dependent Cushing's syndrome. There is a slight male predominance. ACTH may be secreted by a variety of neuroendocrine tumors as shown in Table 9 *(20–24)*. Ectopic CRH secretion,

Table 9
The Incidence and Types of Tumors Causing the Syndrome of Ectopic ACTH Secretion

Tumor	%[a]
Carcinoma of lung (small cell or oat cell)	19–50
Carcinoid of bronchus	2–37
Carcinoid of thymus	8–12
Pancreatic tumors, carcinoid and islet cell	4–12
Pheochromocytoma, neuroblastoma, ganglioma, paraganglioma[2]	5–12
Medullary carcinoma of the thyroid	0–5
Miscellaneous[b]	<1

[a]Data derived from refs. *20–24*.

[b]Miscellaneous tumors reported to secrete ACTH in 1–10 cases, include: carcinoma of ovary, prostate, breast, thyroid, kidney, salivary glands, testes, gallbladder, esophagus, appendix, and gastric carcinoid, renal carcinoid, acute myeloblastic leukemia, melanoma, and cloacogenic carcinoma of anal canal.

with or without ACTH secretion, is a rare cause of ACTH-dependent Cushing's syndrome. The diagnosis cannot be made on the basis of immunohistochemical staining alone, but rather on evidence of tumor secretion of CRH, by demonstration of a CRH gradient across the tumor bed, or by elevated plasma CRH levels. The tumors of the few patients identified with these characteristics include ACTH-secreting bronchial carcinoid, ACTH and CRH-secreting pheochromocytoma, gangliocytoma, and paraganglioma; other patients with small cell carcinoma of the lung, metastatic prostate cancer, and Ewing sarcoma had suggestive but not definitive evidence for CRH secretion *(4)*.

Biochemical Tests

Because imaging of the pituitary is often normal in patients with corticotropinomas (see below), a variety of biochemical tests are used to distinguish between the ACTH-dependent causes of Cushing's syndrome. The NIH group has proposed criteria for interpretation of the biochemical tests that result in 100% specificity, to minimize the chance of misdiagnosing a patient with ectopic ACTH secretion. With this approach, patients with positive responses to ovine CRH (Table 10) *(25)*, 6-d 8-mg dexamethasone (Table 11) *(26)*, overnight 8-mg-dexamethasone (Table 12) *(27)*, or metyrapone stimulation and suppression tests *(28)* would be classified as having Cushing's disease. It is prudent to require that two tests be positive to make this diagnosis. Then, magnetic resonance imaging (MRI) of the pituitary gland may locate the tumor. If it does not, and the surgeon would do a "blind" hemihypophysectomy based on localization data from inferior petrosal sinus sampling (IPSS) (Table 13) *(29)*, and then IPSS may be performed. If the biochemical tests show mixed results, the patient most likely has

Table 10
CRH Stimulation Test for the Differential Diagnosis of ACTH-Dependent Cushing's Syndrome

How

Insert an indwelling line at least 60 min before the first blood draw. Give CRH, 1 μg/kg body weight, intravenously (IV) between 8 and 9 AM. Measure plasma cortisol and/or ACTH 5 and 1 min before and 15 (ACTH), 30 (ACTH and cortisol), and 45 (cortisol), min after CRH.

Interpretation (assuming ACTH-independent forms and non-Cushing's syndrome excluded)

Calculate the percent increase of cortisol using the mean 30 and 45 min values compared to the average of the baseline values (-5, -1 min); calculate the percent increase of ACTH using the mean 15 and 30 min values compared to the mean baseline values.
ACTH increase >34% or cortisol increase >20% = Cushing's disease.
Less increase in both ACTH and cortisol = Cushing's disease or ectopic ACTH secretion.

Table 11
High-Dose (8-mg) 6-Day DST for the Differential Diagnosis of ACTH-Dependent Cushing's Syndrome

How

Collect urine every day for 6 d. Give 0.5 mg dexamethasone every 6 h beginning at 6 AM on d 3, for 8 doses (2 d), and then at 6 AM on d 5, begin 2 mg dexamethasone every 6 h, for 8 doses, ending at midnight of d 6. The urine collection ends the following morning. Measure urine free cortisol, 17-hydroxysteroids (17-OHS) and creatinine on d 1, 2, and 6.

Interpretation (assuming ACTH-independent forms and non-Cushing's syndrome excluded)

Calculate the percent suppression of cortisol and 17-OHS in the last urine collection compared to the average of the baseline collections (day 1 and 2).
UFC suppression 90% or 17-OHS suppression >69% = Cushing's disease.
Less suppression = ectopic ACTH secretion or Cushing's disease.

Caveats

Dexamethasone clearance can be affected by medication; therefore may need to measure dexamethasone (see text). 17-OHS measurements may be altered by renal or liver disease.

Cushing's disease, which can be confirmed by IPSS. Given the difficulty in obtaining metyrapone, and its low diagnostic accuracy, instructions are not given for the performance or interpretation of the test, but can be found in ref. *28*. An algorithm for the differential diagnosis of Cushing's syndrome is shown in Fig. 2.

Table 12
High-Dose (8-mg) Overnight DST for the Differential Diagnosis of ACTH-Dependent Cushing's Syndrome

How

Measure cortisol at 8:30 AM. Give 8 mg dexamethasone that night at midnight. Measure cortisol at 9 AM the next morning.

Interpretation (assuming ACTH-independent forms and non-Cushing's disease excluded)

Calculate the percent suppression of cortisol on the day after compared to the day before dexamethasone.
Cortisol >68% suppresssion = Cushing's disease.
Less suppression = ectopic ACTH secretion or Cushing's disease.

Caveats

Dexamethasone clearance can be affected by medication; therefore may need to measure dexamethasone.

Table 13
Inferior Petrosal Sinus Sampling for the Differential Diagnosis of ACTH-Dependent Cushing's Syndrome

How

Enlist the help of an invasive radiologist. Insert catheters into petrosal sinuses and measure ACTH from samples drawn simultaneously from the right and left petrosal sinuses and a peripheral vein, at 5 and 1 min before and 3, 5, and 10 min after administration of CRH, 1 μg/kg body weight, IV.

Interpretation (assuming ACTH-independent forms and non-Cushing's syndrome excluded)

At each time point, calculate the fold-increase of each petrosal value compared to the peripheral value.
Central to peripheral step-up >2 before CRH = Cushing's disease.
Central to peripheral step-up >3 after CRH = Cushing's disease.
Lesser increases = ectopic ACTH secretion.

Caveats

Abnormal venous drainage may reduce petrosal ACTH values, causing a false negative test. A venogram should be obtained to evaluate venous anatomy.

Caveats Regarding all Biochemical Testing

Tests for the differential diagnosis of Cushing's syndrome must be performed after a 4–6 wk period of sustained hypercortisolism sufficient to suppress normal corticotrope function. Unsuppressed normal corticotropes may have test responses consistent with Cushing disease. Because of this, hypercortisolism

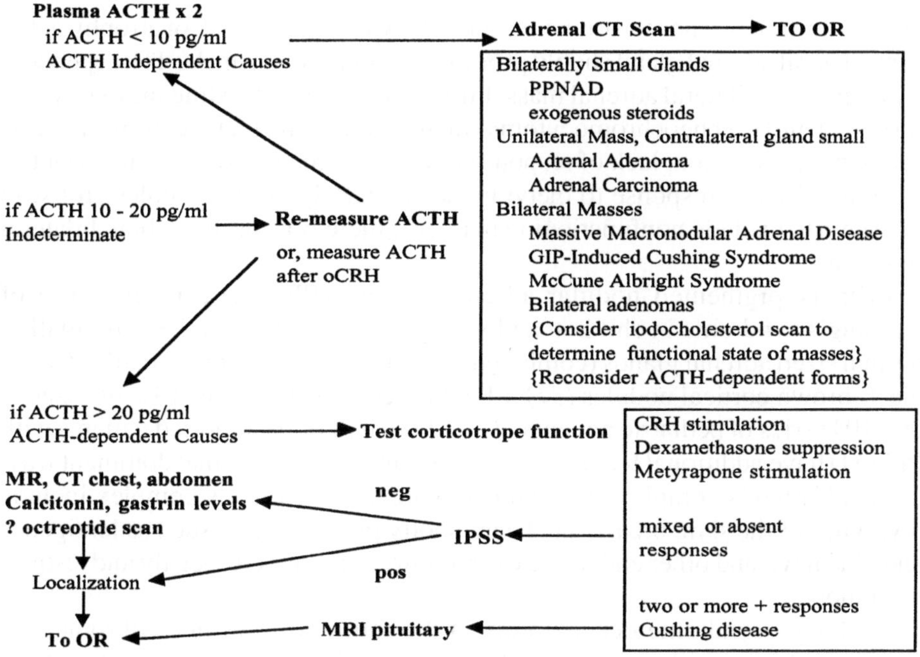

Fig. 2. Algorithm for the differential diagnosis of Cushing's syndrome.

should be confirmed before testing, and adrenal suppressive medication discontinued for at least 4 wk.

It should be noted that CRH is available commercially (ACTHREL), with FDA-approved labeling for the differential diagnosis of Cushing's syndrome, as a peripheral test. Use of the agent in the IPSS test represents, in the strict sense, an off-label use. However, results of the IPSS using CRH have been reported in nearly 500 patients.

Imaging Studies

Imaging in ACTH-Independent Cushing's Syndrome

Nonautonomous adrenal tissue atrophies when ACTH support is subnormal. Because of this, the common ACTH-independent forms of Cushing's syndrome, adrenal adenoma and carcinoma, can be identified as a unilateral adrenal mass, with atrophy of the adjacent and contralateral tissue, on MRI or computed tomography (CT) scan *(30)*. By contrast, the adrenal glands in the ACTH-dependent forms of Cushing's syndrome increase in size as a result of tonically increased ACTH levels. These glands may develop nodules superimposed on this hyperplasia *(19)*. Thus, identification of an adrenal nodule must be accompanied by evaluation of the remaining tissue for either atrophy or hyperplasia.

Demonstration of a normal or increased DHEAS value and lack of atrophy of the contralateral adrenal gland should prompt consideration of an ACTH-dependent etiology of a unilateral adrenal mass. Further biochemical testing may be necessary to identify a pheochromocytoma (increased plasma metanephrine and catecholamine excretion, lack of response to CRH) or the macronodular variant of Cushing disease (response to metyrapone and CRH). An iodocholesterol scan may help to exclude nonfunctioning masses if there is a question about bilateral function.

Primary pigmented nodular adrenal disease (PPNAD), a rare cause of Cushing's syndrome in children and young adults, is characterized by small to normal sized adrenal glands (combined weight <12 g) containing small (<5 mm) black-brown cortical nodules *(31)*. PPNAD accounts for about 10% of cases in the NIH series of pediatric patients *(32)*. About half of the reported patients with PPNAD have additional features, often inherited in an autosomal dominant way, termed Carney's complex. The clinical features of Carney's complex include myxomas of the skin, breast, and heart, spotty pigmentation, such as lentigenes and blue nevi, and other endocrine overactivity, such as acromegaly and testicular tumors.

Cushing's syndrome occurs rarely in the setting of McCune Albright syndrome (MAS), mostly in infants. The adrenal glands show bilateral nodular hyperplasia. MAS tissues carry a mutation in the α-subunit of one of the stimulatory guanine nucleotide-binding proteins (Gs proteins), which causes loss of intrinsic GTPase activity of the Gs protein and autonomous hyperfunction *(33)*.

Autonomous macronodular adrenal disease presents after age 40 with huge adrenal glands *(34,35)*. The etiology of this disorder has, for the most part, remained unclear. However, recent descriptions suggest that aberrant expression of "illicit" receptors for various ligands (gastric inhibitory peptide [GIP], β-adrenergic, vasopressin) in the adrenal glands may be the underlying etiology of this puzzling condition *(36–38)*.

Imaging in ACTH-Dependent Cushing's Syndrome

MRI of the pituitary gland, using a 1.5 T scanner and T1-weighted images, has a sensitivity of about 70% in patients with known Cushing's disease *(39)*. As up to 10% of normal individuals have a pituitary lesion on MRI *(40)*, this modality should not be used to establish the diagnosis of Cushing's disease. However, it may be helpful in guiding the surgical approach. Additionally, the presence of a clear-cut mass on MRI in the setting of positive biochemical tests would abrogate the need for petrosal sinus sampling, so that MRI results may be used to guide this decision.

If endocrine tests suggest ectopic ACTH secretion, imaging of possible sites of tumor is performed. Apart from the small cell carcinomas, ectopic ACTH-producing tumors are most often small bronchial or thymic carcinoids. Thus, we recommend CT and MRI scans of the chest *(24)*. If these are negative, abdominal CT or MRI may identify pancreatic lesions or hepatic metastases. Although octreotide scintigraphy is a promising new option for the detection of larger carcinoid tumors, it does not identify occult tumors not seen by CT or MR *(41,42)*. However, it may be a useful adjunctive test.

Biochemical Testing for Localization of Ectopic ACTH-Secreting Tumors

Measurement of serum calcitonin and gastrin, and urine catecholamines, may identify medullary carcinoma of the thyroid, gastrinoma, and pheochromocytoma. The process may be repeated every 6–12 mo; tumors that make ACTH ectopically have a spectrum of malignant potential, and annual imaging screening should continue, regardless of treatment for hypercortisolism.

CONCLUSION

The clinical diagnosis of Cushing's syndrome is straightforward if classical features—increased supraclavicular fat, truncal obesity, proximal muscle weakness and wide purple striae—are present. Similarly, the biochemical diagnosis is secure if UFC excretion is more than fourfold normal in the presence of clinical signs and symptoms of Cushing's syndrome. Unfortunately, many patients have less distinctive clinical and biochemical signs of hypercortisolism. In these individuals, causes of pseudo-Cushing states should be sought and treated, in which case hypercortisolism may remit. The low-dose (1 mg) dexamethasone suppression test, when interpreted with a low cortisol cut-point (1.16 ug/dL) has nearly 100% sensitivity for Cushing's syndrome, but low specificity. Continued observation for progression of Cushingoid signs and symptoms and the use of adjunctive tests such as midnight cortisol or the 2 mg-2-d dexamethasone suppression test (with or without CRH) may be helpful when the diagnosis is not clear-cut.

Evaluation for the cause of Cushing's syndrome requires consistent hypercortisolism to suppress normal corticotropes. In this setting, the finding of a very low plasma ACTH value identifies patients with ACTH-independent causes, who then undergo imaging of the adrenal glands to identify the autonomous gland(s). Patients with a normal or elevated plasma ACTH concentration have ACTH-dependent disease, and require localization of the tumor to the pituitary gland (Cushing's disease) or elsewhere (ectopic ACTH secretion). Inferior petrosal sinus sampling is the best test to differentiate these disorders, but is not widely available. Other approaches with a lower diagnostic accuracy include the high dose 8 mg-dexamethasone suppression test and the CRH stimulation test. If these tests are used, it is prudent to require that each be positive to make the diagnosis of Cushing's disease, and to refer patients with negative results for petrosal sinus sampling. Imaging of the pituitary gland reveals a tumor in less than 50% of patients with Cushing's disease. Whole body CT and MRI imaging is often needed to localize an ectopic ACTH-secreting tumor.

REFERENCES

1. Plotz CM, Knowlton AI, Ragan C. The natural history of Cushing's syndrome. Am J Med 1952;13:597–614.
2. Ross EJ, Linch DC Cushing's syndrome—killing disease: discriminatory value of signs and symptoms aiding early diagnosis. Lancet 1982;2:646–649.
3. Soffer LJ, Iannaccone A, Gabrilove JL. Cushing's syndrome: a study of fifty patients. Am J Med 1961;300;129–135.
4. Nieman LK, Cutler GB Jr. Cushing Syndrome, In: DeGroot's Textbook of Endocrinology. WB Saunders, Philadelphia, 1994, pp. 1741–1769.
5. Starkman MN, Schteingart DE, Schork MA. Correlation of bedside cognitive and neuropsychological tests in patients with Cushing's syndrome. Psychosomatics 1986;27:508–1.
6. Nugent CA, Warner HR, Dunn JT, Tyler FH. Probability theory in the diagnosis of Cushing's syndrome. J Clin Endocrinol 1964;24:621–629.
7. Melby JC. Assessment of adrenocortical function. N Engl J Med 1971;285:735–739.
8. Crapo, L. Cushing's syndrome: a review of diagnostic tests. Metabolism 1979;28:955–977.
9. Mengden T, Hubmann P, Muller J, Greminger P, Vetter W. Urinary free cortisol versus 17-hydroxycorticosteroids: a comparative study of their diagnostic value in Cushing's syndrome. Clin Investig 1992;70:545–548.
10. Papanicolaou DA, Yanovski JA, Cutler GB Jr, Chrousos GP, Nieman LK. A single midnight serum cortisol measurement distinguishes Cushing's syndrome from pseudo-Cushing states. J Clin Endocrinol Metab 1998;83:1163–1167.
11. Kaye TB, Crapo L. The Cushing's syndrome: an update on diagnostic tests. Ann Intern Med 1990;112,434–444.
12. Newell-Price J, Trainer P, Besser M, Grossman A. The diagnosis and differential diagnosis of Cushing's syndrome and pseudo-Cushing's states. Endocr Rev 1998;19,647–72.
13. Yanovski JA, Cutler GB Jr, Chrousos GP, Nieman, LK. Corticotropin-releasing hormone stimulation following low-dose dexamethasone administration. A new test to distinguish Cushing's syndrome from pseudo-Cushing's states. JAMA 1993;269:2232–2238.
14. Raff H, Raff JL, Findling JW. Late-night salivary cortisol as a screening test for Cushing's syndrome. J Clin Endocrinol Metab 1998;83:2681–2686.
15. Gorges R, Knappe G, Gerl H, Ventz M, Stahl F. Diagnosis of Cushing's syndrome: re-evaluation of midnight plasma cortisol vs urinary free cortisol and low-dose dexamethasone suppression test in a large patient group. J Endocrinol Invest 1999;22:241–249.
16. Montwill J, Igoe D, McKenna TJ. The overnight dexamethasone test is the procedure of choice in screening for Cushing's syndrome. Steroids 1994;59:296–298.
17. Kennedy L, Atkinson AB, Johnston H, Sheridan B, Hadden DR. Serum cortisol concentrations during low dose dexamethasone suppression test to screen for Cushing's syndrome. Br Med J (Clin. Res Ed) 1984;289:1188–1191.
18. Meikle AW. Dexamethasone suppression tests: usefulness of simultaneous measurement of plasma cortisol and dexamethasone. Clin. Endocrinol. (Oxf). 1982;16:401–408.
19. Doppman JL, Miller DL, Dwyer AJ, et al. Macronodular adrenal hyperplasia in Cushing disease. Radiology 1988;166:347–352.
20. Howlett TA, Drury PL, Perry L, et al. Diagnosis and management of ACTH-dependent Cushing's syndrome: comparison of the features in ectopic and pituitary ACTH production. Clin Endocrinol (Oxf) 1986;24:699–713.
21. Jex RK, van Heerden J, Carpenter PC, Grant CS. Ectopic ACTH syndrome. Am J Surg 1985;149:276–282.

22. Odell WD. Ectopic ACTH secretion: a misnomer. Endocrinol Metab Clin N Am 1991;20: 371–379.
23. Grizzle WE, Tolbert L, Pittman CS, Siegel AL, Aldrete, JS. Corticotropin production by tumors of the autonomic nervous system. Arch Pathol Lab Med 1984;108:545–550.
24. Doppman JL, Nieman LK, Miller DL, et al. The ectopic ACTH syndrome: localizing studies in 28 patients. Radiology 1989;172:115–124.
25. Nieman LK, Oldfield EH, Wesley R, et al. A simplified morning ovine corticotropin-releasing hormone stimulation test for the differential diagnosis of ACTH-dependent Cushing's syndrome. J Clin Endocrinol Metab 1993;77:1308–1312.
26. Flack MR, Oldfield EH, Cutler GB, et al. Urine free cortisol in the high dose dexamethasone suppression test for the differential diagnosis of Cushing's syndrome. Ann Int Med 1992;116:211–217.
27. Dichek HL, Nieman LK, Oldfireld EH, et al. A comparison of the standard high-dose dexamethasone suppression test and the overnight 8-mg dexamethasone suppression test for the differential diagnosis of Cushing's syndrome. J Clin Endocrinol Metab 1994;78:418–422.
28. Avgerinos PC, Yanovski JA, Oldfield EH, et al. The metyrapone and dexamethasone suppression tests for the differential diagnosis of Cushing syndrome: a comparison. Ann Intern Med 1994;121:318–27.
29. Oldfield, E.H., Doppman, J.L., Nieman, L.K., et al. (1991) Petrosal sinus sampling with and without corticotropin-releasing hormone for the differential diagnosis of Cushing's syndrome. N. Engl. J. Med. 325, 897-905.
30. Fig, L.M., Gross, M.D., Shapiro, B., et al. (1988) Adrenal localization in the adrenocorticotropic hormone-independent Cushing's syndorme. Ann. Intern. Med. 109, 547-53.
31. Doppman JL, Travis WD, Nieman L, et al. Cushing's syndrome due to primary pigmented nodular adrenocortical disease: findings at CT and MR imaging. Radiology 1989;172:415–420.
32. Magiakou MA, Mastorakos G, Gomez et al. The NIH experience with Cushing syndrome in children and adolescents: presentation, diagnosis and therapy. N Engl J Med 1994;331:629–636.
33. Weinstein LS, Shenker A, Gejman P, et al. Activating mutations of the stimulatory G protein in the McCune-Albright syndrome. N Engl J Med 1991;325:1688–1695.
34. Doppman JL, Nieman LK, Travis WD, et al. CT and MR imaging of massive macronodular adrenocortical disease: a rare cause of autonomous primary adrenal hypercortisolism. J Comput Assist Tomogr 1991;15:773–779.
35. Lieberman SA, Eccleshall TR, Feldman D ACTH-independent massive bilateral adrenal disease (AIMBAD): a subtype of Cushing's syndrome with major diagnostic and therapeutic implications. Eur J Endocrinol 1994;131:67–73.
36. Bertagna X. New causes of Cushing's syndrome. N Engl J Med 1992;327:1024–1025.
37. Lacroix A, Bolte E, Tremblay J, et al. Gastric inhibitory polypeptide-dependent cortisol hypersecretion—a new cause of Cushing's syndrome. N Engl J Med 1992;327:974–980.
38. Lacroix A, N'Diaye N, Mircescu H, Hamtet P, Tremblay J. Abnormal expression and function of hormone receptors in adrenal Cushing's syndrome. Endocr Res 1998;24:835–43.
39. Newton DR, Dillon WP, Norman D, Newton TH, Wilson CB. Gd-DTPA-enhanced MR imaging of pituitary adenomas. Am. J. Neuroradiol. 1989;10:949–954.
40. Hall WA, Luciano MG, Doppman JL, Patronas NJ, Oldfield EH. Pituitary magnetic resonance imaging in normal human volunteers: occult adenomas in the general population. Ann Intern Med 1994;120:817–820.
41. Torpy DJ, Chen CC, Mullen N, et al. Lack of utility of (111) In-pentetreotide scintigraphy in localizing ectopic ACTH producing tumors: follow-up of 18 patients. J Clin Endocrinol Metab 1999;84:1186–1192.
42. Tabarin A, Valli N, Chanson P, et al. Usefulness of somatostatin receptor scintigraphy in patients with occult ectopic adrenocorticotropin syndrome. J Clin Endocrinol Metab 1999;84:1193–1202.

5 Endocrine Hypertension

Jennifer E. Lawrence, MD
and Robert G. Dluhy, MD

CONTENTS

INTRODUCTION

Hypertension, a major risk factor for cardiovascular disease, is a common disorder and occurs in approx 20% of the United States population. The great majority of hypertensives (90%) carry the diagnosis of essential, or primary, hypertension. It is becoming evident that essential hypertension is a polygenic heritable syndrome reflecting a number of disease processes, whereby alterations in different regulatory mechanisms can lead to an increase in blood pressure. On the other hand, although identifiable secondary causes occur in only 10% of hypertensive subjects, this small fraction represents a large number of patients.

Broadly speaking, the secondary causes of hypertension can be divided into renal causes (e.g., parenchymal disease, renovascular disease, Liddle's syndrome) and endocrine causes. The latter etiologies are discussed in this chapter. Although endocrine disorders are uncommon, many patients can be clinically diagnosed, since the signs and symptoms are often distinct. Beyond clinical clues, severity of hypertension or hypertension refractory to conventional antihypertensive agents may prompt the physician to screen for secondary causes. Age and sex of the hypertensive patient may also guide the search. For example, fibromuscular hyperplasia and Cushing's disease occur more commonly in younger females, while primary hypothyroidism is seen predominantly in older

From: *Contemporary Endocrinology: Handbook of Diagnostic Endocrinology*
Edited by: J. E. Hall and L. K. Nieman

female patients. Finally, making a diagnosis of a secondary disorder is gratifying, since it may lead to a cure of the elevated blood pressure.

PRIMARY ALDOSTERONISM

Primary aldosteronism has a variable prevalence ranging between 0.05 and 14.4% of hypertensive patients *(1–5)*. This wide disparity is probably due to different hormone screening techniques and the previous reliance on hypokalemia as a screening criterion. Milder normokalemic forms of primary aldosteronism are now being diagnosed with increasing frequency.

Clinical Features

Aldosterone is regulated by the renin–angiotensin system (RAS) and potassium and, to a lesser extent, by adrenocorticotropin (ACTH). Aldosterone binds to the Type I mineralocorticoid receptor in the cortical collecting tubule principal cells to increase the number of open sodium channels resulting in increased reabsorption of sodium. The reabsorption of sodium produces a negative electrical gradient in the tubular lumen resulting in potassium secretion through potassium channels to maintain electrical neutrality. Volume expansion normally decreases aldosterone production by suppression of the RAS; sodium restriction increases aldosterone secretion by activating the RAS.

Primary hyperaldosteronism results in sodium retention and volume expansion, suppression of the RAS; and renal potassium wasting. As a result of "escape" from the sodium-retaining actions of aldosterone, generalized edema is not a characteristic feature of primary hyperaldosteronism. One fifth of patients with primary hyperaldosteronism have normal serum potassium levels, which may reflect a milder form of hyperaldosteronism and/or a decreased delivery of sodium to distal sites for potassium exchange. Patients may have neuromuscular symptoms such as cramps, paresthesias, or weakness if hypokalemia is severe *(6)*. Hypokalemia-induced nephrogenic diabetes insipidus may lead to nocturia and mild polyuric symptoms (2–5 L urine output/d). Metabolic alkalosis occurs secondary to renal tubule urinary hydrogen ion excretion. Mild hypernatremia (serum sodium concentration in the 145 mEq/dL range) and resetting of the osmostat occurs so that antidiuretic hormone secretion and thirst occur at a higher osmolar (sodium) concentration *(7)*.

Cardiovascular manifestations include increased systemic vascular resistance, hypertension, and cardiac hypertrophy. Hypertension is usually moderate to severe; premature ventricular contractions and electrophysiologic disturbances result from hypokalemia and hypomagnesemia. These clinical features arise from the effects of aldosterone on the kidney. However, there is increasing evidence that aldosterone has direct extra-renal actions producing cardiac and vascular smooth muscle hypertrophy and cardiac fibrosis disproportionate to the elevation in blood pressure *(8–10)*.

Etiologies

The etiologies of primary aldosteronism include aldosterone-producing adenoma (APA), idiopathic hyperaldosteronism (IHA); primary adrenal hyperplasia (PAH), glucocorticoid-remediable aldosteronism (GRA), which is also termed glucocorticoid-suppressible hyperaldosteronism (GSH) or familial hyperaldosteronism type I, familial hyperaldosteronism type II; and adrenal carcinoma. Formerly, it was thought that APA accounted for 65% of cases primary aldosteronism, with IHA accounting for 30–40%, and GRA accounting for 1–3% *(6)*. However, as clinical suspicion and screening for primary aldosteronism has increased, milder forms of aldosterone excess, such as IHA and GRA, are being detected and probably account for higher percentages *(4)*. The biochemical features of hyperaldosteronism, however, are most striking in APA.

APA tumors are small tumors, usually measuring <2 cm in diameter. Surgical removal of the tumor may result in cure or amelioration of the hypertension, but hypokalemia is always reversed. APA tumors are usually angiotensin II (AII) unresponsive, but a small subset are AII responsive. Another form of primary aldosteronism, exhibiting histologic features of unilateral nodular hyperplasia, is referred to as PAH.

In bilateral IHA both adrenal glands are enlarged; microscopically, the zona glomerulosa is hyperplastic and has micro/macro nodule formation. In patients with IHA, the aldosterone response to AII is exaggerated compared with normal individuals.

Screening

A history of hypertension associated with "spontaneous" hypokalemia is suspicious for hyperaldosteronism. Although hypokalemia lacks sensitivity as a screening test for primary aldosteronism, diuretic treatment in these patients often precipitates severe hypokalemia (<3 mmol/L). The finding of an incidentally-discovered adrenal mass also warrants consideration of the diagnosis of hyperaldosteronism in a hypertensive patient. Finally, whenever there is a suspicion for secondary hypertension (e.g., recent onset of hypertension in a previously normotensive patient), primary aldosteronism should be considered.

Evaluation of primary aldosteronism begins with hormonal screening for this disorder (Fig. 1). The initial screening test for primary aldosteronism is usually the plasma aldosterone concentration (PAC) to plasma renin activity (PRA) ratio (PAC/PRA ratio). This ratio is usually <20:1 in normotensive subjects when PAC is measured in ng/dL, and PRA is measured in ng/mL/h. In primary aldosteronism, the aldosterone levels are usually 20–25 ng/dL, and the plasma renin activity is suppressed (usually <0.1ng/mL/h). The sensitivity of the ratio is also increased if the PAC 15 ng/dL. A PAC/PRA >30 is 90% sensitive for primary aldosteronism and 91% specific, while PAC/PRA ratios <20 are seen in essential hypertension *(11)*. The greater the PAC/PRA ratio, the more likely is the diag-

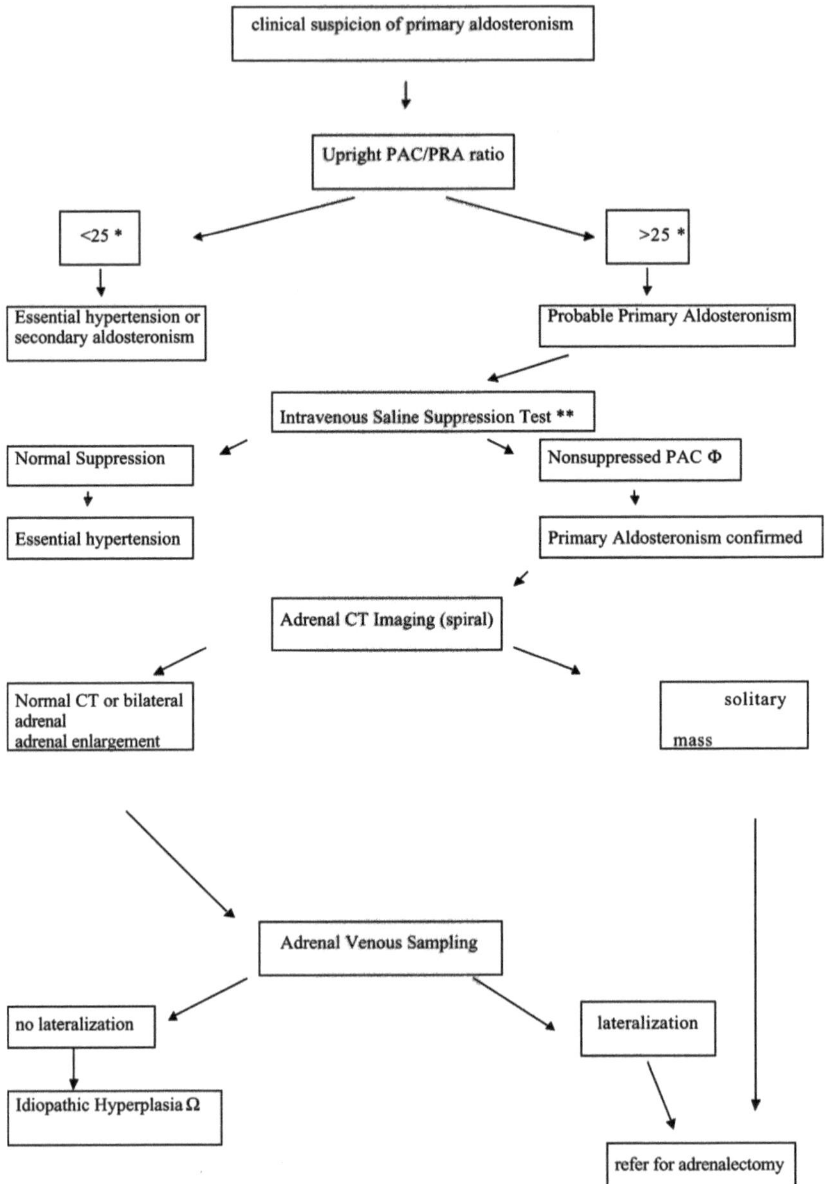

Fig. 1. *, PAC/PRA ratio = Plasma aldosterone concentration (PAC)/plasma renin activity (PRA) ratio. Using conventional units, this ratio is elevated if greater than 25. In SI units, the ratio is considered elevated if greater than 700. **, Intravenous Saline Suppression test: administration of 2 or 3 L of isotonic saline over 4 or 6 h respectively. Plasma aldosterone concentrations should decrease below 166 pmol/L (in SI units) or 6 ng/dl (in

nosis of primary aldosteronism. In secondary hyperaldosteronism, the PAC/PRA ratio should be normal, since aldosterone secretion is increased secondary to activation of the RAS. Measurement of PRA serves to differentiate these forms of hypertension.

To optimize evaluation for primary aldosteronism, factors that might alter PRA or PAC should be avoided. Since hypokalemia reduces aldosterone secretion, potassium levels should be repleted before plasma aldosterone is measured. If possible, the patient should also be withdrawn from angiotensin converting-enzyme inhibitors (ACEI) and β-blockers before evaluation, since levels of PRA will be altered by these medications. However, if the screening test is performed on β-blocker or ACEI therapies, and the PAC/PRA ratio is frankly elevated, then the likelihood of primary aldosteronism is increased since ACEI should increase PRA and decrease aldosterone secretion, while β-blockers should decrease PRA and PAC levels.

Failure to reduce aldosterone levels following the administration of 25 mg of captopril is consistent with autonomous aldosterone production (the so-called captopril test). Normally, aldosterone levels decrease to <15 ng/dL. Prior captopril administration may also improve the diagnostic sensitivity of the PAC/PRA ratio for diagnosing primary aldosteronism. Concommitant cortisol levels should always be obtained when PAC is assessed to exclude a stress or ACTH-mediated increase in aldosterone levels that would serve to exaggerate the PAC/PRA ratio.

Confirming the Diagnosis

If the PAC/PRA ratio is abnormal, but not frankly diagnostic of primary aldosteronism, confirmation of autonomous aldosterone secretion is necessary. Volume expansion should normally suppress the renin–angiotensin–aldosterone system. If suppression is not seen, autonomous secretion is confirmed. Volume-expanding maneuvers include: the saline suppression test, the oral salt-loading test, or the fludrocortisone suppression test (Fig. 1). The saline suppression test involves intravenous isotonic saline administration over 4–6 h (500 mL/h); plasma aldosterone and plasma cortisol levels are measured at the beginning and end of the infusion. In normal subjects, plasma aldosterone levels will decrease below 6 ng/dL following 2 or 3 L intravenous saline. Values between 6 and 10

Fig. 1. *(continued from opposite page)* conventional units). ϕ, Nonsuppressed plasma aldosterone concentration: >280 pmol/L (in SI units) or >10 ng/dl (in conventional units). Ω, Consider screening for GRA if family history is significant for juvenile onset of hypertension (see text). From "Endocrine Hypertension" *Harwood Specialist Series in Medicine: Endocrinology in Clinical Practice*, P. Harris, Ed. Harwood Academic Publishers Reading United Kingdon, with permission

ng/dL are indeterminate, while values greater than 10 ng/dL are diagnostic of autonomous aldosterone production. This procedure should be avoided in patients who have compromised cardiac function. Cortisol levels are obtained to exclude a stress or ACTH-mediated increase in aldosterone levels that would produce a false positive result *(6)*.

In the oral salt suppression test, the patient is instructed to eat a high (200 mmol) sodium diet for 3 d or take 2 1-g NaCl tablets with each meal for 3 d. On the third day of the high sodium diet, a 24-h urine for aldosterone excretion, creatinine, and sodium is collected. A urine sodium excretion of >200 mmol/24 h confirms compliance with the high sodium intake. The normal aldosterone excretion response is 12 μg/24 h.

In the fludrocortisone suppression test, 0.1 mg is given orally every 6 h along with sodium supplementation (20–30 mmol sodium 3x daily [tid]) for 4 d. Plasma aldosterone concentrations should suppress to below 6 ng/dL. This test is less popular, as frequent potassium measurements are needed to ensure that severe hypokalemia does not occur *(11)*.

Features Distinguishing APA from IHA

Biochemical

Distinguishing between APA, IHA, and the less common forms of primary hyperaldosteronism is important. Unilateral adrenalectomy of APA or PAH cures 69% of patients of their hypertension and invariably reverses hypokalemia. On the other hand, bilateral adrenalectomy in IHA cures hypertension in only 19% of patients while also reversing hypokalemia in all patients. Therefore, surgical removal of APA is preferred and pharmacologic therapy of IHA is the treatment of choice.

Features such as young age (age <50 yr), severity of hypokalemia (K <3.0 mmol/L), severity of hypertension and severity of aldosteronism (PAC >25 ng/dL or urinary aldosterone > 30 μg/24 h) favor the diagnosis of APA but lack specificity *(12)*. The posture test (comparing the recumbent level to that obtained after 2–4 h of upright posture) often differentiates APA from IHA, taking advantage of the fact that aldosterone levels characteristically increase in patients with IHA secondary to stimulation by AII. Aldosterone levels in APA are not regulated by AII since the RAS is profoundly suppressed; in fact, in APA, PAC usually declines during the posture test, following the circadian release of ACTH. However, this test lacks specificity, misdiagnosing patients 20% of the time. In addition, it may be misleading; an increase in aldosterone levels in the rare renin-responsive APA may lead to an incorrect diagnosis of idiopathic hyperplasia.

Patients with APA (including the aldosterone-producing renin-responsive tumor subset), often have unique biochemical features. Serum measurements of 18-OH corticosterone (18-OH-B), an intermediate in the aldosterone biosynthetic pathway, are usually >100 ng/dL in APA; patients with IHA have values <100 ng/dL. However, the diagnostic accuracy is reported to be 82% since there is significant overlap between the two patient groups *(6)*.

Radiographic Imaging

Adrenal computed tomography (CT) with thin-slice (3 mm) spiral technique will often anatomically differentiate between APA and IHA *(13)*. If a tumor is imaged in a patient with the characteristic biochemical features of primary aldosteronism, and the contralateral adrenal gland is anatomically normal, the diagnosis of APA is confirmed. Since the size of the APA correlates with aldosterone overproduction and the severity of symptoms, an adenoma >2 cm without hypertension and hypokalemia is more likely a nonfunctioning adrenocortical adenoma (the so-called "incidentaloma"). On the other hand, APA <1 cm in size may not be detected by CT scanning, leading to a misdiagnosis of IHA. Also, because structure as seen by imaging often does not correlate with function, adrenal venous sampling is often necessary and is the definitive test to document lateralization in order to distinguish APA from IHA.

Adrenal Venous Sampling

Adrenal venous sampling should be considered in patients who are surgical candidates, in those whom the adrenal CT scan lacks typical anatomical features of either IHA or APA, or in those where the hormonal testing is not clear cut (Fig. 1) *(14)*. The technique involves sampling the right and left adrenal venous veins using catheters placed in the ipsilateral femoral vein. Peripheral samples are also taken from the inferior vena cava. Accessing the right adrenal vein is difficult, because it commonly arises from the posterior aspect of the inferior vena cava, is short (measuring 5–8 mm in length), and connects directly into the vena cava at an almost 90° angle. Cortisol and aldosterone levels are drawn peripherally and then simultaneously from each adrenal vein, before and every 10 min for 45 min after 250 μg of synthetic ACTH (cosyntropin) is given. Aldosterone/cortisol ratios are calculated for each side and are compared.

In a patient with APA, the aldosterone/cortisol ratio lateralizes to the side of the lesion. In the contralateral adrenal vein, the aldosterone to cortisol ratio is often less than the ratio measured from the peripheral vein since aldosterone production is suppressed. The adrenal vein aldosterone/cortisol ratios are usually 4 to 5:1 from the side with the adenoma compared to the contralateral gland. In bilateral hyperplasia, the aldosterone/cortisol ratios are comparable and are usually < 3.0. Ratios between 3.0 and 4.0 are considered indeterminate.

The rate of successful bilateral adrenal vein catheterization is increasing, especially in large centers where this procedure is frequently performed. With experienced angiographers, the failure rate can be as low as 3% *(12,14)*. Risks of this procedure include renal insufficiency and allergic reactions secondary to the radiocontrast injection as well as direct adrenal injuries incurred from the procedure, such as adrenal infarction and injury to the vein.

Genetic Forms of Primary Aldosteronism

Two heritable forms of hyperaldosteronism are now recognized. GRA (also termed GSH and familial hyperaldosteronism [FH] type I) has an autosomal dominant mode of inheritance *(15)*. In this syndrome, aldosterone production is positively and solely regulated by ACTH. As a result, glucocorticoid administration profoundly suppresses aldosterone production and reverses this mineralocorticoid excess state.

Because the majority of patients with GRA are, paradoxically, not hypokalemic, potassium levels lack sensitivity as a screening test for this disorder. Hemorrhagic stroke at an early age and juvenile hypertension are characteristic of GRA pedigrees. Patients with GRA greatly overproduce the unique hybrid steroid compounds 18-hydroxy and 18-oxocortisol, which share features of both zona fasciculata and zona glomerulosa steroids. Measurement of these compounds in a 24-h urine collection provides a highly sensitive and specific test to diagnose GRA *(15)*.

GRA-affected subjects have two normal copies of genes encoding aldosterone synthase and 11β-hydroxylase, but in addition, they have a novel gene duplication: a hybrid, or chimeric, gene *(16)*. This gene duplication, resulting from an unequal crossing-over between these two homologous genes, contains the 5' regulatory sequences confirming ACTH responsiveness of 11β-hydroxylase fused to more distal coding sequences of aldosterone synthase. In GRA kindreds, the sites of crossing-over are variable, indicating that in different pedigrees, these gene duplications arise independently and do not descend from a single ancestral mutation *(16)*.

Direct genetic screening for the presence of the gene duplication in GRA is 100% sensitive and specific for diagnosing GRA and is recommended for patients with primary aldosteronism without radiographic evidence of tumors, for young hypertensive individuals with suppressed levels of plasma renin activity (especially children), and for at-risk individuals in affected families. Treatment with low-dose glucocorticoids, amiloride, and spironolactone are effective and directed therapies *(15,17)*.

Hyperaldosteronism type II (FH type II) is a subset of familial primary aldosteronism with an autosomal dominant mode of inheritance that has been primarily described in Australian hypertensives. In this disorder, the hyperaldosteronism is not reversed with dexamethasone administration and affected subjects do not have the chimeric gene duplication, which is characteristic of FH type I or GRA. Affected patients within kindreds have unilateral or bilateral adenomas. The molecular basis for this disorder remains unknown, but mutations in the aldosterone synthase and AII receptor genes have been excluded (18–20).

PHEOCHROMOCYTOMA

Pheochromocytoma is a rare cause of hypertension, with an incidence reported to be <1% of patients who are evaluated for hypertension. This may be an underestimate, as exemplified by one autopsy series where up to 50% of the pheochromocytomas were diagnosed at postmortem examination, demonstrating that this disorder is frequently undiagnosed *(21,22)*.

Catecholamine Synthesis and Metabolism

Catecholamines are formed from the amino acid tyrosine by a process of hydroxylation and decarboxylation. This process of amine precursor uptake and decarboxylation (APUD) is a feature of neuroendocrine tissues. Tyrosine is hydrolyzed to L-3,4-dihydroxyphenylalanine (DOPA) by the rate-limiting enzyme, tyrosine hydroxylase, and DOPA is subsequently decarboxylated to dopamine. Dopamine is actively transported into granulated vesicles to be hydroxylated to norepinephrine by the enzyme dopamine β-hydroxylase. These reactions occur in adrenergic neurons in the central and peripheral nervous systems and in the chromaffin cells of the adrenal medulla. In the adrenal medulla, the cytosolic enzyme, phenylethanolamine N-methyltransferase (PNMT), converts norepinephrine into epinephrine. PNMT activity is positively regulated by locally high concentrations of glucocorticoids by a mechanism still not known.

Metabolism of catecholamines occurs via two pathways. The enzyme catechol-o-methyltransferase (COMT), found outside of neuronal tissue, converts epinephrine to metanephrine and norepinephrine to normetanephrine. Metanephrine and normetanephrine are oxidized by monoamine oxidase (MAO) to vanillylmandelic acid (VMA).

In pheochromocytoma, biosynthetic enzymes are increased while the metabolic enzymes are usually decreased. As storage of the catecholamines is limited, and any excess enters into the peripheral circulation, measurement of the unmetabolized catecholamines (so-called "free" catecholamines) and their metabolites are used to confirm the diagnosis of pheochromocytoma.

Clinical Manifestations

Hypertension is the most common manifestation of pheochromocytoma occurring in 90–100% of patients. Hypertension is sustained in approx half of the patients, and paroxysmal in one-third, while normal blood pressure occurs in less than one-fifth *(23)*.

The classic feature of pheochromocytoma is the *paroxysm*, which is a syndrome that includes severe headache, palpitations, and perspiration (the so-called classic triad) *(24)*. Greater than 90% of patients present with two out of the three features of the classic triad. The headaches are often described as rapid in onset, bursting or throbbing, bilateral in nature, and lasting <1 h. Accompanying the headaches are other symptoms such as pallor or nausea. In most patients, these episodes occur abruptly and diminish usually over 1 h. However, in some patients, the episodes may last only a min, while in others, they continue over a wk. Paroxysms may occur daily or as infrequently as every few mo. A diagnostic clue is the random nature of the occurrence of a paroxysm in contrast to a panic attack, which often occurs in a characteristic setting. On the other hand, in pheochromocytoma, certain activities (such as lifting) or medications may precipitate a paroxysm. Symptoms such as palpitations, anxiety, or tremulousness suggest the predominance of epinephrine secretion *(25)*. Orthostatic hypotension may also be the presenting symptom in cases in which epinephrine, DOPA, or dopamine is the predominant hormone secreted *(24)*. Less common symptoms include tremor, Raynaud's phenomenon, livedo reticularis, angina, nausea, and mass effect from the tumor.

Cardiovascular manifestations of pheochromocytoma include dilated cardiomyopathy, which results from long-standing catecholamine excess. Patients may also present with features of acute myocardial infarction from coronary vasospasm or with arrhythmias *(25)*.

Diagnostic Clues and Differential Diagnosis

The diagnosis of pheochromocytoma may be suspected when certain drugs, anesthesia, or surgery precipitate a hypertensive crisis. For example, tricyclic antidepressants, droperidol, metoclopromide, phenothiazines, and naloxone have all been reported to precipitate a hypertensive crisis *(24,25)*. Foods or beverages that contain tyramine, such as certain aged cheeses or red wine, may also precipitate a crisis. Patients with pheochromocytoma may have a paradoxical rise in blood pressure in response to β-blocker therapy.

Several disorders may mimic pheochromocytoma and/or cause elevations in catecholamines. A careful history of ingestion of medications should be taken. Intracranial events including cerebral vasculitis, tumors with increased intracranial pressure, pre-eclampsia with seizures, subarachnoid hemorrhage, migraine, or cluster headache may mimic pheochromocytoma. Patients with pheochromocytoma may be mistaken for having panic attacks or hypoglycemic episodes. Finally, systemic disorders such as mastocytosis and carcinoid in which patients have paroxysmal symptoms may mimic pheochromocytoma *(26–28)* although, in contrast to pheochromocytoma, such patients usually experience vasodilatation and hypotension during an episode.

Most pheochromocytomas occur sporadically, but up to 25% occur within a familial disorder, such as Multiple Endocrine Neoplasia (MEN) type 2A or 2B, Von Hippel-Lindau disease, or neurofibromatosis. The MEN syndromes and Von Hippel-Lindau disease have an autosomal dominant pattern of inheritance with age-related penetrance. In the setting of such familial disorders, pheochromocytomas are usually intra-adrenal and often bilateral. In the MEN syndromes screen-

Table 1
Indications for Screening for Pheochromocytoma

1.	Hypertension in association with symptoms suggesting pheochromocytoma (such as the triad) (see text).
2.	Marked lability of blood pressure.
3.	Hypertension refractory to antihypertensive treatment.
4.	Severe pressor response during anesthesia, surgery, or angiography.
5.	Unexplained circulatory shock during anesthesia, surgery, or pregnancy.
6.	Family history of pheochromocytoma, or familial disorder such as MEN 2, VonHippel-Lindau disease, or neurofibromatosis.
7.	All patients with incidentally-discovered adrenal masses.

ing of at-risk individuals results in the diagnosis of pheochromocytoma at earlier ages compared to sporadic cases. In addition, sporadic cases usually present with hypertension, whereas most patients with a familial syndrome may be diagnosed by biochemical testing often before hypertension is noted *(29)*. At-risk individuals in MEN 2 kindreds should be genetically screened for activating mutations of the RET proto-oncogene at early ages, since affected individuals are at high risk for the development of the lethal medullary carcinoma of the thyroid.

Three to thirteen percent of pheochromocytomas are malignant with a 5-yr survival rate of 23–44%. Tumors metastsize to lung and bone or recur locally. Treatment includes the palliative treatment of pain (such as radiotherapy of bone metastases) or pharmacologic relief of symptoms from excess catechalomines. The tumor response to a variety of chemotherapeutic agents has been disappointing. The indications for biochemically screening for pheochromocytoma tumors are outlined in Table 1.

DIAGNOSIS

Step 1: Biochemical Measurements

The diagnosis of pheochromocytomas is made by demonstrating elevated blood or urinary catecholamines or metabolites. The methods for screening include: (i) 24-h urine collection for excretion of unmetabolized epinephrine and norepinephrine (so-called free catecholamines) or the catecholamine metabolites metanephrine and normetanephrine and vanillymandelic acid; or (ii) plasma catecholamines. The choice of which test to perform often depends on institutional preference, but the clinician is urged to pay strict attention to the conditions of the test selected. When collecting 24-h urines, it is important to measure creatinine to verify the adequacy of the collection and to add a strong acid preservative (such as 6N HCl) to the container. When testing for plasma catecholamines, the patient should have fasted overnight and be lying comfortably in a supine position, with a heparin lock for withdrawing blood inserted 20–30 min before the collection. In the majority of cases of pheochromocytoma, catecholamine levels are persistently elevated, although they rise further during episodic symptomatology; in the uncommon situation, elevated levels are only observed during a paroxysm. Of the 24-h urine metabolites, the measurement of metanephrines is the most sensitive and specific *(30)*. When the upper limit of normal for metanephrines is 1.3 mg/24 h, a value greater than 2.3 mg/24 h is usually considered diagnostic for pheochromocytoma.

There is no single best test for screening, and there is disagreement on the optimum test. Twenty-four-hour urine collection has the advantage of integrating secretion over time, but is more cumbersome for patients. Urinary metanephrine to creatinine ratio can be used as a method to attempt to compensate for over collection (false positives) or under collection (false negatives) *(30)*. The overnight measurements of urine catecholamines, especially norepinephrine, may also be useful in diagnosing pheochromocytoma *(31)*.

With episodic secretion and the very short half-life (min) of catecholamines, random plasma assays may miss the peak catecholamine levels. Conversely, plasma levels are useful, particularly when collected during an episode. A plasma catecholamine level greater than 2000 pg/mL is considered diagnostic of pheochromocytoma. Levels between 1000 and 2000 pg/mL fall in a gray zone. In this situation, a clonidine suppression test can be performed *(32)*. Clonidine, a centrally acting α-2 adrenoceptor agonist, normally suppresses the release of catecholamines from neurons, while the autonomous release of catecholamines from a pheochromocytoma is not affected. Plasma catecholamines are checked before and 3 h after oral administration of 0.3 mg of clonidine. In patients without pheochromocytoma, levels drop below 500 pg/mL. To avoid hypotension, the patient should not be on diuretics (to avoid hypovolemia). Tricyclic antidepressants, β-blockers, and all antihypertensives should also be withheld for 12 h before the test. The clonidine test has high sensitivity (97%) and low specificity (67%).

If the plasma levels are below 1000 pg/mL and the clinical history remains suspicious, a glucagon stimulation test can be performed *(33)*. This test is performed by measurement of catecholamine levels at baseline and 2 min after the intravenous administration of 1 mg glucagon. Patients with pheochromocytoma have a 3-fold increase in plasma catecholamine levels or demonstrate values greater than 2000 pg/ml. Pretreatment with α-blockers (such as prazosin) or calcium channel blockers (such as nifedipine) do not interfere with the results. The glucagon test has high specificity (100%) but low sensitivity (81%). If both the clonidine and glucagon tests are negative, the diagnosis of pheochromocytoma is usually excluded *(33)*.

Measurement of plasma free or unconjugated metanephrines is considered by some to have great diagnostic accuracy, as this is the compound produced by the chromaffin cells. However, measurement of plasma metanephrines is not yet widely available, and experience is limited.

For the initial evaluation of a patient with suspected pheochromocytoma, we recommend a 24-h urine collection for creatinine, "free" or unmetabolized catecholamines, and metanephrines. If the clincial suspicion remains, and the results are normal or equivocal, a repeat 24-h urine or a fractional collection corrected for creatinine is performed when the patient is experiencing characteristic symptomatology. Plasma catecholamines may be needed to confirm the diagnosis. If the plasma catecholamine levels are increased but not diagnostic (1000–2000 pg/mL), a clonidine suppression test may be needed. If, on the other hand, plasma catecholamines are borderline-elevated, and clinical suspicion remains strong, a glucagon stimulation test is performed. Plasma metanephrines may also be helpful at this point. If there is a predominance of epinephrine production, this is likely due to a small intra-adrenal tumor. There is greater metabolism of catecholamines to metanephrines in large tumors compared to smaller ones.

There are a few areas of caution in interpreting catecholamine or metanephrine values, due to the problem of interfering substances using current assays. For example, labetalol, may cause false positive results when catecholamines are measured using fluorometric methods of analysis or metanephrines using spectrophotometric methods *(34)*. In general, drugs that may interfere with testing should be discontinued 4–7 d before collection, and blood pressure should be controlled with medications that do not interfere in the assays (e.g., calcium channel blockers). To provide resolution against interfering substances, our recommendation is to use the reverse phase high-pressure liquid chromatography (HPLC) method and multiple electrochemical detectors. A future direction is to measure these compounds by mass spectroscopy, which should totally eliminate the problem of interfering substances.

Stress from acute events, such as myocardial infarction or cerebral vascular accidents, will cause elevations in catecholamine levels. In renal insufficiency, urinary collections should be expressed in milligrams of creatinine, and plasma levels may be falsely elevated in renal failure *(35)*. From the above, it is evident that catecholamines and metanephrines are not specific markers of pheochromocytoma, but it is the magnitude and/or persistence of the elevations that are diagnostic.

Step 2: Imaging Techniques

After a biochemical diagnosis is made, imaging techniques are used to locate the tumor(s) (see Fig. 2) Pheochromocytomas are usually large (2–5 cm in diameter) and may have areas of hemorrhage or necrosis. Patients with MEN syndromes have tumors that tend to be smaller and bilateral *(36)*. Approximately 98% of pheochromocytomas are located within the abdomen, and 90% are located within adrenal tissue, but pheochromocytomas may occur anywhere within the autonomic nervous system, such as posterior mediastinum,

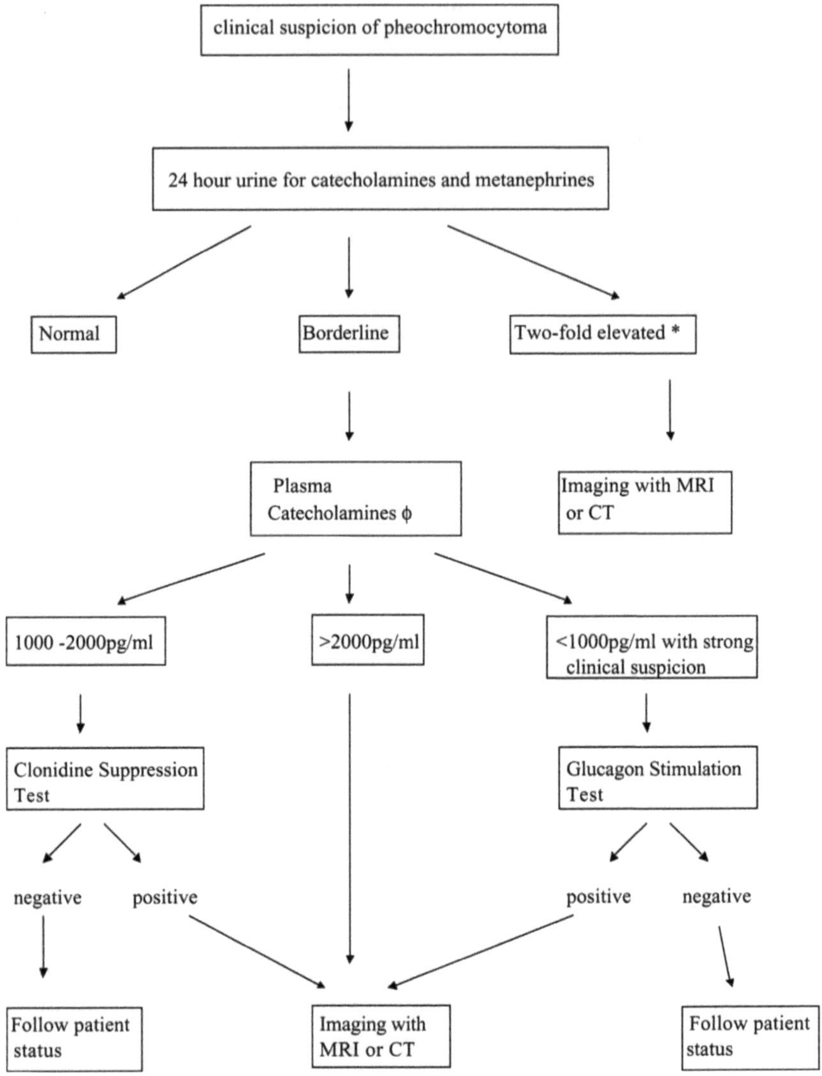

Fig. 2. *See Table 1. ϕ Recumbent levels. (See Text for details.) From "Endocrine Hypertension" *Harwood Specialist in Medicine Endocrinology in Clinical Practice,* P. Harris, Ed. Harwood Academic Publishers Reading United Kingdom, with permission.

pericardium, or bladder. These tumors may be localized by conventional imaging (magnetic resonance imaging [MRI], CT) or by scintigraphic techniques (iodine-labeled meta-iodobenzyl guanidine [MIBG] or octreotide scintigraphy). Due to the size at clinical presentation, most intra-adrenal tumors are easily imaged by CT or MRI. Contrast agents are unnecessary to visualize these tumors due to their size and, in fact, should be avoided since they may precipitate a hypertensive crisis.

MRI is particularly useful for identifying paragangliomas, especially outside of the abdomen, such as intracardiac tumors. On T2-weighted imaging, the tumor is usually 3x as intense as liver, and on T1-weighted images, the tumor is usually iso-intense with the liver. With in-and-out of phasing MRI techniques for determination of fat content, pheochromocytomas can usually be distinguished from lipid-laden cortical adenomas (so-called incidentilomas). However, these radiographic characteristics are not always met, and the pheochromocytomas may appear indistinguishable from other adrenal tumors.

MIBG has chemical similarities to norepinephrine and, therefore, concentrates within intracellular storage granules of catecholamine-secreting tissues *(37)*. Imaging with MIBG is especially useful for localization of extra-adrenal pheochromocytoma and for diagnosing metastatic lesions. Its sensitivity is reported to be greater than 90% with a specificity of 100% *(38,39)*. MIBG labeled with ^{123}I is the preferred isotope, since it is considered to provide greater sensitivity. Thyroid uptake should be blocked with iodine prior to administration of the iodine-labeled MIBG. Medicines that might interfere with catecholamine processing should be discontinued 72 h before MIBG evaluation (e.g., adrenergic receptor blockers and those that deplete the storage vesicle contents, such as labetalol).

Somatostatin receptors are normally expressed in adrenomedullary and paraganglionic tissues *(40)*. Since somatostatin receptor density is increased on pheochromocytoma tissue, the somatostatin analogue octreotide, radiolabled with indium III-labeled diethylenetriamine pentaacetic acid (DTPA), is useful in its detection. Like MIBG, octreotide scanning is most often useful for diagnosing extra-adrenal pheochromocytoma and in the detection of metastases in cases of malignant pheochromocytoma *(41)*.

THYROID HORMONE FUNCTION AND HYPERTENSION

Blood pressure alterations are seen in states of thyroid hormone excess as well as deficiency. In hypothyroidism, the blood pressure typically is characterized by a rise in diastolic blood pressure. In hyperthyroidism, systolic blood pressure is elevated and diastolic is usually lowered as a result of peripheral vasodilatation leading to a widened pulse pressure (so-called isolated systolic hypertension).

Hyperthyroidism

The prevalence of isolated systolic hypertension (ISH) in hyperthyroidism is reported to be between 20 and 30%. This elevation of systolic blood pressure seen in young thyrotoxic patients almost invariably normalizes with treatment. The cardiovascular manifestations of hyperthyroidism include: an increased heart rate, stroke volume, and cardiac output; an increase in blood volume; and a decrease in peripheral vascular resistance to meet increased oxidative demand. These findings appear to reflect increased activation of the sympathetic system. However, catecholamine concentrations have been found to be normal or decreased in hyperthyroidism *(42)*; instead, there appears to be an increased sensitivity to catecholamines with increased density of β-adrenergic receptors. As a result, β-blockers are effective in decreasing blood pressure, heart rate, and many of the other symptoms that occur with hyperthyroidism, such as increased body temperature, perspiration, and anxiety. Definitive treatment is reversal of the hyperthyroid state.

Hypothyroidism

Of more than 4000 patients screened without ascertainment bias for secondary causes of hypertension, 3% were incidentally discovered to have primary hypothyroidism *(1)*. The reversal of hypertension was found in one-third of such hypertensive hypothyroid patients following normalization of thyroid status, allowing discontinuation of antihypertensive treatment. The majority of such hypothyroid subjects are adult women, reflecting the increased prevalence of autoimmune thyroiditis (Hashimoto's disease) in this patient population.

In hypothyroidism, the cardiac manifestations are the converse of those seen in hyperthyroidism: cardiac output, stroke volume and total blood volume are decreased; systemic peripheral resistance is increased; and catecholamine levels are either increased or normal after correction for age *(42,43)*. Treatment for hypertension associated with hypothyroidism is thyroxine replacement, titrating the dosage to bring the thyroid-stimulating hormone (TSH) level into the normal range. With advancing age and more long-standing hypertension, the blood pressure response to treatment of hypothyroidism decreases *(44)*.

HYPERPARATHYROIDISM

Primary hyperparathyroidism is a hypercalcemic disorder resulting from autonomous increased secretion of parathyroid hormone usually from a parathyroid adenoma (80%) or, less commonly, parathyroid hyperplasia (15–20%). This is a common disorder with a prevalence of 100 cases/100,000 population, usually presenting in the fifth and sixth decades of life with a female preponderance *(45)*. However, primary hyperparathyroidism may occur earlier in patients with the MEN type 1 and 2A syndromes, (rarely in type 2B).

Prevalence of hypertension associated with hyperparathyroidism varies from 25–70%, but in most studies exceeds the prevalence of essential hypertension in the general population (approx 20%). The etiology of hypertension associated with primary hyperparathyroidism has been controversial *(46–49)*. Hypotheses include hypercalcemia-related renal parenchymal damage, increased vascular tone and increased activation of the renin–angiotensin or sympathetic systems. There is experimental evidence that release of catecholamines is calcium-dependent *(50)*. Calcium infusions in hypertensive hyperparathyroid patients produced more marked pressor changes compared to normotensive patients *(51)*. These correlations suggest a role of hypercalcemia *per se* and possibly other factors, which enhance sympathetic activation or responsiveness to pressor agents, such as catecholamines. Alternatively, it has been postulated that increased blood pressure results from chronically elevated parathyroid levels *per se*. Although parathyroidectomy typically reverses hypercalcemia, hypertension is not consistently ameliorated. This supports the theory that several factors are likely to be involved in the hypertension associated with primary hyperparathyroidism.

In summary, while the prevalence of hypertension in primary hyperparathyroidism exceeds that seen in the general population, the pathogenesis of hypertension in this disorder remains probably multifactorial. There is also no consensus on the appropriate recommendations for dietary sodium or calcium intake in such patients. However, since many patients with primary hyperparathyroidism may also have essential hypertension, it is important to counsel the patient that the hypertension may not be reversed or ameliorated after surgical cure. In fact, hypertension is not considered a primary indication for surgery in patients with mild asymptomatic primary hyperparathyroidism *(52)*.

ACROMEGALY

Cardiovascular events are the leading cause of mortality in acromegaly, and hypertension is one factor contributing to this increased mortality *(53)*. Hypertension is present in 25–50% of patients with acromegaly, a three- to four-fold increase in prevalence over the general population (54–56). Hypertension is usually mild to moderate, and treatment of acromegaly improves the hypertension, thus supporting a causal link between growth hormone excess and the elevation of blood pressure. Ambulatory blood pressure monitoring in acromegaly has demonstrated an increased frequency (44%) of diastolic hypertension compared with a 19% frequency of systolic hypertension (>132 mmHg) *(57)*. Left ventricular mass index is greater in hypertensive compared to normotensive acromegalics *(58)*. Some acromegalic patients with left ventricular hypertrophy have no history of hypertension; this increased left ventricular mass in such patients is postulated to be the result of an acromegalic cardiomyopathy.

Since exchangeable sodium (Na_E) is increased in both normotensive and hypertensive acromegalics after adjusting for body mass index, volume expansion is probably a key factor in the etiology of the elevated arterial blood pressure *(59,60)*. Growth hormone infusions in human subjects cause increased renal sodium reabsorption and edema is a recognized complication of treatment in growth hormone deficient hypopituitary patients *(61)*. Leukocyte oubain-sensitive sodium pump activity, a model of epithelial sodium transport, is increased in acromegalics, and following treatment, this increased pump activity normalizes *(62)*.

Hyperinsulinemia may be another mechanism that contributes to the volume expansion seen in acromegaly. Insulin resistance is a cardinal feature of acromegaly, and the resulting hyperinsulinemia may result in increased renal sodium reabsorption *(63–65)*. Whether growth hormone *per se* or insulin or both underlie the well-documented volume expansion, sodium retention is seen in both normotensive and hypertensive acromegalics. It is unclear whether the hypertensive subset reflects a greater degree of volume expansion or whether other factors, such as genetic predisposition to hypertension, contribute to the elevation of blood pressure or both.

Volume expansion in acromegaly would be expected to lead to suppression of the rennin–angiotensin–aldosterone system and increased atrial natriuretic peptide (ANP) levels, but findings are inconsistent. There is also evidence that the natriuretic dopamine axis and dopaminergic control of aldosterone secretion is altered in hypertensive patients with acromegaly. Finally, the clinician should note that growth hormone-producing pituitary neoplasms are a feature of the MEN I syndrome, which is also associated with an increased incidence of blood pressure-elevating adrenal neoplasms, including adrenocortical tumors and pheochromocytoma.

Although treatment of hypertension in acromegaly remains empirical, since no randomized studies have been performed, diuretics would logically be considered as first-line agents to treat this volume-expanded condition. Finally, the clinician is cautioned to have a high index of suspicion for secondary hypertensive disorders in acromegalics (such as renovascular hypertension and primary aldosteronism), if hypertension is severe or refractory to antihypertensive therapies.

CUSHING'S SYNDROME

Cushing's syndrome results from glucocorticoid excess. The diagnosis is established by the measurement of increased cortisol production or the demonstration of autonomy of secretion (i.e., failure to suppress cortisol levels when exogenous glucocorticoids are given). The etiologies of Cushing's syndrome can be divided into three types: ACTH-dependent (pituitary or ectopic), ACTH-independent (adrenal adenoma or carcinoma), and iatrogenic.

Regardless of etiology, approx three-fourths of patients with Cushing's syndrome have arterial hypertension. Typically, hypertension is mild, but in some series, 15% of patients with Cushing's syndrome had blood pressures greater than 200/120 mmHg *(66)*. The prevalence of elevated blood pressure is substantially lower (5–25%) with exogenous glucocorticoid intake vs endogenous glucocorticoid excess.

Pathogenesis

The cause of hypertension in Cushing's syndrome is multifactorial and may also vary according to etiology. There are two theories regarding the pathogenesis of hypertension in Cushing's syndrome: increased cardiac output and elevated peripheral vascular resistance, and one is not mutually exclusive of the other. In ACTH-dependent etiologies and in adrenal carcinoma, mineralocorticoids, such as deoxycorticosterone, may be overproduced resulting in sodium retention and volume expansion. However, in glucocorticoid-medidated hypertension, elevated blood pressure can result even if sodium intake is restricted *(67)*. A marked increase in cortisol production, as in ectopic ACTH syndrome and adrenal carcinoma, may exceed the capacity of the renal 11-B-hydroxysteroid dehydrogenase (11-B-HSD), enzyme which converts cortisol to the inactive cortisone. As a result, cortisol binds to mineralocortocoid receptors causing increased sodium retention, extracellular fluid volume expansion, increased cardiac output, and hypertension. Other studies have found that glucocorticoids produce a fluid shift from the intracellular to the extracellular compartment resulting in increased plasma volume *(68)*. Enhanced activation of the sympathetic system secondary to glucocorticoid-mediated increased activity of the PNMT enzyme could result in excess epinephrine production and increased cardiac output.

To explain enhanced peripheral vascular resistance, both increased vasoconstrictor and reduced vasodilator activities have been reported. Glucocorticoids increase production of angiotensinogen within hepatic cells, which should result in increased AII levels due to the kinetics of the renin–substrate reaction *(69)*. Another hypothesis is that the increased tissue production of AII leads to blood pressure elevation. On the other hand, normal or reduced levels of plasma renin activity have been found in patients with Cushing's syndrome. It has been reported that the production of the protein, macrocortin, which inhibits phospholipase A-2 activity, leads to decreased vasodilatory activity by reduction in vasodilator prostaglandins *(70)*. Finally, enhanced vasoconstrictor responsiveness to endogenous vasopressors has been inconsistently noted.

Detection of Cushing's syndrome has major consequences for the patient, since hypertension is often causally associated with increased cardiovascular risk factors, such as hyperlipidemia and diabetes mellitus, which synergistically act to greatly accelerate atherogenic risk. Accordingly, the clinician should have a high index of suspicion for this disorder in hypertensive patients. While the treatment of hypertension in Cushing's syndrome remains empiric, clinicians have usually found good responses to interruption of the RAS usually in combination with diuretics. In certain situations, such as the ectopic ACTH syndrome, where there is a prominent mineralocorticoid action (sodium retention and potassium wasting), mineralocorticoid antagonists, such as spironolactone, have been used with gratifying results.

REFERENCES

1. Anderson GH Jr, Blakeman N, Streeten DH. The effect of age on prevalence of secondary forms of hypertension in 4429 consecutively referred patients. J Hypertens 1994;609:15.
2. Gordon RD. (1994) Mineralocorticoid hypertension. Lancet 1994;344:240–243.
3. Hiramatsu K, Yamada T, Yukimura Y, et al. A screening test to identify aldosterone-producing adenoma by measuring plasma renin activity. Results in hypertensive patients. Arch Intern Med 1981;141:1589–1593.
4. Young WF Jr, Hogan MJ, Klee GG, Grant CS, van Heerden, JA. Primary aldosteronism: diagnosis and treatment. Mayo Clin Proc 1990;65:96–110.
5. Lim PO, Rodgers P, Cardale K, Watson AD and MacDonald TM. Potentially high prevalence of primary aldosteronism in a primary-care population. Lancet 1999;353:40.
6. Litchfield WR, Dluhy RG. Primary aldosteronism. Endocrinol Metab Clin North Am 1995;24:593–612.
7. Ganguly A. Primary aldosteronism. N Engl J Med 1998;339:1828–1834.
8. Young M, Fullerton M, Dilley R, Funder J. Mineralocorticoids, hypertension, and cardiac fibrosis. J Clin Invest 1994;93:2578–2583.
9. Brilla CG, Matsubara LS, Weber KT. Antifibrotic effects of spironolactone in preventing myocardial fibrosis in systemic arterial hypertension. Am J Cardiol 1993;71:12A–16A.
10. Rocha R, Chander PN, Zuckerman A, Stier CT Jr. Role of aldosterone in renal vascular injury in stroke-prone hypertensive rats. Hypertension 1999;33:232–237.
11. Weinberger MH, Fineberg NS. The diagnosis of primary aldosteronism and separation of two major subypes. Arch Intern Med 1993;153:2125–2129.
12. Young WF Jr, Stanson AW, Grant CS, Thompson GB, van Heerden JA. Primary aldosteronism: adrenal venous sampling. Surgery 1996;120:913–919.
13. Sheaves R, Goldin J, Reznek RH, et al. Relative value of computed tomography scanning and venous sampling in establishing the cause of primary hyperaldosteronism. Eur J Endocrinol 1996;134:308–313.
14. Blumenfeld JD, Sealey JE, Schlussel Y, et al. Diagnosis and treatment of primary hyperaldosteronism. Ann Intern Med 1994;121:877–885.
15. Litchfield WR, Dluhy RG, Lifton RP, Rich, GM. Glucocorticoid-remediable aldosteronism. Compr Ther 1995;21:553–558.
16. Lifton RP, Dluhy RG, Powers M, et al. Hereditary hypertension caused by chimaeric gene duplications and ectopic expression of aldosterone synthase. Nat Genet 1992;2:66–74.
17. Williams GH, Dluhy RG. Glucocorticoid-remediable aldosteronism. J Endocrinol Invest 1995;18:512–517.
18. Gordon RD. Primary aldosteronism. J Endocrinol Invest 1995;18:495–511.
19. Torpy DJ, Gordon RD, Lin JP, et al. Familial hyperaldosteronism type II: description of a large kindred and exclusion of the aldosterone synthase (CYP11B2) gene. J Clin Endocrinol Metab 1998;83:3214–3218
20. Stowasser M, Gordon RD, Tunny TJ, Klemm SA, Finn WL, Krek AL. Familial hyperaldosteronism type II: five families with a new variety of primary aldosteronism. Clin Exp Pharmacol Physiol 1992;19:319–322
21. Beard CM, Sheps SG, Kurland LT, Carney JA, Lie, JT. Occurrence of pheochromocytoma in Rochester, Minnesota, 1950 through 1979. Mayo Clin Proc 1983;58:802–804.
22. Sutton MG, Sheps SG, Lie JT. Prevalence of clinically unsuspected pheochromocytoma. Review of a 50-year autopsy series. Mayo Clin Proc 1981;56:354#-360.
23. Bravo EL. Evolving concepts in the pathophysiology, diagnosis, and treatment of pheochromocytoma. Endocr Rev 1994;15:356–368.
24. Sheps SG, Jiang NS, Klee GG, van Heerden JA. Recent developments in the diagnosis and treatment of pheochromocytoma. Mayo Clin Proc 1990;65:88–95.

25. Bravo EL. Pheochromocytoma: new concepts and future trends. Kidney Int 1991;40:544–556.
26. Manger WM, Gifford RW Jr. Pheochromocytoma: current diagnosis and management. Cleve Clin J Med 1993;60:365–378.
27. Werbel SS, Ober KP. Pheochromocytoma. Update on diagnosis, localization, and management. Med Clin North Am 1995;79:131–153.
28. Bouloux PG, Fakeeh M. (1995) Investigation of pheochromocytoma. Clin Endocrinol (Oxf) 1995;43:657–664.
29. Pomares FJ, Canas R, Rodriguez JM, Hernandez AM, Parrilla P, Tebar FJ. (1998) Differences between sporadic and multiple endocrine neoplasia type 2A pheochromocytoma. Clin Endocrinol (Oxf) 1998;48:195–200.
30. Heron E, Chatellier G, Billaud E, Foos E, Plouin, F. The urinary metaneophrine-to-creatinine ratio for the diagnosis of pheochromocytoma. Ann Intern Med 1996;125:300–303.
31. Peaston RT, Lennard TW, Lai LC. Overnight excretion of urinary catecholamines and metabolites in the detection of pheochromocytoma. J Clin Endocrinol Metab 1996;81:1378–1384.
32. Sjoberg RJ, Simcic KJ, Kidd, GS. The clonidine suppression test for pheochromocytoma. A review of its utility and pitfalls. Arch Intern Med 1992;152:1193–1197.
33. Grossman E, Goldstein DS, Hoffman A, Keiser HR. Glucagon and clonidine testing in the diagnosis of pheochromocytoma. Hypertension 1991;17:733–741.
34. Feldman JM. Falsely elevated urinary excretion of catecholamines and metanephrines in patients receiving labetalol therapy. J Clin Pharmacol 1987;27:288–292.
35. Juan D. Pheochromocytoma: clinical manifestations and diagnostic tests. Urology 1981;17:1–12.
36. Korobkin, M, Francis, IR. Adrenal imaging. Semin Ultrasound CT MR 1995;16:317–330.
37. Scott, BA, Gatenby, RA. Imaging advances in the diagnosis of endocrine neoplasia. Curr Opin Oncol 1998;10:37–42.
38. Hanson MW, Feldman JM, Beam CA, Leight GS, Coleman RE. Iodine 131-labeled metaiodobenzylguanidine scintigraphy and biochemical analyses in suspected pheochromocytoma. Arch Intern Med 1991;151:1397–1402.
39. Lauriero F, Rubini G, D'Addabbo F, Rubini D, Schettini F, D'Addabbo A. I-131 MIBG scintigraphy of neuroectodermal tumors. Comparison between I-131 MIBG and In-111 DTPA-octreotide. Clin Nucl Med 1995;20:243–249.
40. Kennedy JW, Dluhy RG. The biology and clinical relevance of somatostatin receptor scintigraphy in adrenal tumor management. Yale J Biol Med 1997;70:565–575.
41. Tenenbaum F, Lumbroso J, Schlumberger M, et al. Comparison of radiolabeled octreotide and meta-iodobenzylguanidine (MIBG) scintigraphy in malignant pheochromocytoma. J Nucl Med 1995;36:1–6.
42. Coulombe P, Dussault JH, Walker P. Plasma catecholamine concentrations in hyperthyroidism and hypothyroidism. Metabolism 1976;25:973–979.
43. Christensen NJ. Increased levels of plasma noradrenaline in hypothyroidism. J Clin Endocrinol Metab 1972;35:359–363.
44. Klein I. Thyroid hormone and the cardiovascular system. Am J Med 1990;88:631–637.
45. al Zahrani A, Levine, MA. Primary hyperparathyroidism. Lancet 1997;349:1233–1238.
46. Fardella C, Rodriguez-Portales JA. Intracellular calcium and blood pressure: comparison between primary hyperparathyroidism and essential hypertension. J Endocrinol Invest 1995;18:827–832.
47. Maheswaran R, Beevers DG. Clinical correlates in parathyroid hypertension. J Hypertens 1989;7(Suppl):S190–S191.
48. Sangal AK, Kevwitch M, Rao DS, Rival, J. Hypomagnesemia and hypertension in primary hyperparathyroidism. South Med J 1989;82:1116–1118.
49. Lind L, Ljunghall S. Parathyroid hormone and blood pressure—is there a relationship? Nephrol Dial Transplant 1995;10:450–451.

50. Lane JD, Aprison MH. Calcium-dependent release of endogenous serotonin, dopamine and norepinephrine from nerve endings. Life Sci 1977;20:665–671.
51. Vlachakis ND, Frederics R, Valasquez M, Alexander N, Singer F, Maronde RF. Sympathetic system function and vascular reactivity in hypercalcemic patients. Hypertension 1982;4:452–458
52. NIH conference. Diagnosis and management of asymptomatic primary hyperparathyroidism: consensus development conference statement. Ann Intern Med 1991;114:593–597
53. Wright, AD, Hill, DM, Lowy, C, and Fraser, TR. (1970) Mortality in acromegaly. Q J Med 1970;39:1–16
54. Balzer R, McCullugh EP. Hypertension in acromegaly. AM J Med Sci 1959;237:449.
55. Molitch ME. Clinical manifestations of acromegaly. Endocrinol Metab Clin North Am 1992;21:597–614.
56. Ezzat S, Forster MJ, Berchtold P, Redelmeier DA, Boerlin V, Harris AG. Acromegaly. Clinical and biochemical features in 500 patients. Medicine (Baltimore) 1994;73:233–240.
57. Terzolo M, Matrella C, Boccuzzi A, et al. Twenty-four hour profile of blood pressure in patients with acromegaly. Correlation with demographic, clinical and hormonal features. J Endocrinol Invest 1999;22:48–54.
58. Lombardi G, Colao A, Ferone D, et al. Cardiovascular aspects in acromegaly: effects of treatment. Metabolism 1996;45:57.
59. Davies DL, Beastall GH, Connell JM, Fraser R, McCruden D, Teasdale GM. (1985) Body composition, blood pressure and the renin-angiotensin system in acromegaly before and after treatment. J Hypertens 1985;3(Suppl):S413–S415.
60. Snow MH, Piercy DA, Robson V, Wilkinson R. An investigation into the pathogenesis of hypertension in acromegaly. Clin Sci Mol Med 1977;53:87–91.
61. Biglieri EG, Watlington CO, Forsham PH. Sodium retention with human growth hormone and its subfraction. J Clin Endocrinol Metab. 1961;21:361–370.
62. Ng LL, Evans DJ. Leucocyte sodium transport in acromegaly. Clin Endocrinol (Oxf) 1987;26:471–480.
63. Ikeda T, Terasawa H, Ishimura M, et al. Correlation between blood pressure and plasma insulin in acromegaly. J Intern Med 1993;234:61–63.
64. Slowinska-Srzednicka J, Zgliczynski S, Soszynski P, Zgliczynski W, Jeske W. High blood pressure and hyperinsulinaemia in acromegaly and in obesity. Clin Exp Hypertens 1989;11:407–425.
65. Muggeo M, Bar RS, Roth J, Kahn CR, Gorden, P. The insulin resistance of acromegaly: evidence for two alterations in the insulin receptor on circulating monocytes. J Clin Endocrinol Metab 1979;48:17–25.
66. Ross EJ, Linch DC. Cushing's syndrome—killing diesase: discriminatory value of signs and symptoms aiding early diagnosis. Lancet 1982;2:646–649.
67. Haak D, Mohring J, Mohring B, et al. Comparative study on development of corticosterone and DOCA hypertension in rats. Am J Physiol 1977;233:F403–F411.
68. Connell JMC, Whitworth JA, Daies DL, et al. Effects of ACTH and cortisol administration on blood pressure, electrolyte metabolism, atrial natriuretic peptide, and renal function in normal man. J Hypertension 1988;6:17–23.
69. Krakoff LR. Measurement of plasma renin substrate by radioimmunoassay of angiotensin I: concentration in syndromes associated with steroid excess. J Clin Endocrinol Metab 1973;37:608–615.
70. Axelrod L. Inhibition of prostacyclin production mediates permissive effect of glucocorticoids on vascular tone. Perturbation of this mechanism contributes to pathogenesis of Cushing's syndrome and Addison's disease. Lancet 1983;1:904–906.

6 Evaluation of Thyroid Function

Anastassios G. Pittas, MD
and Stephanie L. Lee, MD, PhD

Contents

INTRODUCTION

The lifetime prevalence of thyroid dysfunction, hypothyroidism, and hyperthyroidism is about 10% in North America. Thyroid disease occurs in women 2 to 3 times more commonly than men. Thyroid dysfunction may have a variable clinical presentation depending on the age of the patient, degree of dysfunction, and the duration of disease. Thus, its clinical diagnosis is often challenging. Fortunately, the presence of thyroid dysfunction can be easily confirmed biochemically. The clinical picture, together with the judicious use of a limited number of biochemical testing and imaging modalities, can be used to diagnose most of the thyroid illnesses encountered by primary care and family practice physicians, obstetricians, and gynecologists. This chapter will review the basics of thyroid testing, including imaging of the thyroid gland, and will develop a straightforward approach to the diagnosis of hypothyroidism and hyperthyroidism.

MODALITIES OF THYROID EVALUATION

Thyroid Physiology

Thyroid hormones, L-thyroxine (T_4) and the more active form, triiodothyronine (T_3), travel in the circulation bound 99.97 and 99.5%, respectively, to a group of serum thyroid hormone binding proteins synthesized in the liver, which include

From: *Contemporary Endocrinology: Handbook of Diagnostic Endocrinology*
Edited by: J. E. Hall and L. K. Nieman

thyroxine binding globulin (TBG), transthyretin (also known as prealbumin), and albumin. TBG has the highest affinity for thyroid hormone binding and is clinically the most important member of this group. Thyroid hormones bound to a carrier protein are biologically inactive. The thyroid hormones not bound to protein, free T_4 and free T_3, are biologically active. This small quantity of free thyroid hormone can enter a cell and bind to its intranuclear receptor to alter gene expression, which in turn, alters cellular function and determines the thyroid status of the patient. T_3 binds with higher affinity to the thyroid hormone receptor and is approx 15–20 times more biologically active than T_4. L-thyroxine is made exclusively by the thyroid gland, while T_3 is made primarily in peripheral tissues by deiodination of T_4 by a group of enzymes called deiodinases. The activity of the deiodinases and the resulting T_3 level can be reduced by hyperthyroidism, drugs (β-blockers, ipodate, iopanoicacid amiodarone), malnutrition, and severe illness. About 20% of the daily T_3 requirements is directly synthesized and secreted by the thyroid gland.

TSH Assays

Thyroxine stimulating hormone (TSH) stimulates the synthesis and release of thyroid hormone and growth of the thyroid gland. In turn, TSH secretion from the anterior pituitary is inversely regulated by the serum thyroid hormone concentration. For example, when thyroid hormone levels in the circulation are low, TSH rises to increase thyroid hormone production by the thyroid gland to return the system to normal function or equilibrium. The relationship between serum TSH and serum free thyroid hormone level is inverse log-linear, so that small changes in the serum free thyroid hormone levels result in large changes in the serum TSH concentration. Small but significant changes in the patient's thyroid function that may not be clinically apparent nor result in an abnormal thyroid hormone level will be reflected in the serum TSH concentration. The understanding of this relationship and the advent of second and third generation TSH assays have led to the universal conclusion that measurement of serum TSH is the preferred initial and/or screening diagnostic test for evaluation of thyroid function of the ambulatory patient *(1,2)*. In certain situations, however, such as known or suspected pituitary and/or hypothalamic dysfunction, critical illness, starvation, certain medication use (dopamine or high dose glucocorticoid therapy), and thyroid hormone resistance syndromes, measurement of TSH may be deceptive and should not be used alone to determine thyroid function. Fortunately, these conditions are either clinically obvious or exceedingly rare.

TSH assays have evolved considerably over the last 20 yr. The normal range of TSH in most laboratories is approx 0.3–5.5 μU/mL, but depends on the specific assay used. Recent analysis of NHANES III data suggests that of subjects with no historyof thyroid disease or goiter, the normal range for TSH is between 1 and 2.5 μU/mL. *First generation TSH assays* were radioimmunoassays with a detection limit of 1 μU/mL, which were not able to differentiate between euthyroid and hyperthyroid states, as their lower limit of detection was within the normal range for TSH. Currently available *second generation immunometric TSH assays*, which have a detection limit of 0.1 μU/mL, are able to differentiate between euthyroid and hyperthyroid states, but do not indicate the degree of hyperthyroidism. *Third generation immunometric TSH assays*, which utilize a sensitive chemiluminescent detection system, have a detection limit of 0.01 μU/mL and are capable of determining the degree of hyperthyroidism. Most clinical laboratories use a second generation TSH assay, which is adequate for routine thyroid function testing. A third generation TSH assay should be requested only when it is difficult to interpret a suppressed TSH, in conditions such as severe nonthyroidal illness.

Measurement of Thyroid Hormone Levels

A "thyroid panel" is a term commonly used and often misused. The thyroid tests that comprise a thyroid panel are different at each laboratory and often do not include the most important diagnostic test, a TSH. The measurement of TSH should replace any thyroid panel as the initial step in the assessment of thyroid function in the healthy ambulatory patient. However, when the TSH is not believed to be sufficient by itself for diagnosis (first trimester pregnancy, pituitary/hypothalamic dysfunction, critical illness, etc.), or to accurately access the degree of hyperthyroidism when the TSH is low, measurement of thyroid hormone levels must also be obtained.

Total T_4 and total T_3 levels are measured by radioimmunoassay. The total T_4 and total T_3 measure both bound (in active) and free hormone (bioactive) levels. Many clinical conditions and medications alter the quantity of thyroid hormone binding proteins or compete with the binding of T_4 and T_3 to the binding proteins and greatly alter the total thyroid hormone levels. Therefore, the total T_4 or total T_3 should never be used alone as an indication of thyroid function. The majority of patients have relatively normal serum thyroid hormone binding proteins, and the serum free T_4 level can be estimated using the following three assays: (i) free T_4 index (FT_4I); (ii) "direct free" T_4; and (iii) free T_4 detected by equilibrium dialysis. Free T_4 by equilibrium dialysis is the "gold standard" and measures the 0.03% of T_4 that is biologically active and not bound to protein. This assay is available only at specialty laboratories. The levels of free T_4 can have significant interassay variation because of the minute amount of T_4 being measured. Generally, local laboratories use an estimate of free T_4 with either the "direct free" T_4 assay or the calculated FT_4I. The direct free T_4 assay does not measure the free T_4 concentration, but estimates its value with a kit that is dependent on the kinetics of T_4 binding to protein. Under conditions of moderate to severe thyroid hormone binding protein abnormalities, the direct free T_4 assay will not accurately reflect the free T_4 levels. FT_4I is a calculated value that is the product of the total T_4 and thyroid hormone binding ratio (THBR). THBR, derived from the former T_3 resin uptake (T_3RU), seems to be one of the most difficult to understand laboratory tests for the nonendocrinologist. The THBR value is inversely related to the serum thyroid hormone binding protein sites available to bind thyroid hormone, primarily TBG. For example, THBR is low in the setting of a large number of free binding sites that occur either when there is an excess of TBG, such as during estrogen therapy, or because there is a reduction in serum T_4, such as in hypothyroidism. Thus using the equation:

$$T_4 \times \text{THBR} = FT_4I$$

the estimate of free T_4, the FT_4I, is high if TBG is low or low if TBG is high. This concept is illustrated in Table 1. By using the THBR value, which usually falls between 0.8–1.2, the adjusted free T_4 or FT_4I has the same range as the total T_4. When serum thyroid hormone binding protein levels are normal, the FT_4I provides a reliable index of the patient's thyroid status. The binding protein levels markedly change in various conditions (pregnancy, severe illness, malnutrition, dysproteinemia), resulting in changes in the ratio of bound to free hormone, making the FT_4I not an accurate reflection of the free T_4 level. In these cases, TSH alone or in addition to the measurement of the free thyroid hormone level by equilibrium dialysis is required to correctly assess thyroid function. Direct measurement of the TBG level should not routinely be ordered, because its value rarely contributes to the assessment of the patient's thyroid status.

Measurement of serum total T_3 is not part of the initial evaluation of thyroid function. It is used to diagnose and manage patients with thyrotoxicosis and, occasionally, to help with differentiating Graves' disease (higher T_3/T_4 ratio) from subacute thyroiditis (lower T_3/T_4 ratio).

Thyroglobulin

Thyroglobulin (Tg) is the protein precursor and storage form of thyroid hormone. A small portion of it continuously leaks into the circulation. Serum Tg reflects the mass and function of thyroid tissue (including well-differentiated thyroid cancer). Its current primary use is as a tumor marker in patients with thyroid cancer to detect recurrent disease and evaluate efficacy of treatment after thyroidectomy and radioactive iodine (^{131}I). Its clinical value for evaluating thyroid function or thyroid disease (i.e., goiter) is limited and should not be used. The demonstration of suppressed serum Tg levels can be useful in differentiating factitious thyrotoxicosis (from exogenous thyroid hormone ingestion) from overactive thyroid disease of any etiology.

Antithyroid Antibodies

Thyroid dysfunction is often the result of autoimmune disease where immunoglobulinG (IgG) antibodies are formed against thyroid proteins, such as

Table 1
Examples of Thyroid Function Tests

Clinical Condition	*Total* T_4	*THBR*	FT_4I	*TSH*
Euthyroid, Normal T_4 binding proteins	Normal	Normal	Normal	Normal
Euthyroid, High T_4 binding proteins[a]	↑	↓	Normal	Normal
Euthyroid, Low T_4 binding proteins[b]	↓	↑	Normal	Normal
Euthyroid, Normal T_4 binding proteins, Drug displacing T_4 from binding proteins[c]	↓	↑ or Normal	↓	Normal
Hypothyroid, Normal T_4 binding proteins	↓	↓	↓	↑
Hyperthyroid, Normal T_4 binding proteins	↑	↑	↑	↓

[a]Clinical conditions associated with elevation in thyroid hormone binding proteins include active hepatitis, pregnancy, drugs (estrogen, raloxifene, tamoxifen, 5-fluorouracil, perphenazine, clofibrate, heroin, and methadone), acute intermittent porphyria, and hereditary TBG excess.

[b]Clinical conditions associated with reduction in thyroid hormone binding proteins include cirrhosis, nephrotic syndrome, protein losing enteropathies, malnutrition, severe illness, drugs (androgens, glucocorticoids), and hereditary TBG deficiency.

[c]Drugs that can cause displacement of T_4 bound to TBG, reducing the total T_4 level, but maintaining a normal free T_4 level include salicylates, high dose furosemide with renal failure, certain nonsteroidal anti-inflammatory agents (fenclofenac and mefenamic acid), certain anticonvulsants (phenytoin and carbamazepine), and heparin-induced elevation in free fatty acids.

the TSH receptor (TSHRAb), the thyroid peroxidase (TPOAb, previously known as anti-microsomal antibodies), and thyroglobulin (TgAb). TSHRAb is a group of immunoglobulins that can have variable biological activity to either stimulate the TSH receptor (thyroid stimulating immunoglobulins [TSI]) causing Graves' hyperthyroidism or, rarely, to inhibit the receptor from binding TSH (thyroid hormone binding inhibiting immunoglobulins [TBII]) causing hypothyroidism. Thyroid antibodies should rarely be measured clinically except in special circumstances such as hyperthyroidism during pregnancy *(3)* (see section on Pregnancy and Hyperthyroidism).

Almost all patients with autoimmune thyroid disease (Graves' disease and Hashimoto's thyroiditis) will have elevated titers of TPOAb and TgAb. The measurement of TPOAb can be helpful clinically, as it provides additional information regarding the autoimmune nature of the thyroid dysfunction. It is important, however, to remember that TPOAb is not always diagnostic of autoimmune thyroid disease. Elevated titers of thyroid antibodies occur in all types of autoimmune thyroid diseases, but low titers, especially TgAb, can be measured in individuals with normal thyroid function, especially the elderly and patients with other autoimmune conditions. The higher the titer of antithyroid antibody, the more likely the patient has autoimmune thyroid disease. As almost all patients with TPOAb will have TgAb, the measurement of TgAb adds little information to the characterization of thyroid dysfunction and should not be routinely measured.

Thyroid Imaging

Radionuclide imaging of the thyroid gland provides structural as well as functional information about the thyroid gland and can be very helpful in the differential diagnosis of hyperthyroidism. Radioactive iodine (^{123}I) administered orally is often used as the radioisotope, and a scan is obtained 4–24 h later. The radioactive form of iodine is actively accumulated (trapped) by the thyroid follicular cell and covalently incorporated into thyroglobulin (uptake). Alternatively, Technetium-99m pertechnetate (^{99m}Tc) can be administered intravenously, and images are obtained 30–60 min later. Although ^{99m}Tc will be trapped by the thyroid follicular cells, it cannot be attached to thyroglobulin and, therefore, does not absolutely mimic the biological function of iodine. This difference is thought to be the basis of the observation that ^{123}I thyroid scans have fewer false negatives results for the detection of nonfunctional (old) nodules. But because 99mTc scans are easier, faster, more available, and less expensive to perform, they have largely replaced ^{123}I scans. However, if the results of the ^{99m}Tc scan do not match the clinical picture, an ^{123}I scan should be performed. Radionuclide scans are rarely helpful in the diagnosis of hypothyroidism and should not be used for this indication. They are, however, very helpful in the differential diagnosis of hyperthyroidism and to determine the function of a thyroid nodule. Ultrasound, computed tomography (CT) and magnetic resonance imaging (MRI) are structural imaging modalities that provide no functional information about the thyroid gland. They do not have a role in the initial evaluation of thyroid dysfunction, but may be of use in evaluating the thyroid nodule (see Chapter 7).

Modalities of Thyroid Evaluation in Pregnancy

During pregnancy, significant changes in thyroid physiology take place that affect the interpretation of thyroid function tests *(4)*. Notably, TBG markedly increases during pregnancy and greatly elevates the protein-bound levels of T_4 and T_3. These changes result in an apparent elevation of T_4, FT_4I and T_3. The changes in TBG are thought to be due to the direct effect of estrogen on the liver, causing an increase in the synthesis and glycosylation of TBG and resulting in a higher level of circulating TBG. The accuracy of THBR is poor during pregnancy in the setting of extremely elevated TBG. Therefore, the thyroid status of a pregnant woman should be assessed with measurements of a serum TSH and free levels of T_4 and T_3 measured by equilibrium dialysis. Despite the elevation of protein-bound thyroid hormones during pregnancy, the active or free levels of T_4 and T_3 remain normal in euthyroid patients. The euthyroid status of these patients is reflected by a normal serum TSH level. However, as discussed below, caution must be used with a low TSH detected during the first trimester of pregnancy.

There are normal fluctuations in the concentrations of the free T_4, T_3, and TSH during pregnancy that are independent of the changes in binding proteins. During the first trimester, there is an increase in free T_4, which usually remains in the normal range with a decrease in TSH, and is believed to be secondary to the high levels of human chorionic gonadotropin (hCG), which has weak thyrotropic activity. Up to 13% of women during the first trimester have unmeasurable TSH levels (<0.1 μU/mL) and are clinically euthyroid *(4)*. TSH levels can be suppressed in the first trimester because of TSH "receptor cross-over" stimulation by hCG, which peaks approx at the end of the first trimester and then becomes lower in the second and third trimesters. Following the hCG peak, the TSH will usually return to normal levels in the second and third trimester of the euthyroid individual. Therefore, first trimester patients with a suppressed TSH and a normal or even slightly elevated free T_4 and free T_3 level should not be treated for hyperthyroidism. Thyroid testing should be repeated in 4 wk to confirm normalization of the TSH. If the free T_4 or free T_3 is elevated, the patient is thyrotoxic and should have the appropriate treatment (see section on Pregnancy and Hyperthyroidism). If the TSH remains suppressed after the first trimester of pregnancy, the patient should be evaluated by an endocrinologist to confirm hyperthyroidism. Radionuclide imaging with any isotope is contraindicated in pregnancy.

Modalities of Thyroid Evaluation in Nonthyroidal Illness: Euthyroid Sick Syndrome

Severe nonthyroidal illness is accompanied by major alterations in thyroid physiology *(5)*. The total T_4 is decreased primarily because of a decrease in all thyroid binding proteins. Free T_4 measured by equilibrium dialysis should be normal. Total T_3 is decreased secondary to a decrease in the function of the 5' deiodinase, which converts T_4 to T_3. Instead, T_4 is metabolized to the inactive form, reverse T_3 (rT_3). The serum TSH may be low, normal, or high in nonthyroidal illness. Serum TSH is often low secondary to medications (glucocorticoids, dopamine) or a form of acquired central suppression of the hypothalamus, which occurs in nonthyroidal illness. It is difficult to diagnose primary thyroid dysfunction in the setting of nonthyroidal illness. The use of a third generation TSH assay can be helpful in this setting, as the serum TSH will almost always be measurable even if below the normal range. Up to 75% of patients with nonthyroidal illness who have an undetectable third generation serum TSH level are thyrotoxic. In summary, in severe nonthyroidal illness, total T_4, THBR, and

Table 2
Causes of Hypothyroidism

Primary (thyroid failure with elevated TSH)
Hashimoto's thyroiditis (chronic lymphocytic thyroiditis).
Hypothyroid phase of painful subacute thyroiditis (pseudogranulomatous-De Quervain's).
Hypothyroid phase of painless lymphocytic thyroiditis.
Hypothyroid phase of postpartum thyroiditis.
Radioactive iodine.
Thyroidectomy.
Head and neck radiation.
Drugs: lithium, amiodarone, interleukin, interferon, propylthiouracil, methimazole, iodine excess in patients with thyroiditis.
Iodine deficiency (uncommon in the U.S.).
Biosynthetic defects (rare and presents in childhood).
Agenesis of the thyroid (rare and presents in childhood).
Secondary (hypothyroidism with low or inappropriately normal TSH)
Pituitary dysfunction (uncommon).
Tertiary (hypothyroidism with low or inappropriately normal TSH)
Hypothalamic dysfunction (rare).

FT_4I are usually low, total T_3 is relatively lower than expected for the total T_4 level, but the serum TSH measured by a third generation assay is almost always measurable. During recovery from the acute illness, the TSH tends to rise to levels slightly above normal for a short period of time prior to returning to normal.

EVALUATION OF HYPOTHYROIDISM

Excluding surgical thyroidectomy and radioactive iodine (^{131}I) ablation of the thyroid, the most common causes of hypothyroidism in the adult are Hashimoto's thyroiditis and the hypothyroid phase of subacute thyroiditis, including postpartum thyroiditis. The clinician must be able to differentiate between these disorders, because the long-term treatment is very different. Less common causes of hypothyroidism can be found in Table 2.

Symptoms and Signs of Hypothyroidism

Symptoms and signs of hypothyroidism are listed in Table 3. These are nonspecific, and not all patients will have all symptoms. Symptoms depend on the degree and duration of thyroid dysfunction, but most frequently include weight gain, fatigue, constipation, and menstrual irregularities/infertility. This makes the clinical diagnosis of mild to moderate hypothyroidism challenging, and a high level of suspicion must be maintained. This is especially true in women with

Table 3
Symptoms and Signs of Hypothyroidism

General	*Reproductive*
Fatigue	Irregular menstrual cycles
Weight gain	Menorrhagia
Cold intolerance	Amenorrhea
Hypothermia	Galactorrhea with elevated prolactin
	Infertility
Musculoskeletal	*Gastrointestinal*
Myalgias	Constipation
Carpel Tunnel Syndrome	
Muscle Cramps	
Skin	*Head and neck*
Dry skin	Hoarseness
Yellow skin	Enlarged tongue
Pretibial myxedema (nonpitting edema)	Goiter
Hair loss	
Nervous system	*Cardiovascular*
Decreased concentration	Bradycardia
Depression	Diastolic hypertension
Dementia	Hypercholesterolemia
	Pericardial effusion

increased risk for thyroid dysfunction, because of a strong family history of thyroid disease (hypothyroidism as well as hyperthyroidism), and during the postpartum period.

Thyroid Functions Tests in the Evaluation of Hypothyroidism

The recommended initial test for hypothyroidism is a serum TSH, measured by a second or third generation assay, if the patient has any of the symptoms or signs shown in Table 3 or any of the risk factors shown in Table 4. As mentioned previously, measurement of TSH is a very sensitive and specific method to diagnose hypothyroidism. It is almost always elevated in primary hypothyroidism, and the TSH rise occurs prior to a fall in the T_4 or T_3 levels. Measurement of TSH is not a good initial test for secondary hypothyroidism and should not be used to assess the thyroid status of a patient with known or suspected hypothalamic or pituitary disease or severe nonthyroidal illness. Fortunately, these disorders are uncommon and often clinically apparent. It would be extremely rare to miss an unsuspected case of central hypothyroidism with a single measurement of TSH.

Table 4
Risk Factors for Hypothyroidism

Female, age over 45.
Male, age over 60.
Family history of autoimmune thyroid disease.
Infertility, miscarriage.
History of thyroid disease.
Goiter.
Other autoimmune disease (Type 1 diabetes mellitus, vitiligo, Addison's disease, pernicious anemia).
History of head and neck radiation.
Drugs: lithium, amiodarone, kelp supplements, iodine-containing expectorants.
Dyslipidemia.

An algorithm for thyroid testing for the diagnosis of hypothyroidism can be followed in Fig. 1. If the TSH is within normal limits, the patient does not have hypothyroidism and can be followed periodically. If the TSH is over 10, we recommend initiating treatment with synthetic T_4, L-thyroxine, for hypothyroidism, as most of these patients will be symptomatic or will have a subnormal free T_4 level if checked. An exception to this is during recovery from an acute illness, when the TSH may rise to slightly elevated levels for a short period of time prior to returning back to normal.

If the TSH level is between 5.5 and 10, we recommend repeating the TSH and adding an estimate of free T_4 level, most commonly done with a FT_4I, about 1 mo later. Measurement of total or free T_3 level is not indicated, as the T_3 level is maintained within the normal range for long periods of time in mild hypothyroidism because of increased conversion of T_4 to T_3 by deiodinases. If the free T_4 level (FT_4I) is subnormal, we recommend initiating treatment for hypothyroidism.

Subclinical Hypothyroidism

When the TSH is between 5.5 and 10 and the free T_4 level (FT_4I) is normal, the patient has subclinical hypothyroidism. This is defined as an elevated TSH with normal free thyroid hormone levels. The optimal management of subclinical hypothyroidism has been a matter of controversy. There is some objective physiological data that has shown benefit of treating subclinical hypothyroidism. However, small well-controlled studies have suggested a benefit in patients' sense of well being and reduction in cholesterol levels when treated with L-thyroxine *(6,7)*. In general, the decision to treat patients with subclinical hypothyroidism depends on the presence of signs and/or symptoms of hypothyroidism (Table 3) or increased risk of progression to overt hypothyroidism, as indicated by a positive risk factor (Table 4), presence of goiter and/or significant titers of antithyroid antibodies. Our approach to subclinical hypothyroidism has

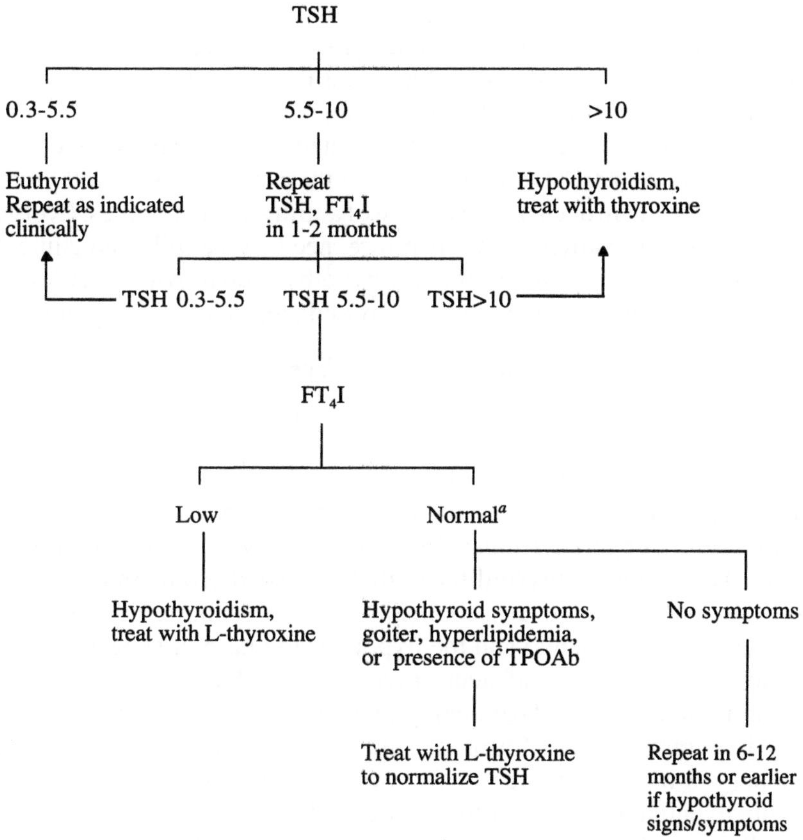

Fig. 1. Evauation of hypothyroidism. [a]Management of subclinical hypothyroidism is controversial. The American College of Physicians (ACP) does not have an official recommendation for treatment. The American Association of Cinical Endocrinologists (AACE) and the American Thyroid Association (ATA) favors treatment with L-thyroxine to normalize the TSH.

been the following: if the patient has symptoms or signs attributable to hypothyroidism, hypercholesterolemia, or risk for progression to clinical hypothyroidism, then treatment with L-thyroxine is indicated. If the patient is asymptomatic, the most conservative approach is to follow the patient clinically and repeat the TSH in 6–12 mo or earlier as directed by symptoms and/or signs. About 15% of the population over 60 will have a TSH level between 5 and 10 *(8)*. If one follows these individuals over time, approx one-third of them regress to a normal TSH over a 4-yr period. If one treats all patients with a TSH between 5 and 10, one-third of patients might be treated unnecessarily. Some clinicians would get additional data to determine the risk of progression to overt hypothyroidism by confirming a family history of autoimmune thyroid disease and by checking for the presence of anti-TPOAb. If present, the patient is at risk for developing clinical hypothyroidism in the future at a rate of 5%/yr *(9,10)*. The higher the antithyroid antibody titer, the more likely it is that the patient will develop clinically evident hypothyroidism. It is reasonable to consider treatment in a young patient who has mildly elevated TSH, elevated TPOAb, and a goiter on exam. However, patients may have progression of their subclinical hypothyroidism to overt hypothyroidism even in the absence of antithyroid antibodies. Every patient with subclinical hypothyroidism, therefore, needs to be followed clinically and biochemically for progression to overt hypothyroidism with TSH levels measured every 6–12 mo or sooner if hypothyroid signs and/or symptoms develop.

Etiology of Hypothyroidism

Once the diagnosis of clinical or subclinical hypothyroidism is established, the etiology needs to be identified. Often the patient is found to have an elevated TSH with or without symptoms of hypothyroidism and is treated unnecessarily for life with L-thyroxine for presumed Hashimoto's thyroiditis, which is the most common cause of hypothyroidism in the adult. However, it is extremely important that Hashimoto's thyroiditis is distinguished from transient forms of hypothyroidism, such as excess iodine intake (from contrast administration and kelp/seaweed supplements) and the hypothyroid phase of subacute thyroiditis. There are three forms of subacute thyroiditis, including postpartum, painful pseudogranulomatous, and painless lymphocytic subacute thyroiditis. A careful history is paramount. All forms of subacute thyroiditis are characterized by transient (4–8 wk) thyrotoxicosis, followed by transient (2–4 mo) hypothyroidism, with eventual return to euthyroid state, although not all patients will experience all phases. Postpartum thyroiditis occurs 1–12 mo following a miscarriage, therapeutic abortion, or delivery. Subacute painful thyroiditis is associated with an enlarged and very painful thyroid gland, flu-like symptoms, including high fever, myalgias, and a high erythrocyte sedimentation rate (ESR). Painless or silent lymphocytic subacute thyroiditis is associated with an enlarged thyroid with the typical thyroid dysfunction of subacute thyroiditis described previously. This is the most difficult to recognize of the three types of thyroiditis and can be diagnosed only with a low radioactive iodine uptake (see section on Thyroid Imaging in Hyperthyroidism). If the history and testing is consistent with the hypothyroid phase of subacute thyroiditis, we recommend observation if the patient has no signs or symptoms of hypothyroidism. If symptomatic, the patient should be placed on L-thyroxine treatment to normalize the TSH. After 6 mo, the L-thyroxine should be stopped, and a serum TSH measured 3 to 4 wk later. Patients with Hashimoto's with permanent thyroid dysfunction will have an elevated TSH, while the patients who have recovered from subacute thyroiditis will have a normal TSH. Alternatively, the L-thyroxine dose may be cut in half or tapered more slowly prior to repeating serum TSH measurements if there are concerns that the patient may not tolerate hypothyroidism. This approach may also be followed in patients on thyroxine replacement seen for the first time when the diagnosis of hypothyroidism is in doubt.

Antithyroid Antibodies in Hypothyroidism

Measurement of antithyroid antibodies in the differential diagnosis of primary hypothyroidism should be interpreted with extreme caution and always in correlation with the clinical history. TPOAb and/or TgAb are positive in 90–95% of patients with autoimmune thyroiditis (Hashimoto's thyroiditis), but should not be measured routinely, because the presence or absence of thyroid antibody titers will not alter therapy of hypothyroidism. However, in subacute thyroiditis, the release of thyroid antigens into the circulation often leads to the development of low levels of antibodies (TPOAb, TgAb). Very high levels of antibodies are more likely to be secondary to autoimmune thyroiditis. Postpartum thyroiditis, a transient autoimmune thyroid disorder, is also associated with the presence of antibodies. The history, however, will be illuminating. If antibodies are measured, then only TPOAb are needed, as almost all patients with TPOAb will also have TgAb.

Thyroid Imaging in Hypothyroidism

Imaging of the thyroid is almost never helpful for the diagnosis of hypothyroidism. Thyroid ultrasound and/or radionuclide imaging should be performed only to evaluate suspicious structural abnormalities, such as a dominant nodule in the thyroid gland in the hypothyroid patient (see Chapter 7).

Monitoring of Patients with Hypothyroidism

Hypothyroidism is treated with supplementation with the synthetic form of L-thyroxine (Levothroid™, Forest Pharmaceuticals, Inc., St. Louis, MO; Levoxyl™, Jones PharmaIncorporated, St. Louis, MO; Synthroid™, Abbott Laboratories Inc., North Chicago, IL). Thyroid extracts should never be used because of the variable amount of thyroid hormone in different lots of medication. In patients with primary hypothyroidism (the majority of patients), adjustments in their dose should be made based on a serum TSH measured every 6–8 wk. The goal of treatment is to normalize the serum TSH level. Once the TSH has normalized, the patient is followed with TSH determination every 6–12 mo. Adjustments in dose may be required during pregnancy (see section on Pregnancy and Hyperthyroidism) or with institution of hormone replacement therapy. In secondary hypothyroidism, TSH levels will not reflect the thyroid hormone levels, and direct measurement of free thyroid hormone level is needed to assess thyroid function.

A recent report suggests that patients may have symptomatic improvement when the L-thyroxine dose is supplemented with small amounts of the short-acting and more potent T_3. Although some animal data may support the need for

T_3 supplementation, there is no case controlled clinical studies showing a significant physiological benefit. At the present time, hypothyroidism should not be routinely treated with T_3 alone or in combination with L-thyroxine.

EVALUATION OF HYPERTHYROIDISM

The most common cause of adult hyperthyroidism in North America is Graves' disease, an autoimmune thyroid hyperfunction. Other common causes of hyperthyroidism include toxic multinodular goiter (MNG), toxic adenoma, and the thyrotoxic phase of subacute thyroiditis including postpartum thyroiditis. Other less common causes can be found in Table 5. The diagnosis and management of hyperthyroidism is somewhat more involved and time-consuming for the physician than that of hypothyroidism. The evaluation and treatment of the patient with hyperthyroidism is often best managed by the endocrinologist.

Symptoms and Signs of Hyperthyroidism

Hyperthyroidism is approx 10 times less common than hypothyroidism at any age, and its presentation is not as ambiguous as hypothyroidism except in the elderly. Symptoms and signs of hyperthyroidism are listed in Table 6. Hyperthyroid elderly patients often have more cardiac symptoms but less systemic manifestations of thyrotoxicosis. Patients should be evaluated for signs and or symptoms, of weight loss, heat intolerance, tremor, palpitations, anxiety, menstrual abnormalities, and new onset atrial fibrillation. Evaluation should be considered, especially in patients with increased risk of hyperthyroidism, including a strong family history of thyroid dysfunction (hypothyroidism and hyperthyroidism), other autoimmune conditions, or long-standing goiter. Routine screening of asymptomatic patients for hyperthyroidism is not recommended.

Thyroid Function Tests in the Evaluation of Hyperthyroidism

Measurement of serum TSH is the most sensitive way to diagnose hyperthyroidism, as it is almost always suppressed in the most common form, primary hyperthyroidism. Patients with hyperthyroidism will almost always have a serum TSH concentration of <0.1 and often under 0.05 μU/mL. The use of a second generation TSH assay with a functional sensitivity of 0.1 μU/mL is sufficient for the diagnosis and management of hyperthyroidism. Secondary hyperthyroidism from a TSH-secreting pituitary adenoma is extremely rare, but should be suspected when the patient has symptoms suggestive of hyperthyroidism with an inappropriately "normal" TSH. This rare clinical condition should be referred to an endocrinologist for further diagnosis and management.

When interpreting low TSH values, the clinician must remember that not all suppressed TSH values are associated with hyperthyroidism. Certain medical conditions (severe nonthyroidal illness, acute psychiatric illness, weight loss,

Table 5
Causes of Hyperthyroidism

Primary (thyroid hyperfunction with a low TSH)
Graves' disease.
Toxic multinodular goiter.
Toxic adenoma.
Hyperthyroid phase of painful subacute thyroiditis (pseudogranulomatous-De Quervain's).
Hyperthyroid phase of painless lymphocytic thyroiditis (silent thyroiditis).
Hyperthyroid phase of postpartum thyroiditis.
Excessive ingestion of thyroid hormone.
Metastatic thyroid carcinoma.
Struma ovarii.
Iodine-induced.
Secondary (Thyrotoxicosis with an elevated or inappropriately normal TSH)
TSH-producing pituitary adenoma.
Thyroid hormone resistance syndromes.

Table 6
Symptoms and Signs of Hyperthyroidism

General	*Reproductive*
Weight loss Heat intolerance Insomnia	Irregular menstrual cycles Menorrhagia Amenorrhea Infertility Gynecomastia (males)
Skin	*Gastrointestinal*
Excess perspiration Palmar erythema	Diarrhea
Nervous sustem	*Musculoskeletal*
Tremor Nervousness Anxiety Hyperkinesis	Myalgias Large muscle weakness Hypokalemic periodic paralysis (intermittent severe muscle weakness)
Cardiovascular	*Head and neck*
Palpitations Tachycardia Dypsnea on exertion Atrial fibrillation	Ophthalmopathy of Graves' disease (proptosis, chemosis, and conjuctival injection) Goiter

aging, pregnancy) and medications (glucocorticoids, dopamine), in addition to hypothalamic or pituitary disease, can result in low TSH. If any of these conditions are suspected, the help of an endocrine specialist is invaluable for determining the thyroid status of the patient.

An algorithm of thyroid function testing for hyperthyroidism is shown in Fig. 2. The discussion in the following section refers to the ambulatory otherwise healthy patient, who has a low suspicion for any of the medical conditions mentioned above that may falsely lower the serum TSH.

If the TSH is within normal limits, the patient does not have hyperthyroidism and no further work-up is indicated. Thyroid function tests should be repeated as clinically indicated. If the TSH is less than 0.3, thyroid hormone levels should be determined in addition to repeat measurement of TSH. As mentioned previously, the relationship between TSH and thyroid hormone level is inverse log-linear, so that small increases of the thyroid hormone level will cause a disproportionate suppression of TSH. The degree of hyperthyroidism cannot be assessed by looking at the TSH alone, especially when using a second generation assay. Although a third generation assay can better differentiate between the degrees of hyperthyroidism, routine laboratory measurement of total T_4, THBR, FT_4I, and total T_3 can easily and accurately assess the degree of hyperthyroidism. Measurement of total T_3 is needed in the evaluation of hyperthyroidism, as some primary thyroid hyperfunction states, such as Graves' disease, secrete predominantly T_3 in excess of T_4.

If serum TSH is less than 0.3, and FT_4I and total T_3 is low, hypothalamic or pituitary disease needs to be considered. More often, however, this constellation of values will be associated with other conditions that result in low TSH concentration, such as nonthyroidal illness.

Subclinical Hyperthyroidism

If serum TSH is less than 0.3, and FT_4I and total T_3 is within normal limits, the patient has subclinical hyperthyroidism. These patients have few or no symptoms of hyperthyroidism. If the patient is taking thyroid hormone, the dose should be adjusted to normalize the TSH. The only clinical situation, in which L-thyroxine suppression of TSH below the normal range is acceptable, is in patients with thyroid cancer, where the goal of treatment is subclinical hyperthyroidism to suppress tumor growth.

Subclinical hyperthyroidism (suppressed TSH, normal FT_4I, and normal total T_3) must be distinguished from nonthyroidal illness and malnutrition. Generally, a careful review of systems, past medical history, medications, history of dieting for weight loss, and a physical examination will identify patients with a systemic nonthyroidal cause of a suppressed TSH. The optimal management for subclinical hyperthyroidism has not been established. Most elderly patients with a slightly suppressed second generation TSH will not progress to overt hyperthyroidism, and about half of them will revert to biochemical euthyroidism within 1 yr *(11,12)*.

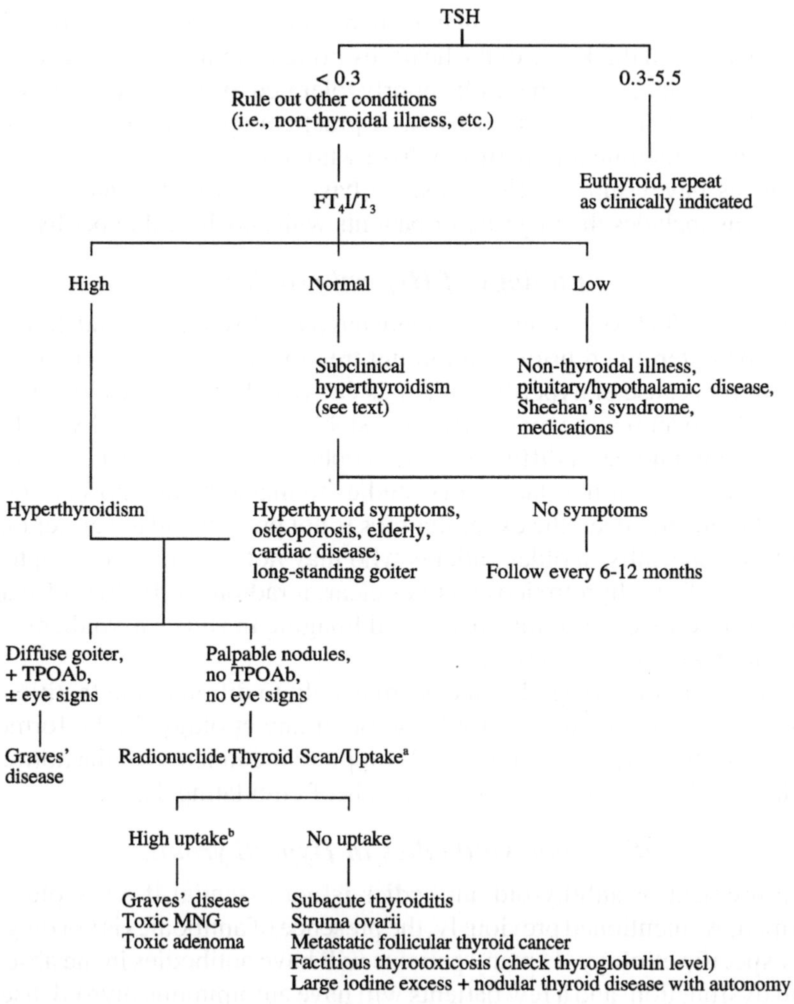

Fig. 2. Evaluation of hyperthyroidism. [a]Contraindicated in women who are pregnant or breast feeding. [b]See Table 7 for typical scintigraphy image for each type of thyrotoxicosis.

These are often elderly patients, who may present with a slightly low TSH that remains unchanged for years. In general, the lower the TSH, the more likely it is that the patient will develop overt hyperthyroidism. The clinical importance of subclinical hyperthyroidism is its potentially adverse effects on bone and heart. Excess thyroid hormone is associated with cortical bone loss, especially in postmenopausal women not on estrogen replacement therapy. However, there is no evidence that patients with subclinical hyperthyroidism have excess fractures. More convincing evidence exists that subclinical hyperthyroidism has a number of adverse effects on the heart, such as increasing the risk of atrial fibrillation, increasing the wall thickness of the heart resulting in abnormal contractility, and diastolic dysfunction, which may be poorly tolerated by elderly patients or those with established heart disease *(13,14)*. A practical approach has been to treat patients with subclinical hyperthyroidism who have symptoms, are at risk for osteoporosis, have established heart disease, have an enlarged nodular goiter, or are elderly. This includes the majority of patients with subclinical hyperthyroidism.

Etiology of Hyperthyroidism

If the FT_4I or T_3 level is high, the patient has hyperthyroidism, and the etiology needs to be determined prior to initiating treatment. As mentioned above, the most common cause of hyperthyroidism is Graves' disease. The clinical history and a careful examination may suffice to establish the etiology of hyperthyroidism. A patient who has a diffuse goiter, exophthalmos, and biochemical thyrotoxicosis needs no further laboratory studies to make the diagnosis of Graves' disease. Often, however, the exophthalmos is not present and the goiter may not be evident, especially in older patients who may not have classic symptoms. If the etiology of the thyrotoxicosis is not clear, a radionuclide thyroid scan and uptake, as described in section on Thyroid Imaging in Hyperthyroidism, will be helpful in making the diagnosis.

Measurement of thyroglobulin (Tg) may help to differentiate factitious thyrotoxicosis from overactive thyroid disease of any etiology. In the former, the self-administered thyroid hormone will suppress the function of the normal thyroid gland and will result in very low levels of circulating Tg.

Antithyroid Antibodies in Hyperthyroidism

Measurement of antithyroid antibodies is not essential if a thyroid scan is performed. As mentioned previously, the presence of antibodies is not diagnostic for any specific etiology, as many patients will have antibodies in the absence of thyroid dysfunction, and a few patients will have autoimmune thyroid disease in the absence of antibodies. Measurement of antibodies or a thyroid scan can be used to confirm the diagnosis in a patient who is suspected of having Graves' disease. A high titer correlates well with clinically important autoimmune thyroid disease. If antibodies are measured, only TPO Abs should be done, as their presence highly correlates with the presence of other antibodies, and they are elevated at presentation in 95% of patients with Graves' thyrotoxicosis.

Thyroid Imaging in Hyperthyroidism

The etiology of thyrotoxicosis is often determined after a detailed past medical and family history and physical exam are performed. If the etiology remains unclear, a thyroid scan can be an invaluable tool in the differential diagnosis of hyperthyroidism, as it can easily differentiate between the most common etiolo-

Table 7
Thyrotoxicosis and Radioactive Iodine Thyroid Scan and Uptake Results

Diagnosis	*Degree of thyrotoxicosis*	*Radioactive iodine uptake*	*Scintigraphy image*
Graves' disease	++++	++++	Enlarged gland with homogenous uptake.
Toxic multinodular goiter	+/++	normal or +/++	Enlarged gland with multiple "hot" and "cold" nodules.
Thyrotoxic phase of subacute thyroiditis[a]	++++	<1% at 4 or 24 h	Absent isotope uptake.
Toxic adenoma	+/++	normal or +/++	Dominant "hot" nodule with low or absent uptake in the surrounding normal gland.

[a]Similar results with no radioactive iodine uptake in the neck can be seen with exogenous excess administration of thyroid hormone, ectopic thyroid hormone synthesis by a struma ovarii, metastatic thyroid carcinoma, or large excess ingestion of nonradioactive iodine.

gies. Either an ^{123}I scan with uptake or ^{99}Tc thyroid scan with trapping is the preferred diagnostic study to determine the etiology of the biochemical evidence of thyrotoxicosis, as shown in Table 7.

It is important to remember that the uptake depends not only on the autonomy of the thyroid gland but also on the nonradioactive iodine intake of the patient. The nonradioactive iodine can compete with the radioactive iodine tracer, resulting in a reduced iodine uptake. Thus, in patients with a very high intake of iodized salt, the thyroid uptake may be normal or even low despite an excessive production of thyroid hormone and thyrotoxicosis. Thyroid scans are contraindicated during pregnancy and lactation.

Monitoring of Patients with Hyperthyroidism

Treatment modalities for primary hyperthyroidism include radioactive ablation, antithyroid medications, and thyroidectomy. Radioactive ablation provides definitive treatment and is the preferred modality by endocrinologists in the U.S. Methimazole and propylthiouracil block thyroid hormone synthesis and are the two medications approved in the U.S. for treatment of hyperthyroidism. β-blockers are also used initially to ameliorate the cardiovascular and neuromuscular symptoms of thyrotoxicosis. Cold iodine is not recommended for the routine treatment of thyrotoxicosis. Monitoring of thyroid status is done by measurement of TSH, total T_4, an estimated free T_4, and T_3, with adjustment of antithyroid medication every 1 to 2 mo until euthyroid. Thyroid hormone levels tend to frequently fluctuate because of the effect of the antithyroid treatment and the inherent variability of the thyroid disease. It is recommended that the management of the patient with hyperthyroidism is done by the endocrinologist.

PREGNANCY AND THYROID DYSFUNCTION

Pregnancy and Hypothyroidism

Hypothyroidism is associated with menstrual irregularities and infertility. Therefore, the new diagnosis of hypothyroidism during pregnancy is uncommon. When diagnosed, hypothyroidism is almost always mild and almost always due to Hashimoto's thyroiditis. It is very important to make the diagnosis early, as hypothyroidism has been associated with maternal and fetal morbidity. Diagnosis of hypothyroidism is confirmed by an elevated TSH level. We recommend screening for hypothyroidism with TSH in pregnant women with a history of thyroid disease, goiter, other autoimmune disease, recurrent miscarriage, or family history of autoimmune thyroid disease. During pregnancy, the thyroid hormone requirements in the majority of patients may increase up to 50% compared to the patient's pre-pregnancy L-thyroxine dose. Frequent monitoring and adjustment of the L-thyroxine is needed during all three trimesters of pregnancy to maintain a TSH within the normal range *(15)*. The presence of antithyroid antibodies in the absence of thyroid dysfunction is associated with an increased risk for miscarriage. However, we do not recommend measuring antithyroid antibodies in all euthyroid pregnant women, as no established treatment modalities exist that would prevent miscarriage.

Pregnancy and Hyperthyroidism

Many signs and symptoms of hyperthyroidism occur in normal pregnancy. Therefore, a high degree of clinical suspicion is needed to diagnose hyperthyroidism during pregnancy. A search for more specific signs of hyperthyroidism are needed, such as failure of the mother or fetus to gain weight, resting tachycardia, an enlarged thyroid gland, exophthalmos, lid lag, muscle weakness, diarrhea, or tremor. The most common cause is Graves' disease, which often has clinical exacerbations during the first trimester of pregnancy. Toxic MNG is an uncommon cause. It usually occurs in women older than 40 yr with a history of MNG. Other causes of hyperthyroidism listed in Table 5 are much less common during pregnancy. The diagnosis of hyperthyroidism during pregnancy is made by demonstrating a suppressed TSH with an elevated free T_4 or free T_3 by equilibrium dialysis. The routine FT_4I may not be an accurate measure because of the high TBG levels of pregnancy (see section on Modalities of Thyroid Evaluation in Pregnancy). Measurement of TSH alone cannot be used to diagnose thyroid dysfunction in early pregnancy because of the cross-over stimulation of the thyroid by high hCG levels (see section Modalities of Thyroid Evaluation in

Pregnancy). Measurement of TPOAb can confirm the autoimmune nature of the thyroid dysfunction if other signs associated with Graves' disease are not present. TSI is measured during the third trimester, because high titers increase the risk of fetal goiter and hyperthyroidism due to TSI transfer across the placenta. If the TSI is high, a third trimester fetal ultrasound should be considered to determine if the fetal goiter will prevent a vaginal delivery. Radionuclide tests are contraindicated during pregnancy. The preferred antithyroid medication is propylthiouracil (PTU), because it is highly protein bound and less able to cross the placenta than methimazole. Generally, the PTU is given at a total dose of <200 mg/d to maintain the free thyroid hormone levels just above the normal range to reduce the exposure of the fetus to PTU. Often, the PTU dose can be reduced and stopped as the pregnancy progresses, as Graves' thyrotoxicosis and other autoimmune conditions usually improve in the second and third trimesters. Hyperemesis gravidara is associated with a low TSH without elevated thyroid hormone levels. Without elevated thyroid hormone, it is not recommended to treat with antithyroid medications. The diagnosis and management of hyperthyroidism during pregnancy is best managed by an endocrinologist.

Postpartum Thyroid Disease

Thyroid dysfunction occurs more commonly during the postpartum period than in pregnancy. It represents an exacerbation of autoimmune thyroid disorders. The most common cause of postpartum thyroid dysfunction is postpartum subacute thyroiditis, followed by exacerbation of or new onset Graves' thyrotoxicosis or Hashimoto's hypothyroidism. Postpartum thyroiditis is a form of transient autoimmune lymphocytic thyroiditis. It is painless, affects about 8% of North American postpartum women, and may occur up to 1 yr postpartum. The peak prevalence is 6 mo postpartum. Similar to other forms of subacute thyroiditis, it is associated with transient thyrotoxicosis, followed by transient hypothyroidism with eventual return to the euthyroid state in 90% of women. Only 50–60% of patients will experience all phases of postpartum thyroiditis. The diagnosis can be difficult, as the symptoms are often mild, and a high degree of clinical suspicion is required. The evaluation is done by measurement of serum TSH. Screening for postpartum thyroiditis is controversial because of the self-limiting nature of the disease. We recommend a screening TSH in women with symptoms suggestive of thyroid dysfunction or a personal history of postpartum thyroiditis (as it will reoccur after each pregnancy) or a family history of autoimmune thyroid disease. Given the autoimmune origin of postpartum thyroiditis, women who recover from this form of transient thyroiditis are at risk for developing clinical hypothyroidism at some time in the future. Therefore, lifelong follow-up is required. Postpartum hyperthyroidism should be evaluated with a thyroid scan/uptake when possible. Radionuclide tests are contraindicated in mothers who are breast-feeding.

Postpartum hypothyroidism may rarely be due to a central (secondary) etiology, such as to Sheehan's syndrome or lymphocytic hypophysitis. Measurement of TSH and free T_4 levels are required for diagnosis.

NONTHYROIDAL ILLNESS: EUTHYROID SICK SYNDROME

Euthyroid sick syndrome refers to the abnormalities seen in thyroid function tests in the setting of nonthyroidal illness (see section on Modalities of Thyroid Evaluation in Nonthyroidal Illness: Euthyroid Sick Syndrome). It is not considered a primary thyroid disorder, and its pathophysiology is not clear. The evaluation of a chronically ill or hospitalized patient with abnormal thyroid function tests can often be confusing. Our recommendation is to avoid measuring thyroid function tests during illness, unless thyroid dysfunction is thought to contribute to the illness. Measurement of serum TSH, total T_4, THBR, FT_4I, total T_3, and free level of T_4 by equilibrium dialysis should be done. It is important that the diagnosis of primary thyroid dysfunction is not established during severe illness based on an abnormal serum TSH. Typically in nonthyroid illness, TSH may be low, normal, or high, T_4 is low or normal, and T_3 is reduced proportionately more than T_4. Free levels of T_4 are usually normal. rT_3, although not routinely done, may be measured. It is usually increased in nonthyroidal illness. When possible, thyroid evaluation after recovery from the acute illness is recommended in patients suspected of having thyroid disease.

REFERENCES

1. Singer PA, Cooper DS, Levy EG, et al. Treatment guidelines for patients with hyperthyroidism and hypothyroidism. Standards of Care Committee, American Thyroid Association [see comments]. JAMA 1995;273:808–812.
2. Chopra IJ, Hershman JM, Pardridge WM, Nicoloff JT. Thyroid function in nonthyroidal illnesses. Ann Intern Med 1983;98:946–957.
3. Feldt-Rasmussen U, Schleusener H, Carayon P. Meta-analysis evaluation of the impact of thyrotropin receptor antibodies on long term remission after medical therapy of Graves' disease. J Clin Endocrinol Metab 1994;78:98–102.
4. Glinoer D. Thyroid hyperfunction during pregnancy. Thyroid 1998;8:859–864.
5. Chopra IJ. Clinical review 86: euthyroid sick syndrome: is it a misnomer? J Clin Endocrinol Metab 1997;82:329–334.
6. Cooper DS, Halpern R, Wood LC, Levin AA, Ridgway EC. L-Thyroxine therapy in subclinical hypothyroidism. A double-blind, placebo-controlled trial. Ann Intern Med 1984;101:18–24.
7. Nystrom E, Caidahl K, Fager G, Wikkelso C, Lundberg PA, Lindstedt G. A double-blind cross-over 12-month study of L-thyroxine treatment of women with 'subclinical' hypothyroidism. Clin Endocrinol (Oxf) 1988;29:63–75.
8. Sawin CT, Castelli WP, Hershman JM, McNamara P, Bacharach P. The aging thyroid. Thyroid deficiency in the Framingham Study. Arch Intern Med 1985;145:1386–1388.
9. Tunbridge WM, Brewis M, French JM, et al. Natural history of autoimmune thyroiditis. Br Med J (Clin Res Ed) 1981;282:258–262.
10. Vanderpump MP, Tunbridge WM, French JM, et al. The incidence of thyroid disorders in the community: a twenty-year follow-up of the Whickham Survey. Clin Endocrinol (Oxf) 1995;43:55–68.

11. Parle JV, Franklyn JA, Cross KW, Jones SC, Sheppard MC. Prevalence and follow-up of abnormal thyrotrophin (TSH) concentrations in the elderly in the United Kingdom. Clin Endocrinol (Oxf) 1991;34:77–83.
12. Sawin CT, Geller A, Kaplan MM, Bacharach P, Wilson PW, Hershman JM. Low serum thyrotropin (thyroid-stimulating hormone) in older persons without hyperthyroidism. Arch Intern Med 1991;151:165–168.
13. Sawin CT, Geller A, Wolf PA, et al. Low serum thyrotropin concentrations as a risk factor for atrial fibrillation in older persons [see comments]. N Engl J Med 1994;331:1249–1252.
14. Woeber KA. Thyrotoxicosis and the heart. N Engl J Med 1992;327:94–98.
15. Mandel SJ, Larsen PR, Seely EW, Brent GA. Increased need for thyroxine during pregnancy in women with primary hypothyroidism [see comments]. N Engl J Med 1990;323:91–96.

7 Thyroid Nodules and Thyroid Cancer

M. Regina Castro, MD
and Hossein Gharib, MD, FACE, FACP

Contents

INTRODUCTION

Thyroid nodules are a common problem in clinical practice. The majority are benign lesions, predominantly follicular adenomas, although other common causes of benign lesions include cysts, multinodular goiters, colloid goiters, benign Hürthle cell neoplasms, and thyroiditis *(1,2)*. However, some thyroid nodules may, in fact, represent thyroid cancer. The frequency of thyroid cancer in patients presenting with a solitary thyroid nodule has been estimated to be around 5% *(2)*, but the overall prevalence of cancer in all patients with solitary nodules has been estimated to be 0.1–0.2% *(3)*. Because thyroid nodules are so common, but, in general, only malignant nodules or benign ones large enough to cause compressive symptoms require operation, a cost-effective approach to the evaluation of thyroid nodules is important to minimize the number of unnecessary operations.

THYROID NODULES

Prevalence/Incidence

Thyroid nodules are seen frequently in the general population. The prevalence of this common disorder depends, to a great extent, on the method of screening and the population being evaluated. However, regardless of the screening method used, increasing age, female sex, iodine deficiency, and a

From: *Contemporary Endocrinology: Handbook of Diagnostic Endocrinology*
Edited by: J. E. Hall and L. K. Nieman

history of head and neck irradiation seem to increase consistently the overall risk of development of thyroid nodules *(4,5)*. A palpable nodule is more likely to be malignant in men (2:1 compared with women), in patients with a history of head and neck irradiation, when the nodule is hard, and when it is fixed to surrounding tissues *(1,4)*.

Palpation of the thyroid during routine physical examination is the easiest and least expensive screening method, albeit also the least sensitive. The prevalence of thyroid nodules detected by this method ranges from 4.7–51/1000 subjects in the adult population (Table 1) *(6–9,15)*. Probably the 2 studies that give the best estimates of the prevalence of thyroid nodules by palpation in the general population are described by Vander et al. *(7)* in the Framingham, MA, population, with an estimated prevalence of 4.2%, and the study by Tunbridge et al. *(8)* in a randomly sampled population in Whickham, England, where the overall prevalence was 3.2%.

High-resolution ultrasound can detect nodules as small as 2 mm. With this sensitive screening method, several studies have estimated that the prevalence of thyroid nodules in the general population ranges from 190–347/1000 subjects (Table 1) *(9–11,15)*. The overall prevalence obtained by pooling data from many of these studies is 280/1000 *(16)*. Although high-resolution ultrasound is a sensitive method for detecting thyroid nodules, it cannot definitively distinguish between benign and malignant lesions. Therefore, its specificity for this disorder is low.

The standard for determining the true prevalence of thyroid nodules is autopsy data. Several such studies have been performed in nonendemic and endemic areas and estimate the prevalence at between 82 and 650/1000 autopsies (Table 1) *(12–14)*. This variability depends, at least in part, on the thoroughness of the examination. Mortensen et al. *(14)* at the Mayo Clinic studied thyroid glands for macroscopic lesions from 821 consecutive autopsies in patients with no history of thyroid disease and found a prevalence of 495/1000. Schlesinger et al. *(12)* evaluated autopsy specimens from 3 teaching hospitals in the Boston area and noted a prevalence of 82/1000. In this study, however, only lesions measuring at least 1 cm were recorded, and this probably underestimates the true prevalence of thyroid nodules.

The incidence rate of thyroid nodules has been less well studied. The best data come from the Framingham study *(7)* and estimated the annual incidence rate, by palpation, at 0.09%. This means that about 275,000 new nodules will be discovered in the U.S. in 2002. The fact that the prevalence rate is much higher than the incidence rate suggests that once thyroid nodules are formed, they tend to remain present for long periods. Because palpation is a relatively insensitive method for detection of thyroid nodules, the incidence rate would probably be significantly higher if ultrasonography were used for detection.

Table 1
Prevalence of Thyroid Nodules per 1000 Subjects in the Community

Method of detection (yr)	*Investigator (reference)*	*Subjects (no.)*	*Prevalence*	*Country*	*Age (yr)*
Palpation					
1965	Matovinovic et al. *(6)*	8641	4.7	U.S.	0–70
1968	Vander et al. *(7)*	5127	42.0	U.S.	30–59
1977	Tunbridge et al. *(8)*	2979	32.0	England	18–75
1991	Brander et al. (9)	253	51.0	Finland	19–50
Ultrasonography					
1985	Woestyn et al. (10)	300	190.0	Belgium	0–90
1991	Brander et al. *(9)*	253	273.0	Finland	19–50
1994	Bruneton et al. *(11)*	1000	347.0	France	Adults
Autopsy[a]					
1938	Schlesinger et al. *(12)*	1373	82.0	U.S.	0–89
1955	Hull *(13)*	221	646.0	U.S.	20–100
1955	Mortensen et al. *(14)*	821	495.0	U.S.	0–99

[a]Autopsy series report all nodules seen by microscopic examination, except for the study by Schlesinger et al. *(12)* who reported only nodules 1 cm or larger.

U.S., United States.

Modified from Wang and Crapo *(15)*, by permission of WB Saunders Company.

Evaluation

Thyrotropin

The majority of patients with a palpable single nodule are euthyroid. However, about 5% of all solitary thyroid nodules are hyperfunctioning on scintigraphy, and up to 25% of patients harboring these so-called hot nodules or autonomously functioning thyroid adenomas may be clinically hyperthyroid *(17)*. Therefore, in any patient with a single nodule on palpation, a subnormal or suppressed serum thyrotropin (TSH) value, measured by current sensitive assays, should lead to the suspicion of a hyperfunctioning nodule. Because hyperfunctioning nodules are seldom malignant *(18)*, in the presence of a suppressed TSH value, confirmation of the functional status of a palpable thyroid nodule by scintigraphy is important. In these patients, observation alone may be sufficient. A suppressed TSH also indicates the need to monitor the patient for the possible development of hyperthyroidism and indicates that there is no point in attempting further suppression of TSH with thyroxine therapy *(19)*. An increased TSH value, on the other hand, indicates hypothyroidism and suggests Hashimoto thyroiditis.

Radioisotope Scanning

Scintigraphy is the standard method for functional imaging of the thyroid. The two isotopes most commonly used are ^{123}I and ^{99m}Tc pertechnetate, the latter being the agent of choice, because of lower cost and greater availability. Scanning provides a measure of the iodine-trapping function in a nodule compared with the surrounding thyroid tissue. Normally, there is uniform tracer uptake throughout both lobes and sometimes even in the isthmus (Fig. 1A). On the basis of tracer uptake, nodules may be classified as hypofunctioning (cold), indeterminate (warm), or hyperfunctioning (hot). Most are cold (decreased uptake, 80–85%) (Fig. 1B) or warm (uptake similar to surrounding tissue, 10%), including cancers and benign nodules *(18)*. Only the finding of a hot nodule (increased nodular uptake with suppression of uptake in the surrounding tissue), occurring in <5% of cases, is helpful in suggesting autonomously hyperfunctioning adenomas. Multinodular glands exhibit a heterogeneous patchy uptake, with increased uptake suggestive of toxic (Fig. 1C) or nontoxic (Fig. 1D) multinodular gland.

The sensitivity of ^{123}I scanning is about 83% *(1)*, whereas that of technetium scanning is about 91% *(18)*. The specificity of thyroid scans is low: 25% for radioiodine scans and 5–15% for technetium scans, and this low specificity is mostly because other thyroid lesions interfere with uptake of the radioisotopes *(1,18)*. Because, as stated previously, most solitary thyroid nodules are cold on scanning and only a fraction of these nodules are malignant (5–15%) *(19,20)*, a large proportion of positive scans are falsely positive. Because of its low diagnostic accuracy, the utility of thyroid scintigraphy in the evaluation of thyroid nodules is limited, and at present, its major role is in confirming the functional status of a suspected autonomously functioning thyroid nodule.

Ultrasonography

Current ultrasound technology, using high-resolution (5–10 MHz) transducers, is an excellent method for detection of thyroid nodules as small as 1 to 2 mm. Its sensitivity approaches 95% *(1)*, which is better than any other available method, including radioisotope scanning, computed tomography, and magnetic resonance imaging. It has replaced radionuclide scanning as the procedure of choice for imaging thyroid nodules. It provides a precise and reproducible measurement of nodule size and demonstrates whether a nodule is cystic, solid, or mixed (complex) *(21)* (Fig. 2). Because cystic nodules are seldom malignant, the finding of such a lesion on ultrasonography is, in general, reassuring evidence against malignancy (Fig. 3A). However, purely cystic thyroid nodules are extremely rare, representing only 1 in 550 thyroid nodules in a large series *(22)*. On the other hand, ultrasonographic findings of a hypoechoic pattern, incomplete peripheral halo, irregular margins, or internal microcalcifications in thyroid nodules are features that suggest malignancy *(23–25)* (Fig. 3B). However, none

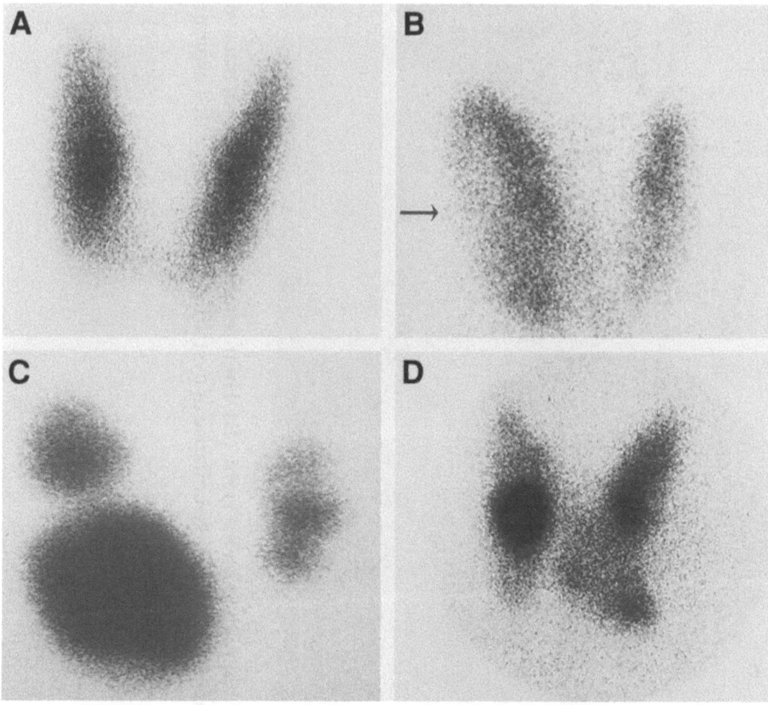

Fig. 1. Diagnostic thyroid radioisotope scans (^{99m}Tc). **(A)** Normal scan shows symmetrical uptake with butterfly pattern. **(B)** Scan reveals no uptake in the right lobe nodule (arrow). **(C)** Intense and patchy uptake in a patient with toxic multinodular gland, suppressed thyrotropin level, and radioactive iodine uptake of 54%. **(D)** Irregular uptake in a euthyroid patient with a small multinodular gland.

of these sonographic features is specific enough to guide the selection of patients for surgical treatment, hence the central role of fine-needle aspiration (FNA).

Ultrasonography is useful in confirming the presence of a mass, determining whether it is of thyroidal or extrathyroidal origin, assessing whether the lesion is single or multiple, and guides FNA. It has been suggested that, in the setting of multinodularity, a dominant palpable thyroid nodule is most often benign *(22)*. However, Tan et al. *(26)* at the Mayo Clinic reported that, in 151 patients with a clinically solitary nodule, high-resolution ultrasound showed that 73 (48%) had one or more nodules. Nodules not palpated were smaller than 1 cm in diameter. Importantly, a study by Belfiore et al. *(27)* found that the frequency of thyroid malignant tumors in patients with a solitary nodule (4.7%) does not differ from that in patients with a nontoxic multinodular goiter (4.1%). Therefore, detection of multiple lesions in patients with a clinically solitary nodule is not a reliable sign for excluding malignancy.

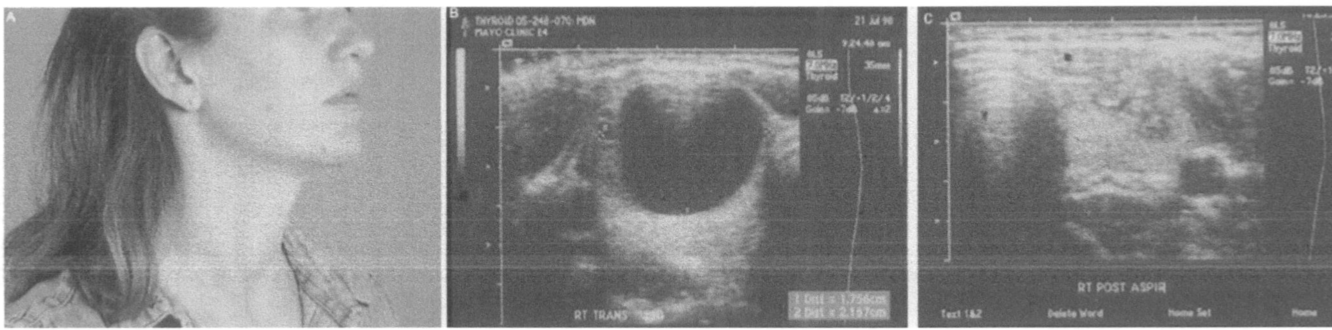

Fig. 2. Thyroid cyst. **(A)** A 36-yr-old woman with a recent 2.0-cm nodule on the right. **(B)** High-resolution ultrasound in transverse plane reveals a lesion with mostly cystic and little solid component. **(C)** Complete collapse of cyst after ultrasound-guided aspiration, which yielded 4-mL clear amber-colored fluid.

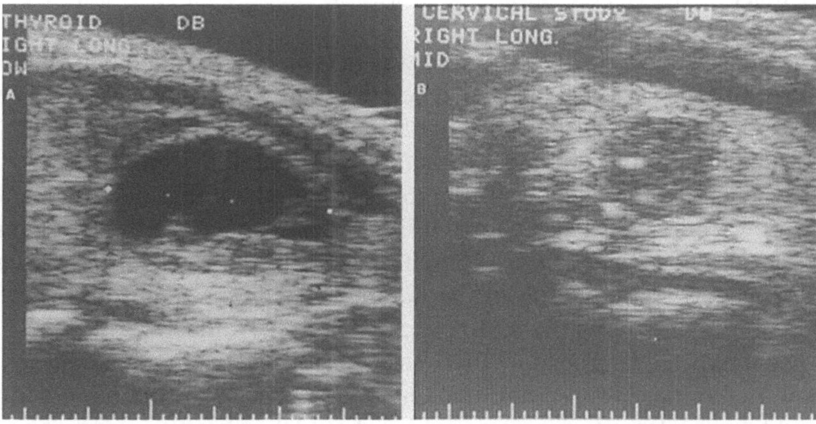

Fig. 3. Diagnostic thyroid ultrasound. **(A)** Longitudinal sonogram of the right thyroid lobe in a 17-yr-old girl reveals a 1.5-cm solid-cystic lesion, which by ultrasound-guided FNA was benign. **(B)** Sonogram in a patient with a familial medullary thyroid cancer syndrome reveals a thyroid nodule containing calcifications. Thyroidectomy confirmed medullary thyroid cancer.

The incidental finding of thyroid nodules during the course of ultrasonographic examination of the neck for evaluation of carotid or parathyroid disease is not uncommon. These lesions, referred to as "thyroid incidentalomas", are <1.5 cm, nonpalpable, and often pose a management problem to the clinician, who must then decide about their significance and subsequent course of action. Reading et al. *(28)*, using a high-frequency ultrasound system, found unsuspected thyroid nodules in 40% of patients examined for suspected parathyroid disease, and Carroll *(16)* reported incidental thyroid nodules in 13% of patients undergoing carotid ultrasound examination. Although the clinical significance of thyroid incidentalomas is uncertain, it is known that most of these lesions are benign *(29)*. Therefore, in the absence of features suggestive of malignancy, observation has been recommended for incidentalomas smaller than 1.5 cm and ultrasound-guided FNA for larger nodules *(29)*.

Because of the high prevalence of thyroid nodules, the fact that most (80%) thyroid malignancies are noncystic (solid and mixed) lesions and most noncystic thyroid nodules are benign, the specificity of thyroid ultrasonography in accurately diagnosing malignancy is only about 18% *(1)*. Ultrasonography by itself has a limited role in the initial evaluation of thyroid nodules, but is an important tool in the follow-up of both benign and malignant lesions. However, ultrasonographic guidance is extremely helpful in assisting FNA biopsy of suspicious thyroid nodules, and its use increased the diagnostic accuracy of the procedure and reduced the rate of false-positive results and inadequate specimens *(30)*.

FNA Biopsy

Although FNA biopsy of the thyroid was first described more than 60 yr ago, it was not until the early 1980s when it began to gain general clinical acceptance in the U.S. This procedure represents a major advance in the diagnosis and management of thyroid nodules and is now considered the most effective test currently available to distinguish benign from malignant thyroid nodules, with a diagnostic accuracy that approaches 95% *(31)*. Its influence in the management of thyroid nodules cannot be overemphasized. Most centers using FNA have achieved a 35–75% reduction in the number of patients requiring operation, while doubling or tripling the malignancy yield at thyroidectomy *(32–35)*. It is a safe and inexpensive procedure that can be performed in the outpatient setting, with minimal or no serious complications. Experience of the operator is important to obtain an adequate specimen, which should then be reviewed by an experienced cytopathologist.

FNA is an office procedure. Although it is relatively simple, experience and good technique are required for obtaining satisfactory results. Proper cytologic interpretation also requires special training in thyroid cytopathology. FNA results are divided into satisfactory (diagnostic) and unsatisfactory (nondiagnostic) *(31,36)*. Benign diagnoses include colloid nodule (Fig. 4A), cyst, lymphocytic thyroiditis (Fig. 4B), and granulomatous thyroiditis. Malignant cytology includes papillary thyroid cancer (Fig. 4C), anaplastic cancer (Fig. 4D), medullary thyroid cancer, lymphoma, and metastatic carcinoma *(36)*. Papillary thyroid cancer is the most common thyroid cancer and easily diagnosed by FNA. The suspicious (indeterminate) diagnoses include Hürthle or follicular cell neoplasms (Fig. 5), with findings suggestive of but not conclusive for malignancy *(36,37)*.

One major limitation of this procedure is the inadequate or insufficient result, which tends to occur in about 15% of cases *(31,36)*. Factors that contribute to insufficiency rates for FNA include operator experience, nodule vascularity, criteria used to judge adequacy, and the cystic component of the nodule *(4)*. Aspirates with too few epithelial cells are nondiagnostic or inadequate. The criteria to judge adequacy of aspirates are somewhat arbitrary and tend to vary among laboratories. We consider a satisfactory specimen one containing a minimum of six groups of well-preserved cells, each composed of at least 10 cells. Inadequate specimens are often collected from cystic lesions with degenerative foam cells but may also be the result of too much blood, excessive air-drying, or inadequate experience with FNA technique *(2)*. Repeat aspirations, particularly if done under ultrasonographic guidance, usually increase the biopsy yield. However, those nodules in which repeat aspirates fail to provide an adequate specimen should be excised if >4 cm, solid, or suggestive of malignancy *(2)*.

The other problem associated with FNA biopsy is the dilemma of suspicious or indeterminate cytologic findings, when cytologic criteria are equivocal

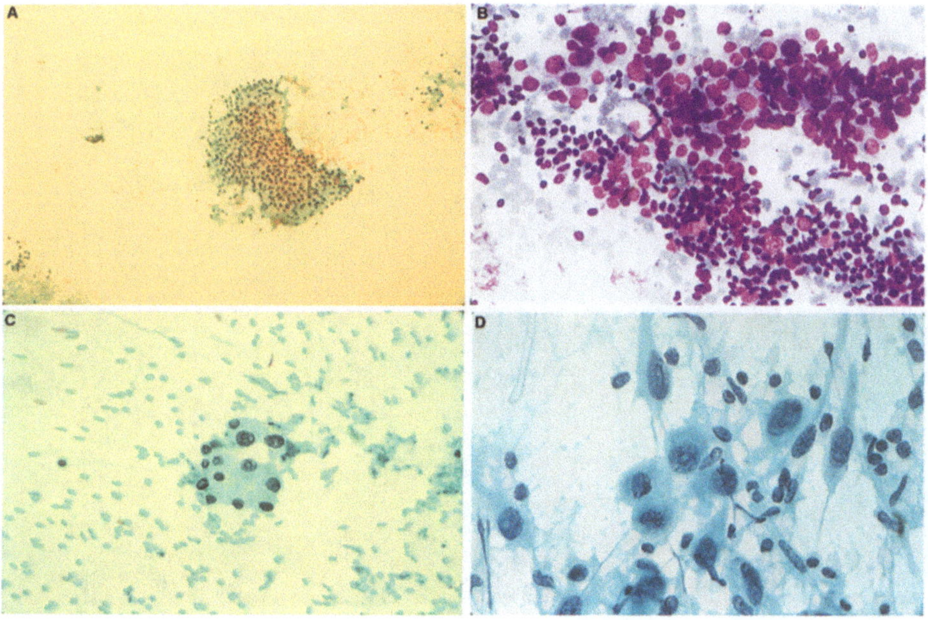

Fig. 4. Diagnostic thyroid cytology. **(A)** Benign nodule. Sheets of benign follicular cells mixed with background colloid. (Papanicolaou [PAP]; ×100.) **(B)** Hashimoto thyroiditis. Aspirate shows numerous lymphocytes and cells with abundant oxyphilic cytoplasm and large nuclei. There is no colloid. (May-Grunwald-Giemsa; ×250.) **(C)** Papillary thyroid carcinoma. Tumor cells with large irregular nuclei marked by lack of colloid. (PAP; ×250.) **(D)** Anaplastic thyroid carcinoma. Abundance of abnormal cells with large irregular nuclei is seen in aspirate. (PAP; ×400.)

(37,38). This is usually owing to the presence of Hürthle or follicular cell neoplasms or findings suggestive but not conclusive for malignancy (Fig. 5). About 20% of satisfactory specimens belong to this category *(31)*.

A review of more than 18,000 biopsies from seven different institutions showed that 69% were benign, 27% were suspicious or nondiagnostic, and 4% were malignant *(36)*. Analysis of the data revealed that the sensitivity of FNA ranged from 65–98% (mean, 83%), and the specificity from 72–100% (mean, 92%). The predictive value of a positive or suspicious cytologic result was about 50%. The false-negative rate was 1–11% (mean, 5%), and false positive rates ranged from 0–10% (mean, 3%). The overall accuracy for cytologic diagnosis approaches 95% *(36)*. Recently, it was suggested that repeat FNA in nodules with initially benign cytologic features may reduce the false-negative rate from an average of 5% to <1.3% *(39)*.

The current diagnostic work-up using TSH and FNA as initial tests is outlined in Fig. 6.

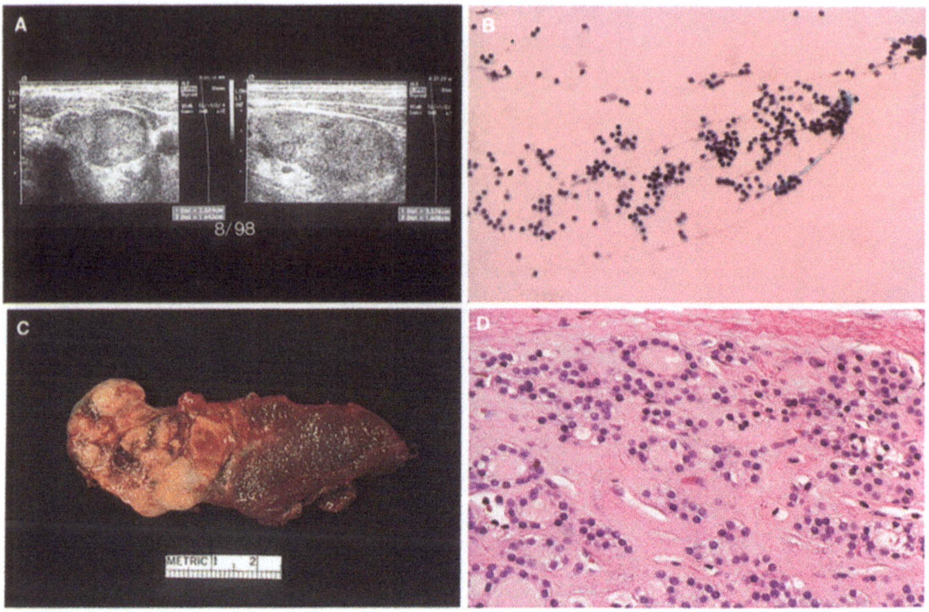

Fig. 5. Suspicious cytology. A 52-yr-old man with a 3.5-cm thyroid nodule on left. **(A)** High-resolution ultrasonography showed nodule to be solid. **(B)** Fine-needle aspiration biopsy was suspicious for malignancy, showing follicular neoplasm. (Papanicolaou; ×50.) **(C)** Thyroidectomy revealed a 3.8 x 2.2 x 1.0-cm follicular adenoma. **(D)** Histology showed a benign follicular lesion. (Hematoxylin and eosin; ×125.)

THYROID CANCER

Thyroid nodules, the most frequent presenting feature of thyroid cancer, are common in clinical practice. By contrast, clinically diagnosed thyroid cancer is a rarity. The challenge for the clinician, therefore, is to define accurately the small minority of patients with nodular thyroid disease who are at increased risk of having thyroid cancer. In the following section, we present the diagnostic studies that might help make this important distinction and guide further management and therapy. The pivotal role of FNA in the diagnosis of thyroid cancer was discussed in the previous section.

Prevalence /Incidence

Approximately 17,000 new cases of thyroid cancer are diagnosed in the U.S. each year, and about 1200 deaths occur annually as a consequence of this disease *(40)*. Thyroid cancer constitutes only about 1–2% of all malignant neoplasms in most populations *(6)*. The annual incidence of thyroid cancer is 0.5 to

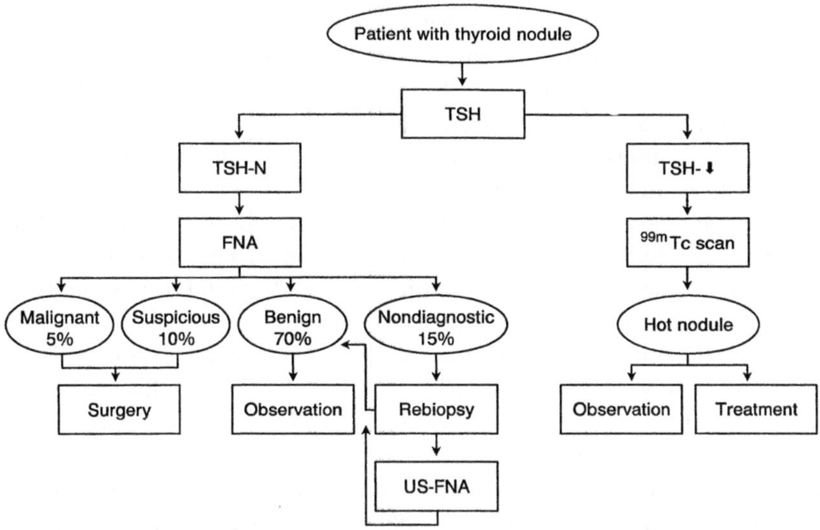

Fig. 6. Schematic approach to a patient with a solitary thyroid nodule. Initial test is for TSH, followed by FNA if TSH is normal and radioisotope scan if TSH is suppressed. Management is based on results of cytology. See text for discussion. US, ultrasound. (From Gharib, H. [2000] Thyroid fine needle aspiration biopsy, in *Thyroid Ultrasound and Ultrasound-Guided FNA* Biopsy [Baskin, H. J., ed.], Kluwer Academic Publishers, Norwell, MA, pp. 103–123. By permission of Kluwer Academic Publishers.)

10/100,000 in the world *(41)*, and it is three times more common in women than in men *(6)*.

Occult thyroid cancer was originally defined as any tumor 1.5 cm in diameter *(42)*. At present, it is defined as any inapparent tumor found on a specimen by a pathologist *(43)*. Several autopsy studies performed in the U.S. have found a mean prevalence of 3.6%, with a range between 0.5–13% *(44–46)*. In each of these studies, 1- to 3-mm slices of thyroid were evaluated for the presence of microscopic malignancies.

A study by Giuffrida and Gharib *(20)*, combining a series of FNA studies from the Mayo Clinic and the University of Catania (Italy), involving a total of 16,576 cases, calculated the prevalence of thyroid malignancy by FNA of 4%. The prevalence of thyroid cancer in children with clinically detectable nodules seems to be somewhat higher than in adults, averaging 18% *(47)*.

The mortality rate from thyroid cancer is low, despite the high prevalence of occult thyroid cancer. Transformation of benign thyroid nodules to thyroid carcinomas is extremely rare, occurring in <1% of cases, as shown in a 6-yr follow-up study of 439 nodules by Grant et al. *(48)*. It is thought that the 1% conversion rate most likely represents false-negative results of the initial biopsy.

Classification and Prognostic Factors

Thyroid cancer includes four primary histologic types. Papillary and follicular cancers arise from the follicular thyroid cells and are the well-differentiated forms of thyroid cancer. Other follicular cell-derived thyroid cancers include the oxyphilic or Hürthle cell variant and the undifferentiated anaplastic carcinoma. Medullary thyroid cancer (MTC), on the other hand, originates in the calcitonin (CT)-secreting parafollicular (C) cells. Other thyroid tumors include those arising from mesenchymal elements (sarcomas and angiomatoid thyroid neoplasms), which are extremely rare, and lymphoid cells (malignant lymphomas) as well as metastatic tumors to the thyroid gland.

Papillary thyroid cancer is, by far, the most common histologic type, accounting for about 80% of thyroid cancers in the U.S. *(49)*, followed by follicular thyroid cancer with 10– 15%. The histologic hallmarks are papillary fronds composed of stalks of fibroconnective tissue, containing blood vessels, characteristic hypochromatic nuclei with absent nucleoli, nuclear grooves and eosinophilic intranuclear cytoplasmic invaginations, and psammoma bodies (Fig. 4C). Papillary thyroid cancer is also recognized for its infiltrative pattern of growth, multicentricity, and spread to regional lymph nodes *(49)*. It usually grows slowly, and the prognosis, in general, is good. Different subtypes of papillary thyroid cancer may have somewhat different prognoses: papillary microcarcinoma, which comprises tumors 1.0 cm or smaller has an excellent prognosis *(50)*; in encapsulated papillary carcinoma mortality is extremely rare; follicular variant and tall cell and columnar cell variants have more aggressive behavior and higher mortality rates; and Hürthle cell variant has higher rates of local and distant metastases and 10-yr mortality of 18% *(51)*.

Besides the histologic subtype, additional prognostic risk factors in papillary thyroid cancer include histologic tumor grading, tumor size, multicentricity, vascular invasion, thyroid capsular and extrathyroidal invasion, local and distant metastases, and age at diagnosis (increased tumor-specific mortality in older age groups). Many different scoring systems have been devised to determine the risk of mortality in patients with thyroid cancer. TNM is a widely used international classification system that evaluates the size of the **t**umor, **n**odal involvement, and distant **m**etastases. Other scoring systems include AMES (based on **a**ge, distant **m**etastases, **e**xtent of the primary tumor, and **s**ize of the primary tumor) *(52)* and MACIS (distant **m**etastases, **a**ge at time of surgery, **c**ompleteness of surgery, **i**nvasion of extrathyroidal tissues, and **s**ize of the primary tumor) *(53)*.

For the most part, risk factors in follicular thyroid cancer are the same as for papillary thyroid cancer. Brennan et al. *(54)*, in a Mayo Clinic study, found that distant metastases at presentation, with patient age older than 50 yr, tumor size of 4 cm or more, marked vascular invasion, and higher grade histotype predicted a poor outcome. Five-year survival rate was 99% if none of these factors were present, but only 47% if 2 or more of these factors were present.

MTC accounts for about 10% of all thyroid neoplasms *(55,56)*. It originates in the C cells of the thyroid, which are interspersed among the follicular cells and which produce CT, a 32-amino acid peptide that functions as a calcium-lowering hormone. Seventy-five percent of patients with MTC have sporadic disease, and 25% present with the hereditary or familial form *(57)*. Four variants of the hereditary form have been identified: multiple endocrine neoplasia (MEN) IIA, MEN IIB, familial MTC (FMTC) without other components of MEN IIA, and MEN II associated with cutaneous lichen amyloidosis *(58)*. The male-to-female ratio is 1:1 in hereditary and familial forms. MEN IIA and MEN IIB are autosomal dominant syndromes, in which MTC is associated with pheochromocytoma in about 50% of cases. Parathyroid neoplasia is the third component of MEN IIA, whereas in MEN IIB, ganglioneuromas, which may be clinically obvious or subtle, are present (Fig. 7). In this form of the disease, MTC is usually more aggressive.

Several prognostic markers have been described in MTC. The clinical course in MTC is variable, and patients with MEN IIA and FMTC have a better long-term outcome than patients with MEN IIB or sporadic tumors *(59)*. Factors predictive of outcome include tumor stage, plasma CT levels, DNA ploidy, CT and somatostatin immunohistochemistry, and carcinoembryonic antigen (CEA) values *(59,60)*.

Anaplastic carcinoma of the thyroid is the most aggressive solid tumor of any organ; tends to affect predominantly older patients (mean age, 57–67 yr); and presents as a rapidly growing thyroid mass, causing hoarseness, dyspnea, dysphagia, or cervical pain *(61,62)*. The clinical course is rapid and relentless, despite most therapeutic interventions, and most patients die of local progression or distant metastases, often within weeks of diagnosis *(62)*. According to the Surveillance, Epidemiology and End Results (SEER) program, this type of cancer constitutes 1.6% of thyroid cancers in the U.S. *(63,64)*.

Primary thyroid lymphomas are rare, representing 1–5% of thyroid malignancies *(65)*. The majority of these tumors originate in glands with autoimmune thyroiditis and almost all are B-cell type *(65)*. Nearly all patients present with a preexisting goiter, and almost 80% show a sudden rapid growth of the goiter—13% with hoarseness, 7% with dysphagia, and 7% with fever *(65)*. The finding of stridor on presentation is highly associated with death from this disease *(66)*. Mean age at diagnosis is 60–68 yr, and the vast majority of patients are women *(65)*.

Evaluation

Tumor Markers

Thyroglobulin. Thyroglobulin (Tg) is a 660,000-kDa glycoprotein that serves as the prohormone for thyroid hormone production. Serum Tg concentrations reflect three factors: (*i*) the mass of differentiated thyroid tissue present; (*ii*) any physical damage to, or inflammation of, the thyroid gland; and (*iii*) the level of

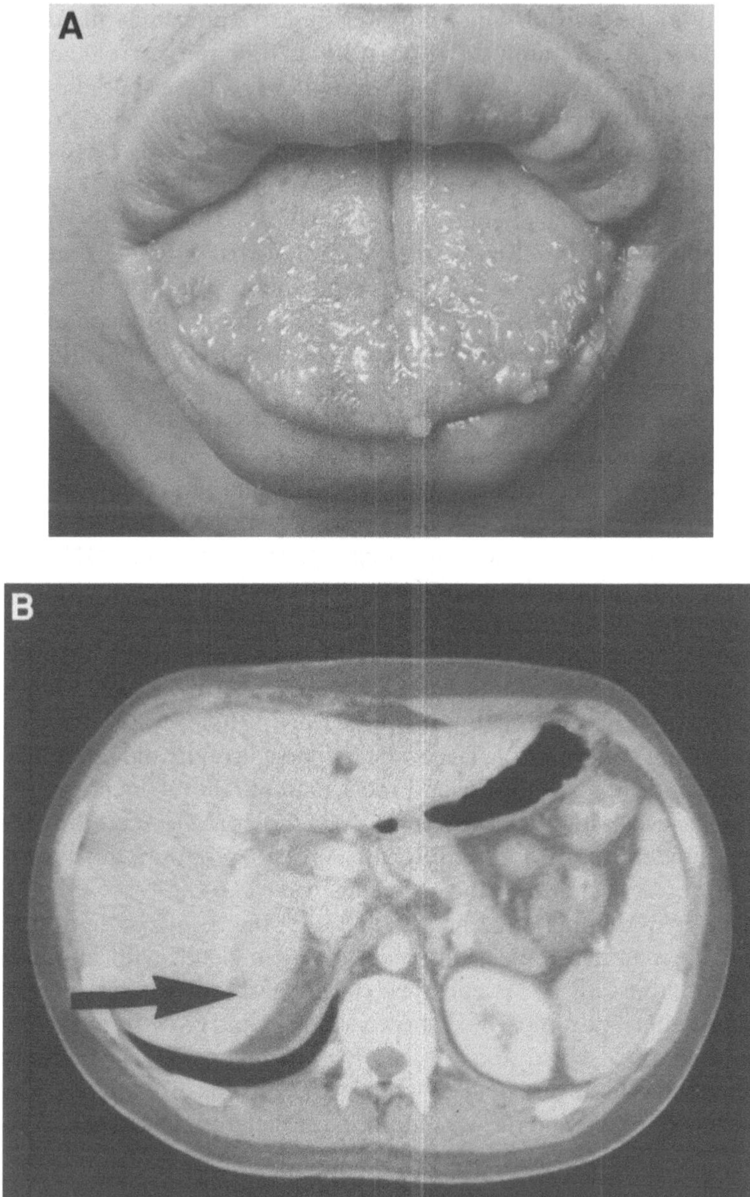

Fig. 7. A 19-yr-old male with MEN IIB. **(A)** Note the thick bumpy lips and tongue characteristic of mucosal neuromas. Basal calcitonin was 2100 pg/mL, consistent with metastatic disease. **(B)** Computed tomographic scan of the abdomen of same patient shows hepatic lesion (arrow), which proved to be medullary thyroid cancer deposits on biopsy.

TSH-receptor stimulation, because most steps in Tg biosynthesis and secretion are TSH-dependent *(67)*. Because Tg is a normal tissue component, it can only be used reliably as a tumor marker after total thyroid ablation, such as after thyroidectomy ablative ^{131}I therapy. In these cases, serum Tg is a reliable marker for the local recurrence of thyroid cancer, lymph node metastases, and distant-site metastases *(68)*. Some current assays have difficulty detecting Tg when levels are low, during TSH suppression of normal or lobectomized patients. The clinical sensitivity of Tg measurement for detecting small amounts of thyroid tissue is greatest (>90%) when endogenous TSH levels are elevated before ^{131}I imaging *(68)*.

On the other hand, the clinical value of serum Tg measurements is limited in the presence of Tg autoantibody (TgAb) interference, which can lead to underestimation or overestimation of the serum total Tg concentration *(67)*. When sensitive TgAb immunoassay methods are used, TgAb is detected in the serum of 4–27% of healthy individuals, 51–97% of patients with Graves disease or Hashimoto thyroiditis, respectively, and between 15 and 30% of patients with thyroid carcinoma *(67)*. TgAb concentrations generally decline or disappear over time after initial surgical treatment for differentiated thyroid cancer in patients who are judged clinically disease free, but they remain relatively unchanged or increase in patients with persistent or progressive disease *(69,70)*. TgAb interference is the most serious specificity problem affecting serum Tg measurement. Because of this, when measuring Tg levels in the follow-up of patients with a history of differentiated thyroid cancer, serum needs to be screened for TgAbs with a sensitive immunoassay and, if positive, results must be interpreted with caution and with consideration to any changes in TgAb levels *(67)*. In the absence of TgAb, detectable Tg levels in a patient who has been treated with total thyroid ablation suggest recurrence or persistent thyroid cancer *(71)*. The value of serum Tg measurement as a tumor marker in patients who have not had ablation of residual thyroid tissue after surgery is less clear, but it appears that in this group of patients, Tg levels are still of value but need to be interpreted in relation to the amount of thyroid tissue left and to the consistency of the results with time *(72)*. A Tg level of 10 ng/mL or less during suppressive therapy in patients with thyroid remnants significantly decreases, but does not eliminate, the possibility of recurrent disease *(73)*.

More recently, detection of circulating Tg mRNA from peripheral blood by amplification using reverse transcription-polymerase chain reaction has been shown to be a more sensitive method than the standard immunoassay for serum Tg, particularly in patients treated with thyroid hormone and in those who have circulating antithyroglobulin antibodies *(74)*. Its diagnostic accuracy of about 80% compares favorably to that of the standard immunoassay (about 70%) *(74)*.

Calcitonin. Plasma CT, the 32-amino acid secretory product of the para-follicular C cells, is the most sensitive marker for the diagnosis and monitoring of MTC, because the majority of patients with MTC have elevated basal CT levels. High basal plasma CT values may already be found in microscopic MTC. Moreover, the injection of CT secretagogues, such as calcium and pentagastrin (Pg), causes an increase in the CT level in MTC, whatever the stage, and this increase also allows C-cell hyperplasia to be detected before development of MTC *(75,76)*.

Rarely, basal plasma CT levels can be increased during normal childhood and pregnancy, after vigorous exercise, and in small cell lung cancers, breast cancers, hepatomas, pancreatic tumors, gastrinomas, pernicious anemia, thyroiditis, and end-stage renal failure. However, patients with these conditions usually have a blunted or absent response to provocative testing with CT secretagogues *(55)*.

Pentagastrin (0.5 µg/kg) is given by intravenous bolus injection, and blood is sampled before injection (baseline) and at 1.5 and 5 min *(77)*. Calcium gluconate (2 mg calcium/kg) is infused intravenously over 5 min, and blood is sampled at 0 (baseline), 5, and 10 min. The normal ranges for basal and Pg-stimulated CT levels vary among different laboratories using different assays, but most laboratories report higher basal as well as stimulated values in men than in women *(77)*. CT radioimmunoassays vary considerably in their sensitivity and specificity. A sensitive radioimmunoassay that uses an extraction technique has been developed at the Mayo Clinic *(78)*. Pg is generally regarded as the most effective CT secretory discriminator in patients with MTC and is currently the most widely used test. In patients who have undergone total thyroidectomy for MTC, detectable basal and stimulated CT suggests persistent or recurrent MTC *(79,80)*. In addition, provocative testing with Pg stimulation has been used to screen first-degree relatives of patients with MTC in the setting of FMTC syndromes *(81)*. Gagel et al. *(82)* reported that abnormal Pg test results are seen in 50% of carriers of MEN IIA by age 12 yr, 80% by age 20 yr, and about 95% by age 35 yr.

Carcinoembryonic Antigen. CEA was first described in 1965 by Gold and Freedman *(83)* as a marker of colorectal cancer. High concentrations of this tumor marker have since been found in patients with malignant tumors of the gastrointestinal tract, lung, breast, genitourinary tract, and nervous system *(84)*. However, CEA is now a well-recognized biochemical tumor marker of MTC, and increased levels of this antigen have been reported in a large percentage of patients with this thyroid malignancy *(84,85)*. In combination with CT, CEA is an excellent method of monitoring MTC, because persistent increase of these markers after primary curative surgery suggests residual or metastatic disease *(86)*. The levels seem to correlate positively with tumor burden, being higher in patients with clinically evident MTC than in those with occult disease *(84)*.

A study by Behr et al. *(87)* using anti-CEA monoclonal antibodies showed that these had a sensitivity for detection of occult MTC and staging of known MTC superior to that of conventional modalities. ^{131}I-labeled anti-CEA monoclonal antibodies have been shown in recent years to be helpful tools for targeting metastatic MTC and in an early study appear to be a promising therapeutic option *(88)*.

IMAGING

Ultrasound. High-resolution ultrasound can detect thyroid nodules as small as 2 to 3 mm. Even though thyroid nodules are relatively common, the frequency of malignancy in these nodules is small, on the order of 5–10%. It is also well known that many glands with apparent solitary nodules by palpation, when screened with ultrasonography, are shown to be, in fact, multinodular *(24,26)*. Certain echosonographic features of a thyroid nodule or mass tend to suggest a benign nature of the disease, such as anechoic nodule, anechoic with floating debris, hyperechoic, or eggshell calcifications *(89)*. On the other hand, malignant nodules are likely to be hypoechoic, have irregular or poorly defined margins, or have microcalcifications *(21,25)*.

Pure cysts, which are extremely rare, are defined by their smooth, featureless walls and no internal echoes and are always benign *(90)*. However, complex cysts, containing both fluid and solid material, can harbor malignancy in up to 14% of cases *(91)*.

Ultrasonography is useful for detecting thyroid cancer recurrences (sensitivity of 96% and specificity of 83%) in the thyroid bed and in local lymph nodes *(92)*, which may be enlarged yet nonpalpable. Localization of enlarged lymph nodes can be used to direct subsequent biopsy *(89)*. As with the study of thyroid nodules, certain echosonographic characteristics of lymph nodes may indicate their benign or malignant nature. Normal lymph nodes are usually flattened, whereas malignant ones tend to be more rounded or bulging; normal and hyperplastic lymph nodes usually exhibit an echogenic line through the center called a hilus line, which is seldom seen in malignant lymph nodes *(21)*. However, ultrasonography cannot definitively distinguish benign from malignant disease, but is of key importance in guiding FNA biopsy to further evaluate the suspicious nodes.

^{131}I Scan. Radioiodine has an important role in the treatment of well-differentiated forms of thyroid cancer and in the evaluation of metastatic disease *(90)*. Because metastases, in general, are less efficient at iodine uptake than normal thyroid tissue, they are not visualized until all normal tissue has been removed, which may be accomplished by complete surgical resection or a combination of surgery and ^{131}I ablation. After successful ablation, between 50 and 67% of well-differentiated forms of thyroid cancer and about 50% of metastases to lung and bones can be imaged with ^{131}I *(93)* (Fig. 8). Increased TSH concentration increases uptake in both benign and malignant thyroid tissue, and this elevation may be accomplished by withholding levothyroxine for at least 6 wk before a follow-up scan. More recently, however, recombinant human TSH (rTSH) has become available for injection and may be given in preparation for a scan while the patient remains on thyroid hormone replacement *(94)*. A study by Ladenson et al. *(94)* demonstrated that rTSH was equivalent to or better than conventional withdrawal scanning in 83% of the cases studied, and it has the advantage of avoiding the unpleasant effects of hypothyroidism that occur after prolonged withdrawal of thyroid hormone replacement.

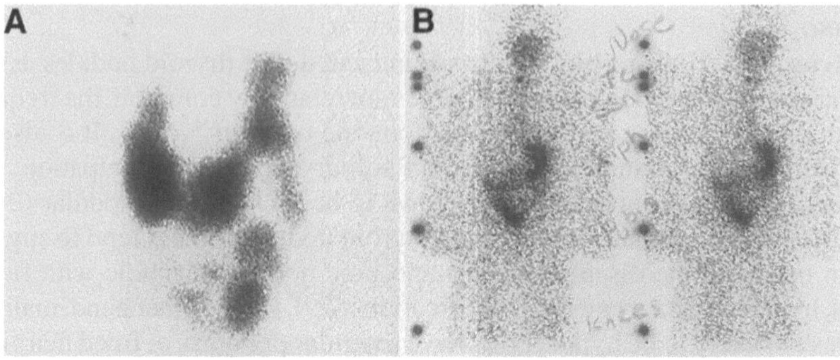

Fig. 8. Radioisotope imaging in thyroid cancer. **(A)** Technetium thyroid scan demonstrates uptake in thyroid gland and neck nodes on left. Neck exploration confirmed the presence of metastatic papillary thyroid cancer. **(B)** ^{131}I whole body scan in post-thyroidectomy patient shows tiny uptake in thyroid bed and normal uptake in the gastrointestinal tract and bladder.

The specificity of radioiodine scanning is high and approaches 100% *(93,95)*. However, its sensitivity is more variable, ranging from 48–84%, depending on several factors, including tumor size, histologic type, primary vs metastatic disease, and sites of metastases *(90,95)*. False-positive results are usually due to body secretions, pathologic transudates and exudates, infection or inflammation, and nonthyroidal tumors *(96)* and occur most frequently in salivary glands, nasopharyngeal area or thymus, and more rarely, in many other sites *(90)*. A low or undetectable Tg value and abnormalities that occur in a single image view may occasionally be a clue that a positive scan could, in fact, be a false-positive study.

Computed Tomography. Computed tomographic scans are useful in the evaluation of thyroid cancer recurrence, especially in delineating the extent of retrosternal involvement and defining the presence and extent of lymph node metastases, tracheal invasion, compression or displacement, and vascular invasion *(19)*. These scans are also helpful in assessing tumors not clearly arising from the thyroid and bulky tumors with possible invasion of local structures *(19)*. It is not useful, however, in differentiating benign from malignant nodules *(90)*. If a contrast agent containing a large amount of iodine is used for image enhancement, subsequent radioiodine scanning or therapy should be delayed *(90)*.

Positron Emission Tomography Scanning. [^{18}F]fluorodeoxyglucose (FDG) is a radioactively labeled glucose derivative, which is concentrated in metabolically active tissues, including heart, kidney, brain, and malignant and inflammatory tissues. The main utility of this relatively new imaging modality in the evaluation of thyroid cancer is in detecting metastatic deposits of thyroid cancer in patients with elevated Tg levels but negative post-therapy ^{131}I scans. Its sensitivity ranges from 71–95%, and its specificity ranges from 81–95% *(97,98)*. Diffuse thyroidal uptake of FDG has been described in autoimmune thyroid disease such as Hashimoto thyroiditis and Graves disease.

Genetic Testing

MTC, which accounts for about 10% of thyroid malignancies, may occur either as a sporadic disease (75%) or as a familial disorder (25%) *(57)*. The familial form of MTC can present as isolated thyroid malignancy (FMTC) or as part of MEN II. The clinical characteristics of each of these 2 forms of MEN have been described above. The familial forms of MTC (FMTC, MEN IIA, and MEN IIB) have long been recognized to have an autosomal dominant mode of inheritance. However, because the clinical penetrance of the MEN II gene is not complete, a negative family history in a patient presenting with MTC is not sufficient to exclude familial disease. Family screening should, therefore, be considered for all new cases of MTC, including those with apparent sporadic disease.

The recent development of genetic testing has been one of the major advances in the evaluation and management of patients with MTC. With genetic linkage analysis in 1987, the gene for MEN IIA was mapped to the *ret* proto-oncogene, located in the centromeric region of chromosome 10 *(99,100)*. Subsequently, germline mutations in the *ret* proto-oncogene were identified in patients with MEN IIA, MEN IIB, and FMTC *(101,102)*. The mutations in MEN IIA have been found in exons 10, 11, and 13 and involve a cysteine residue *(57,101,103–105)*, whereas in MEN IIB, mutations in exon 16, involving substitution of threonine for methionine, have been found in 95% of the subjects studied *(106,107)*. In FMTC, mutations involving exon 14 of the *ret* proto-oncogene have been described in addition to those found in MEN IIA *(57)*. The *ret* proto-oncogene, on chromosome 10q11.2, is a transmembrane tyrosine kinase with a cysteine-rich extracellular domain, expressed normally in thyroid tissue, medullary thyroid carcinoma, and pheochromocytoma *(108)*.

Every patient with MTC, sporadic or familial, should undergo direct DNA analysis to identify mutations in the *ret* proto-oncogene. If a mutation is identified, all family members should be tested for the same mutation as early as possible. Once gene carriers are identified, prophylactic total thyroidectomy should be offered, which in most patients is curative. Family members without the *ret* mutation have essentially the same risk as the general population for future MTC and should be reassured and informed that no further tests are necessary for them or their offspring. When familial MTC is suspected, but no mutation is identified in a given patient, genetic linkage analysis should be done to evaluate family members at risk *(108)*. Our current management strategy, as described by Ledger et al. *(108)*, is shown in Fig. 9.

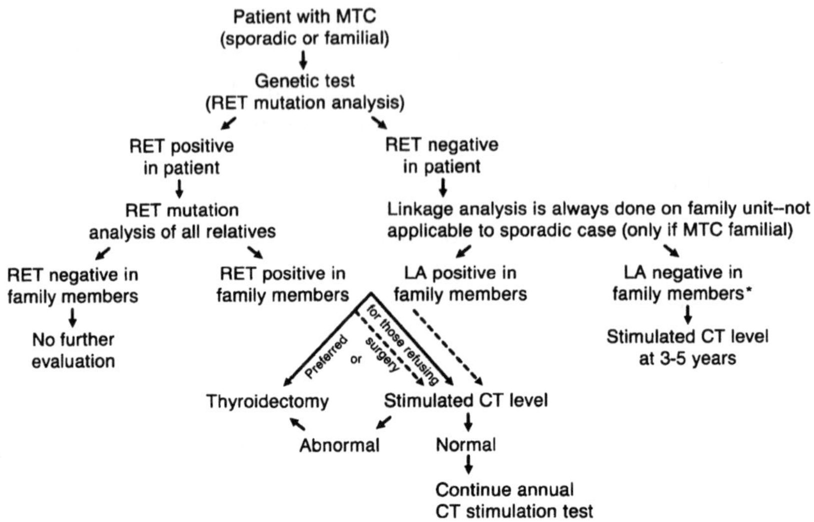

Fig. 9. Algorithm suggests sequence of tests in a patient with MTC, family screen, and management based on results of genetic testing. Thyroidectomy is recommended for all predicted gene carriers by either direct DNA mutation analysis or linkage-based testing. Dashed line represents an alternative, less desirable course, when surgical decision is based on follow-up evaluation with Pg tests. *Indicates further evaluation dictated by adequacy of markers to exclude gene carriers. CT, calcitonin; LA, linkage analysis. (From Ledger et al. [108]. By permission of American College of Physicians.)

CONCLUSIONS

Thyroid nodules are a common clinical problem. The majority of them are benign lesions, which require only observation. Thyroid cancer, on the other hand, is an infrequent malignancy, which often presents as a nodule. Cost-effective evaluation of thyroid nodules should be able to distinguish benign from malignant lesions; benign nodules are followed medically, whereas malignant ones should be surgically excised. FNA plays a key role in this differential diagnosis and has been the single most important advance in the diagnosis and management of thyroid nodules. Other imaging modalities including ultrasound, ^{99m}Tc scan, and radioiodine scan are adjunctive diagnostic methods, which, together with tumor markers, such as Tg, CT, and CEA, are useful in the preoperative evaluation and postoperative follow-up of patients with thyroid cancer to detect evidence of recurrence and guide further management.

REFERENCES

1. Dolan JG. Thyroid nodules. In: Panzer RJ, Black ER, Griner PF, eds. Diagnostic Strategies for Common Medical Problems. The American College of Physicians, Philadelphia, 1991, pp. 385–393.

2. Gharib H. Changing concepts in the diagnosis and management of thyroid nodules. Endocrinol Metab Clin North Am 1997;26:777–800.
3. Klonoff DC, Greenspan FS. The thyroid nodule. Adv Intern Med 1982;27:101–126.
4. Burch HB. Evaluation and management of the solid thyroid nodule. Endocrinol Metab Clin North Am 1995;24:663–710.
5. Schneider AB, Recant W, Pinsky SM, Ryo UY, Bekerman C, Shore-Freedman E. Radiation-induced thyroid carcinoma. Clinical course and results of therapy in 296 patients. Ann Intern Med 1986;105:405–412.
6. Matovinovic J, Hayner NS, Epstein FH, Kjelsberg MO. Goiter and other thyroid diseases in Tecumseh, Michigan: studies in a total community. JAMA 1965;192:234–240.
7. Vander JB, Gaston EA, Dawber TR. The significance of nontoxic thyroid nodules. Final report of a 15-year study of the incidence of thyroid malignancy. Ann Intern Med 1968;69:537–540.
8. Tunbridge WM, Evered DC, Hall R, et al. The spectrum of thyroid disease in a community: the Whickham survey. Clin Endocrinol (Oxf) 1977;7:481–493.
9. Brander A, Viikinkoski P, Nickels J, Kivisaari L. Thyroid gland: US screening in a random adult population. Radiology 1991;181:683–687.
10. Woestyn J, Afschrift M, Schelstraete K, Vermeulen A. Demonstration of nodules in the normal thyroid by echography. Br J Radiol 1985;58:1179–1182.
11. Bruneton JN, Balu-Maestro C, Marcy PY, Melia P, Mourou MY. Very high frequency (13 MHz) ultrasonographic examination of the normal neck: detection of normal lymph nodes and thyroid nodules. J Ultrasound Med 1994;13:87–90.
12. Schlesinger MJ, Gargill SL, Saxe IH. Studies in nodular goiter: incidence of thyroid nodules in routine necropsies in nongoitrous region. JAMA 1938;110:1638–1641.
13. Hull OH. Critical analysis of 221 thyroid glands: study of thyroid glands obtained at necropsy in Colorado. Arch Pathol 1955;59:291–311.
14. Mortensen JD, Woolner LB, Bennett WA. Gross and microscopic findings in clinically normal thyroid glands. J Clin Endocrinol Metab 1955;15:1270–1280.
15. Wang C, Crapo LM. The epidemiology of thyroid disease and implications for screening. Endocrinol Metab Clin North Am 1997;26;189–218.
16. Carroll BA. Asymptomatic thyroid nodules: incidental sonographic detection. Am J Roentgenol 1982;138:499–501.
17. Ridgway EC. Clinical review 30: clinician's evaluation of a solitary thyroid nodule. J Clin Endocrinol Metab 1992;74:231–235.
18. Meier DA, Kaplan MM. Radioiodine uptake and thyroid scintiscanning. Endocrinol Metab Clin North Am 2001;30:291–313.
19. Shulkin BL, Shapiro B. The role of imaging tests in the diagnosis of thyroid carcinoma. Endocrinol Metab Clin North Am 1990;19:523–543.
20. Giuffrida D, Gharib H. Controversies in the management of cold, hot, and occult thyroid nodules. Am J Med 1995;99:642–650.
21. Haber RS. Role of ultrasonography in the diagnosis and management of thyroid cancer. Endocr Pract 2000;6:396–400.
22. Simeone JF, Daniels GH, Mueller PR, et al. High-resolution real-time sonography of the thyroid. Radiology 1982;145:431–435.
23. Koike E, Noguchi S, Yamashita H. Murakami T, Ohshima A, Kawamoto H. Ultrasonographic characteristics of thyroid nodules: prediction of malignancy. Arch Surg 2001;136:334–337.
24. Brander A, Viikinkoski P, Tuuhea J, Voutilainen L, Kivisaari L. Clinical versus ultrasound examination of the thyroid gland in common clinical practice. J Clin Ultrasound 1992;20:37–42.
25. Solbiati L, Ballarati E, Cioffi V, Poerio N, Croce F, Rizzatto G. Microcalcifications: a clue in the diagnosis of thyroid malignancies [abstract]. Radiology 1990;177:140.

26. Tan GH, Gharib H, Reading CC. Solitary thyroid nodule. Comparison between palpation and ultrasonography. Arch Intern Med 1995;155:2418–2423.
27. Belfiore A, La Rosa GL, La Porta GA, et al. Cancer risk in patients with cold thyroid nodules: relevance of iodine intake, sex, age, and multinodularity. Am J Med 1992;93:363–369.
28. Reading CC, Charboneau JW, James EM, et al. High-resolution parathyroid sonography. Am J Roentgenol 1982;139:539–546.
29. Tan GH, Gharib H. Thyroid incidentalomas: management approaches to nonpalpable nodules discovered incidentally on thyroid imaging. Ann Intern Med 1997;126:226–231.
30. Solymosi T, Toth GL, Bodo M. Diagnostic accuracy of fine needle aspiration cytology of the thyroid: impact of ultrasonography and ultrasonographically guided aspiration. Acta Cytol 2001;45:669–674.
31. Gharib H. Fine-needle aspiration biopsy of thyroid nodules: advantages, limitations, and effect. Mayo Clin Proc 1994;69:44–49.
32. Werk EE Jr, Vernon BM, Gonzalez JJ, Ungaro PC, McCoy RC. Cancer in thyroid nodules. A community hospital survey. Arch Intern Med 1984;144:474–476.
33. Pepper GM, Zwickler D, Rosen Y. Fine-needle aspiration biopsy of the thyroid nodule. Results of a start-up project in a general teaching hospital setting. Arch Intern Med 1989;149:594–596.
34. Asp AA, Georgitis W, Waldron EJ, Sims JE, Kidd GS II. Fine needle aspiration of the thyroid. Use in an average health care facility. Am J Med 1987;83:489–493.
35. Hamburger JI. Consistency of sequential needle biopsy findings for thyroid nodules. Management implications. Arch Intern Med 1987;147:97–99.
36. Gharib H, Goellner JR. Fine-needle aspiration biopsy of the thyroid: an appraisal. Ann Intern Med 1993;118:282-289.
37. Gharib H, Goellner JR, Zinsmeister AR, Grant CS, van Heerden JA. Fine-needle aspiration biopsy of the thyroid. The problem of suspicious cytologic findings. Ann Intern Med 1984;101:25–28.
38. Gharib H, Goellner JR, Johnson DA. Fine-needle aspiration cytology of the thyroid. A 12-year experience with 11,000 biopsies. Clin Lab Med 1993;13:699–709.
39. Chehade JM, Silverberg AB, Kim J, Case C, Mooradian AD. Role of repeated fine-needle aspiration of thyroid nodules with benign cytologic features. Endocr Pract 2001;7:237–243.
40. Parker SL, Davis KJ, Wingo PA, Ries LA, Heath CW Jr. Cancer statistics by race and ethnicity. CA Cancer J Clin 1998;48:31–48.
41. Franceschi S, La Vecchia C. Thyroid cancer. Cancer Surv 1994;19-20:393–422.
42. Woolner LB, Lemmon ML, Beahrs OH, Black BM, Keating FR Jr. Occult papillary carcinoma of the thyroid gland: a study of 140 cases observed in a 30-year period. J Clin Endocr 1960;20:89–105.
43. Mazzaferri EL, de los Santos ET, Rofagha-Keyhani S. Solitary thyroid nodule: diagnosis and management. Med Clin North Am 1988;72:1177–1211.
44. Mortensen JD, Bennett WA, Woolner LB. Incidence of carcinoma in thyroid glands removed at 1000 consecutive routine necropsies. S Forum 1954;5:659-663.
45. Sampson RJ, Woolner LB, Bahn RC, Kurland LT. Occult thyroid carcinoma in Olmsted County, Minnesota: prevalence at autopsy compared with that in Hiroshima and Nagasaki, Japan. Cancer 1974;34:2072–2076.
46. Nishiyama RH, Ludwig GK, Thompson NW. The prevalence of small papillary thyroid carcinomas in 100 consecutive necropsies in an American population. In: DeGrott LJ, ed. Radiation-Associated Thyroid Carcinoma. Grune and Stratton, New York, 1977; pp. 123–135.
47. Raab SS, Silverman JF, Elsheikh TM, Thomas PA, Wakely PE. Pediatric thyroid nodules: disease demographics and clinical management as determined by fine needle aspiration biopsy. Pediatrics 1995;95:46–49.
48. Grant CS, Hay ID, Gough IR, McCarthy PM, Goellner JR. Long-term follow-up of patients with benign thyroid fine-needle aspiration cytologic diagnoses. Surgery 1989;106:980–985.

49. Robbins J, Merino MJ, Boice JD, Jr, et al. Thyroid cancer: a lethal endocrine neoplasm. Ann Intern Med 1991;115:133–147.
50. Hay ID, Grant CS, van Heerden JA, Goellner JR, Ebersold JR, Bergstralh EJ. Papillary thyroid microcarcinoma: a study of 535 cases observed in a 50-year period. Surgery 1992;112:1139–1146.
51. Herrera MF, Hay ID, Wu PS, et al. Hürthle cell (oxyphilic) papillary thyroid carcinoma: a variant with more aggressive biologic behavior. World J Surg 1992;16:669–674.
52. Cady B, Rossi R. An expanded view of risk-group definition in differentiated thyroid carcinoma. Surgery 1988;104:947–953.
53. Hay ID, Bergstralh EJ, Goellner JR, Ebersold JR, Grant CS. Predicting outcome in papillary thyroid carcinoma: development of a reliable prognostic scoring system in a cohort of 1779 patients surgically treated at one institution during 1940 through 1989. Surgery 1993;114:1050–1057.
54. Brennan MD, Bergstralh EJ, van Heerden JA, McConahey WM. Follicular thyroid cancer treated at the Mayo Clinic, 1946 through 1970: initial manifestations, pathologic findings, therapy, and outcome. Mayo Clin Proc 1991;66:11–22.
55. McDermott MT. Calcitonin and its clinical applications. Endocrinologist 1992;2:366–373.
56. Vasen HF, Vermey A. Hereditary medullary thyroid carcinoma. Cancer Detect Prev 1995;19:143–150.
57. Giuffrida D, Gharib H. Current diagnosis and management of medullary thyroid carcinoma. Ann Oncol 1998;9:695–701.
58. Dottorini ME, Assi A, Sironi M, Sangalli G, Spreafico G, Colombo L. Multivariate analysis of patients with medullary thyroid carcinoma. Prognostic significance and impact on treatment of clinical and pathologic variables. Cancer 1996;77:1556–1565.
59. Moley JF. Medullary thyroid cancer. Surg Clin North Am 1995;75:405–420.
60. Gilliland FD, Hunt WC, Morris DM, Key CR. Prognostic factors for thyroid carcinoma. A population-based study of 15,698 cases from the Surveillance, Epidemiology and End Results (SEER) program 1973-1991. Cancer 1997;79:564–573.
61. Nel CJ, van Heerden JA, Goellner JR, Gharib H, McConahey WM, Taylor WF, Grant CS. Anaplastic carcinoma of the thyroid: a clinicopathologic study of 82 cases. Mayo Clin Proc 1985;60:51–58.
62. Ain KB. Rare forms of thyroid cancer. In: Fagin J, ed. Thyroid Cancer. Kluwer Academic Publishers, Boston, 1998, pp. 319–340.
63. Aldinger KA, Samaan NA, Ibanez M, Hill CS Jr. Anaplastic carcinoma of the thyroid: a review of 84 cases of spindle and giant cell carcinoma of the thyroid. Cancer 1978;41:2267–2275.
64. Venkatesh YS, Ordonez NG, Schultz PN, Hickey RC, Goepfert H, Samaan NA. Anaplastic carcinoma of the thyroid. A clinicopathologic study of 121 cases. Cancer 1990;66:321–330.
65. Matsuzuka F, Miyauchi A, Katayama S, et al. Clinical aspects of primary thyroid lymphoma: diagnosis and treatment based on our experience of 119 cases. Thyroid 1993;3:93–99.
66. Sasai K, Yamabe H, Haga H, et al. Non-Hodgkin's lymphoma of the thyroid. A clinical study of twenty-two cases. Acta Oncol 1996;35:457–462.
67. Spencer CA, Wang CC. Thyroglobulin measurement. Techniques, clinical benefits, and pitfalls. Endocrinol Metab Clin North Am 1995;24:841–863.
68. Grunwald F, Menzel C, Fimmers R, Zamora PO, Biersack HJ. Prognostic value of thyroglobulin after thyroidectomy beforc ablative radioiodine therapy in thyroid cancer. J Nucl Med 1996;37:1962–1964.
69. Rubello D, Girelli ME, Casara D, Piccolo M, Perin A, Busnardo B. Usefulness of the combined antithyroglobulin antibodies and thyroglobulin assay in the follow-up of patients with differentiated thyroid cancer. J Endocrinol Invest 1990;13:737–742.

70. Rubello D, Casara D, Girelli ME, Piccolo M, Busnardo B. Clinical meaning of circulating antithyroglobulin antibodies in differentiated thyroid cancer: a prospective study. J Nucl Med 1992;33:1478–1480.
71. Pachucki J, Burmeister LA. Evaluation and treatment of persistent thyroglobulinemia in patients with well-differentiated thyroid cancer. Eur J Endocrinol 1997;137:254–261.
72. Van Wyngaarden K, McDougall IR. Is serum thyroglobulin a useful marker for thyroid cancer in patients who have not had ablation of residual thyroid tissue? Thyroid 1997;7:343–346.
73. Torrens JI, Burch HB. Serum thyroglobulin measurement. Utility in clinical practice. Endocrinol Metab Clin North Am 2001;30:429–467.
74. Ringel MD, Ladenson PW, Levine MA. Molecular diagnosis of residual and recurrent thyroid cancer by amplification of thyroglobulin messenger ribonucleic acid in peripheral blood. J Clin Endocrinol Metab 1998;83:4435–4442.
75. Gagel RF, Tashjian AH Jr, Cummings T, et al. The clinical outcome of prospective screening for multiple endocrine neoplasia type 2a. An 18-year experience. N Engl J Med 1988;318:478–484.
76. Barbot N, Calmettes C, Schuffenecker I, et al. Pentagastrin stimulation test and early diagnosis of medullary thyroid carcinoma using an immunoradiometric assay of calcitonin: comparison with genetic screening in hereditary medullary thyroid carcinoma. J Clin Endocrinol Metab 1994;78:114–120.
77. Gharib H, Kao PC, Heath H III. Determination of silica-purified plasma calcitonin for the detection and management of medullary thyroid carcinoma: comparison of two provocative tests. Mayo Clin Proc 1987;62:373–378.
78. Kao PC, Gharib H. Clinical performance of an extraction calcitonin radioimmunoassay. Mayo Clin Proc 1993;68:1165–1170.
79. Wells SA Jr, Chi DD, Toshima K, et al. Predictive DNA testing and prophylactic thyroidectomy in patients at risk for multiple endocrine neoplasia type 2A. Ann Surg 1994;220:237–247.
80. Dunn JM, Farndon JR. Medullary thyroid carcinoma. Br J Surg 1993;80:6–9.
81. Calmettes C, Ponder BA, Fischer JA, Raue F. Early diagnosis of the multiple endocrine neoplasia type 2 syndrome: consensus statement. European community concerted action: medullary thyroid carcinoma. Eur J Clin Invest 1992;22:755–760.
82. Gagel RF, Jackson CE, Block MA, et al. Age-related probability of development of hereditary medullary thyroid carcinoma. J Pediatr 1982;101:941–946.
83. Gold, P., Freedman, SO. (1965) Specific carcinoembryonic antigens of the human digestive system. J Exp Med 1965;122:467–481.
84. Wells SA Jr, Haagensen DE Jr, Linehan WM, Farrell RE, Dilley WG. The detection of elevated plasma levels of carcinoembryonic antigen in patients with suspected or established medullary thyroid carcinoma. Cancer 1978;42(Suppl 3):1498–1503.
85. Juweid M, Sharkey RM, Behr T, et al. Targeting and initial radioimmunotherapy of medullary thyroid carcinoma with ^{131}I-labeled monoclonal antibodies to carcinoembryonic antigen. Cancer Res 1995;55(Suppl):5946S–5951S.
86. Juweid M, Sharkey RM, Behr T, et al. Improved detection of medullary thyroid cancer with radiolabeled antibodies to carcinoembryonic antigen. J Clin Oncol 1996;14:1209–1217.
87. Behr TM, Gratz S, Markus PM, et al. Anti-carcinoembryonic antigen antibodies versus somatostatin analogs in the detection of metastatic medullary thyroid carcinoma: are carcinoembryonic antigen and somatostatin receptor expression prognostic factors? Cancer 1997;80(Suppl):2436–2457.
88. Juweid ME, Hajjar G, Stein R, et al. Initial experience with high-dose radioimmunotherapy of metastatic medullary thyroid cancer using ^{131}I-MN-14 F(ab)2 anti-carcinoembryonic antigen MAb and AHSCR. J Nucl Med 2000;41:93–103.
89. Solbiati L, Cioffi V, Ballarati E. Ultrasonography of the neck. Radiol Clin North Am 1992;30:941–954.

90. Galloway RJ, Smallridge RC. Imaging in thyroid cancer. Endocrinol Metab Clin North Am 1996;25:93–113.
91. Cusick EL, McIntosh CA, Krukowski ZH, Matheson NA. Cystic change and neoplasia in isolated thyroid swellings. Br J Surg 1988;75:982–983.
92. Simeone JF, Daniels GH, Hall DA, et al. Sonography in the follow-up of 100 patients with thyroid carcinoma. Am J Roentgenol 1987;148:45–49.
93. Lubin E, Mechlis-Frish S, Zatz S, et al. Serum thyroglobulin and iodine-131 whole-body scan in the diagnosis and assessment of treatment for metastatic differentiated thyroid carcinoma. J Nucl Med 1994;35:257–262.
94. Ladenson PW, Braverman LE, Mazzaferri EL, et al. Comparison of administration of recombinant human thyrotropin with withdrawal of thyroid hormone for radioactive iodine scanning in patients with thyroid carcinoma. N Engl J Med 1997;337:888–896.
95. Haugen BR, Lin EC. Isotope imaging for metastatic thyroid cancer. Endocrinol Metab Clin North Am 2001;30:469–492.
96. Mitchell G, Pratt BE, Vini L, McCready VR, Harmer CL. False positive ^{131}I whole body scans in thyroid cancer. Br J Radiol 2000;73:627–635.
97. Wang W, Macapinlac H, Larson SM, et al. [^{18}F]-2-fluoro-2-deoxy-D-glucose positron emission tomography localizes residual thyroid cancer in patients with negative diagnostic ^{131}I whole body scans and elevated serum thyroglobulin levels. J Clin Endocrinol Metab 1999;84:2291–2302.
98. Chung JK, So Y, Lee JS, et al. Value of FDG PET in papillary thyroid carcinoma with negative ^{131}I whole-body scan. J Nucl Med 1999;40:986–992.
99. Mathew CG, Chin KS, Easton DF, et al. A linked genetic marker for multiple endocrine neoplasia type 2A on chromosome 10. Nature 1987;328:527–528.
100. Simpson NE, Kidd KK, Goodfellow PJ., et al. Assignment of multiple endocrine neoplasia type 2A to chromosome 10 by linkage. Nature 1987;328:528–530.
101. Mulligan LM, Kwok JB, Healey CS, et al. Germ-line mutations of the *ret* proto-oncogene in multiple endocrine neoplasia type 2A. Nature 1993;363:458–460.
102. van Heyningen V. Genetics. One gene—four syndromes. Nature 1994;367:319–320.
103. Mulligan LM, Eng C, Healey CS, et al. Specific mutations of the *ret* proto-oncogene are related to disease phenotype in MEN 2A and FMTC. Nat Genet 1994;6:70–74.
104. Tsai MS, Ledger GA, Khosla S, Gharib H, Thibodeau SN. Identification of multiple endocrine neoplasia, type 2 gene carriers using linkage analysis and analysis of the *ret* proto-oncogene. J Clin Endocrinol Metab 1994;78:1261–1264.
105. Donis-Keller H, Dou S, Chi D, et al. Mutations in the RET proto-oncogene are associated with MEN 2A and FMTC. Hum Mol Genet 1993;2:851-856.
106. Eng C. Seminars in medicine of the Beth Israel Hospital, Boston. The RET proto-oncogene in multiple endocrine neoplasia type 2 and Hirschsprung's disease. N Engl J Med 1996;335:943–951.
107. Hofstra RM, Landsvater RM, Ceccherini I, et al. A mutation in the RET proto-oncogene associated with multiple endocrine neoplasia type 2B and sporadic medullary thyroid carcinoma. Nature 1994;367:375–376.
108. Ledger GA, Khosla S, Lindor NM, Thibodeau SN, Gharib H. Genetic testing in the diagnosis and management of multiple endocrine neoplasia type II. Ann Intern Med 1995;122:118–124.

8 Diagnosis and Management of Diabetes

Allison B. Goldfine, MD

CONTENTS

INTRODUCTION

Diabetes mellitus represents a heterogeneous group of metabolic disorders characterized by decreased insulin secretion, insulin action, or both (Table 1). Diabetes affects over 16 million Americans, such that about 10% of the U. S. population above the age of 60 yr has diabetes, including a disproportionate number of nonwhites *(1)*. Type 1 diabetes is characterized by autoimmune destruction of the insulin secreting pancreatic β-cells and represents <10% of all diabetes. Type 2 diabetes is the predominant disorder and is characterized by insulin resistance and a relative reduction in insulin production. It is estimated that fully half of the population with diabetes remains undiagnosed. Diabetes mellitus is associated with significant morbidity and mortality from acute complications of hypoglycemia and chronic complications including the microvascular diseases of retinopathy and nephropathy, macrovascular manifestations of coronary artery disease, myocardial infarction, and stroke, and neuropathies. As safe and effective medical therapies are available to improve metabolic control and large-scale clinical trials have demonstrated reduced complications with treatments for both types 1 and 2 diabetes, diagnostic procedures are very important.

From: *Contemporary Endocrinology: Handbook of Diagnostic Endocrinology*
Edited by: J. E. Hall and L. K. Nieman

Table 1
Characteristics of Diabetes Mellitus

Types of diabetes	*Characteristic*
Type 1 diabetes	Previously referred to as insulin-dependent diabetes mellitus (IDDM): characterized by low or absent endogenous insulin production; and exogenous insulin dependence to prevent ketoacidosis. Onset is usually in youth or young adulthood, but can occur at any age. Patients are usually lean. Frequently initiated by autoimmune destruction of the insulin-producing pancreatic β-cells, this group can include idiopathic cases, but does not include forms of β-cell dysfunction which can otherwise be ascribed (see Secondary).
Type 2 diabetes	Previously referred to as non-insulin dependent diabetes mellitus (NIDDM): insulin-resistant condition with an impaired insulin secretory component. Onset usually older in age, and often associated with obesity. Insulin may be required for glucose control, however patients are ketosis resistant. Approximately 90% of diabetes is type 2.
Secondary	Pancreatitis (recurrent pancreatitis, cystic fibrosis, carcinoma, hemochromatosis). Pheochromocytoma, Acromegaly, Cushing's disease or syndrome, glucagonoma, somatostatinoma, thyrotoxicosis, medications (i.e., glucocorticoids, oral contraceptives, thiazides), etc.
Maturity onset diabetes of the young (MODY)	Nonketotic form of diabetes with very strong genetic determination. Several single gene defects with autosomal dominance pattern of inheritance have been identified including the glucokinase gene and several members of the hepatic nuclear factor (HNF) family proteins. Mitochondrial DNA mutations have also been demonstrated to produce diabetes, but are associated with maternal transmission.
Gestational diabetes mellitus (GDM)	Glucose intolerance with onset or first recognition during pregnancy.
Malnutrition-related diabetes mellitus	Diabetes associated with fibrocalcific pancreatitis, occurring in tropical countries. This disorder has not definitively been linked to protein malnutrition.

DIAGNOSIS OF DIABETES

The pathophysiology of both types 1 and 2 diabetes include a preclinical period of a variable duration where subtle disturbances in glucose metabolism may be detected. Although laboratory evaluations differ during the preclinical period, the definitive diagnosis of diabetes is based on demonstration of hyperglycemia. In the absence of unequivocal hyperglycemia accompanied by metabolic compromise, diagnosis should depend upon two tests with confirmatory measurement of hyperglycemia on separate days. Diagnostic testing includes the fasting plasma glucose (FPG) of 126 mg/dL (7.0 mmol/L), where fasting is defined as without caloric intake for 8 h; a random plasma glucose of 200 mg/dL (11.1 mmol/L), defined as without regard to time since last meal; or the 75-g oral glucose tolerance test (OGTT) with the 2-h plasma glucose 200 mg/dL. In patients with or without the classical symptoms of hyperglycemia, including polyuria, polydipsia, and polyphagia with unexplained weight loss, documentation of elevated glucose should be made on different days to confirm a diagnosis. Additionally, a random glucose >160 mg/dL (8.9 mmol/L) is considered suspicious for diabetes, and warrants additional testing. These glucose levels have been defined based on enzymatic assays of plasma glucose.

The diagnostic criteria for diabetes were revised to lower levels in 2000 (Table 2), by the American Diabetes Association Expert Committee on the Diagnosis and Classification of Diabetes Mellitus *(2)*, from previous criteria defined by the National Diabetes Data Group (NDDG) *(3)*. Plasma glucose concentrations follow a continuous distribution in the population, and the threshold identifying persons at substantially increased risk of specific diabetes-related complications is under continuous review. The lower glycemic cutpoints in the amended criteria are largely supported by studies specific to microvascular complications that demonstrate a higher prevalence of retinopathy above these more restricted glycemic limits *(4)*.

Screening with either the fasting or 2-h post-load plasma glucose should be considered in persons at high risk for the development of type 2 diabetes, including persons with: (*i*) a previous diagnosis of abnormal glucose levels; (*ii*) a positive family history of diabetes (such as parents or siblings); (*iii*) obesity (body mass index [BMI] = weight [kg]/height [m^2] 27, or 20% above ideal body weight [IBW]); (*iv*)history of gestational diabetes mellitus (GDM) or delivery of an infant >9 lbs; (*v*) age (>45 yr); and (*vi*) hypertension or hyperlipidemia. Individuals of Native American, African-American, or Hispanic ethnicity are at risk and should be screened. The appropriate interval for repeated screening has not been clearly defined but should be between 1–5 yr depending on the number of risk factors. In general, screening every 3 yr is reasonable, as there is little likelihood of developing complications of diabetes within this interval of a negative test. Glycated hemoglobin measurements are valuable to monitor overall glucose control, but are not yet accepted as either a screening or diagnostic test owing to a high false negative rate.

Impaired Fasting Glucose and Impaired Glucose Tolerance

Impaired fasting glucose (IFG) and impaired glucose tolerance (IGT) refer to more moderate elevations in glucose and are associated with increased risk of progression over time to overt diabetes. However, some individuals with these designations do not progress and may even revert to normal glucose tolerance.

Table 2
Revised Criteria for Diabetes Mellitus

	Fasting glucose	*Random glucose*	*2-h post 75-g load glucose*
Normal glucose tolerance	110 mg/dL	140 mg/dL	140 mg/dL
Impaired fasting glucose	110mg/dL, 126 mg/dL		
Impaired glucose tolerance			140 mg/dl, 200 mg/dL
Diabetes	126 mg/dL (nonpregnant adults)[a]	200 mg/dL	200 mg/dL

[a]Diagnosis requires confirmatory test on separate day

The rates of progression vs reversion differ in different ethnic populations and are related to the underlying prevalence of the disease. IFG is present if the fasting glucose is 110 mg/dL (6.1 mmol/L) but 126 mg/dL, and IGT is present if the 2-h post OGTT level is 140 mg/dL (7.8 mmol/L) but 200 mg/dL. Daily blood glucose and glycohemoglobin levels may be near normal in these patients, however these metabolic designations are important, as individuals with even low levels of glucose impairment are at considerable risk of cardiovascular disease *(5)* and may warrant counseling and medical therapy of classical cardiovascular risk factors.

Gestational Diabetes Mellitus

See Chapter 9 for an in-depth discussion of this subject. Insulin sensitivity and action is reduced during the physiologic changes that accompany pregnancy, particularly during the third trimester. Gestational diabetes is defined as any degree of glucose intolerance with onset or first recognition during pregnancy, and complicates approx 4% of pregnancies in the U.S., with a prevalence that varies from 1–14% depending on the population studied *(6)*. It does not exclude the possibility that glucose intolerance anteceded conception, nor is it specific for an underlying genetic, molecular, or immunologic basis for the disease.

Elevations in maternal glucose during early pregnancy are associated with congenital malformations in the fetus. During late pregnancy elevated maternal glucose is associated with neonatal macrosomia, increasing the frequency of cesarean section for delivery, and the metabolic complications of hypoglycemia, hyperbilirubinemia, hypocalcemia, and erythremia in the fetus. Thus, due to the frequency in the population and importance of detection, all pregnant women should be considered for screening. However, there are a few factors placing women at lower risk, including age <25 yr, normal body weight, without a first degree relative with diabetes, with no history of an abnormal glucose measurement or poor obstetric outcome, and not of a racial/ethnic group with a high prevalence for diabetes. Risk assessment should occur at the first prenatal visit. If a woman meets all of these criteria, screening for diabetes during pregnancy is optional. Women at high risk should undergo screening procedures as soon as feasible. If glucose tolerance is normal early in pregnancy, retesting should be performed between 24–28 wk gestation, the interval recommended for women of moderate risk. Screening involves an initial plasma or serum glucose measurement 1 h following a 50-g oral glucose load, the glucose challenge test (GCT), performed at any time of day and regardless of time since last meal. A value of 140 mg/dL (7.8 mmol/L) identifies 80% of women with GDM, and a threshold of 130 mg/dL (7.2 mmol/L) increases the sensitivity to 100%. However, this testing also identifies women who do not have abnormal glucose tolerance during the 75-g OGTT, which is required for the diagnosis of gestational diabetes. Thus, in high risk women, the GCT may be omitted for a 1-step diagnostic approach using the OGTT. Over the years, several diagnostic variations of the OGTT have been used and modified. Currently, either the 100-g or 75-g glucose load are acceptable *(2)*, although diagnostic criteria are more stringent with the 100-g load, as the glucose levels are the same despite the higher carbohydrate stimulus administered with 100 g. Both tests assess the glucose response fasting (between 8 and 14 h) and at 1 and 2 h after the glucose load. Additionally, the 100-g test includes a 3 h glucose assessment. In either test, two or more of the venous plasma concentrations must be exceeded to be positive. Normal values include a fasting plasma glucose level 95 mg/dL (5.3 mmol/L), 1-h 180 mg/dL (10.0 mmol/L), 2-h 155 mg/dL (8.6 mmol/L), and for the 100-g load 3-h 140 mg/dL (7.8 mmol/L). Although an abnormal GCT in the presence of a normal OGTT, or a single abnormal glucose value on the OGTT are not classified as gestational diabetes, this mild degree of glucose intolerance may be associated with increased risk of cesarean section or need for special neonatal care *(7–9)*.

Screening for Type 1 Diabetes

Clinically, type 1 diabetes usually presents abruptly with the symptoms of polyuria, polydipsia, polyphagia, and/or weight loss of several days to weeks duration. Hyperglycemia may be extreme and is often associated with ketoacidosis. However, there is a period of slowly progressive inflammatory destruction of the insulin-producing pancreatic islet β-cells. This preclinical period can last for a variable amount of time, over months to more than 10 yr. More than 80% of the β-cells have been destroyed by the time type 1 diabetes becomes manifest by hyperglycemia and/or ketosis. Genetic factors contribute to the development of type 1 diabetes, and both high risk and protective loci have been identified in the human leukocyte antigen (HLA) alleles. In Caucasians, the HLA DR4 DQBI *0302 alleles and DR3 DQBI *02 are associated with increased risk, and DQB1*0602, *0603, and *0301 are protective *(10)*. However, the at-risk alleles are frequent in the population, and thus, the presence of the gene is insufficient for development of disease, and identification of the presence of the gene in an unaffected individual has low specificity for prediction of disease development.

A series of auto-antigens have been identified that are predicitive for the development of type 1 disease. The first prediabetic marker identified was the cytoplasmic islet cell antibodies (ICAs), measured by indirect immuno-flourescence on sections of normal human pancreas. However, the assay is semiquantitative and difficult to standardize due to the need for subjective scoring of the sections for positivity and a wide variability with pancreatic tissue from different donors *(11)*. Radioassay for antibodies against islet auto-antigens has replaced ICA testing. The most well-characterized antibodies include insulin auto-antibody (IAA), the γ-amino butyric acid (GABA)-synthesizing enzyme glutamic acid decarboxylase (GAD), and amino acid residues of the intracellular domain on the protein IA-2 (ICA512/IA-2). There is a significant increase in the risk of development of diabetes with an increasing number of auto-antibodies present, such that the 5-yr risk for a first degree relative of a type 1 diabetic person is about 68% if two antibodies are positive, but approaches 100% if all three are elevated *(12)*. In the setting of one or two antibody positivity, a low first-phase insulin release to an intravenous glucose load would help determine risk. Wide-spread use of these tests in asymptomatic individuals is not yet recommended. The incidence of type 1 diabetes is small in the general population, so testing of healthy children would identify only a small number (<0.5%) who may be in the early stages of developing the disease, and there is no clearly effective treatment to halt the progression to overt diabetes *(13)*. Clinical studies of high-risk persons with a first degree relative for type 1 diabetes to find effective preventive treatments are ongoing. These studies may justify such screening in the future. In clinical practice, antibody testing may be useful to distinguish between early autoimmune type 1 or type 2 diabetes.

MONITERING GLYCEMIA IN THE PATIENT WITH DIABETES

For years, the role of hyperglycemia in the development of complications of diabetes remained controversial. Results of two recent large-scale clinical trials in patients with both types 1 and 2 diabetes, the Diabetes Control and Complication Trial (DCCT) and United Kingdom Prospective Diabetes Study (UKPDS), respectively, have clearly demonstrated the importance of glycemic control to reduce the risk of development or slow progression of microvascular complications of diabetes. In the DCCT, intensive insulin therapy with the goal of near-normalization of blood glucose levels could delay the onset or slow the progression of clinically important retinopathy, nephropathy, and neuropathy by 35–70% *(14)*. Any improvement in glycemia that was achieved was associated with a decreased risk of complications, and no glycemic target could be demonstrated below which there was no additional benefit to the patient. However, this intensive insulin treatment was associated with an approximate three-fold

Table 3
Safe Glycemic Goals

Glycemic goals by co-morbid risk	*Fasting*	*1-h Postprandial*	*2-h Postprandial*	*Premeal*
Pregnancy and/or low risk	<95 mg/dL	<120–140 mg/dL	<120 mg/dL	80–100 mg/dL
Moderate risk	<120 mg/dL	<160 mg/dL	<140 mg/dL	100–120 mg/dL
High risk	<150 mg/dL	<200 mg/dL	<180 mg/dL	<150 mg/dL

increase in the risk of significant hypoglycemia, defined as hypoglycemia in which assistance was required for treatment and included coma and seizures *(15)*. Similarly, in the UKPDS the intensive control cohort demonstrated a 10–12% lower risk for combined diabetes-related endpoints or diabetes-related death *(16)*. Most risk reduction, however, was found in microvascular endpoints. Thus, a clear rationale exists for the intensive treatment of patients with diabetes, with the goal of normalization or near-normalization of blood glucose levels. To determine safe glycemic ranges for individual patients, physicians must consider their age, coexisting medical problems, degree of hypoglycemia awareness, and ability to follow a labor-intensive treatment program (Table 3).

Home Blood Glucose Monitoring

To achieve near-normalization of blood glucose levels, each patient may require a different regimen, including multiple daily injections of insulin, subcutaneous insulin pumps, oral hypoglycemic or insulin sensitizing agents, exercise, and/or diet. The more information available about a patient's glucose profile and the impact of exercise and meal content on this profile, the better one can tailor the medical therapy. Several companies market small meter devices that accurately measure blood glucose levels and can be carried in a purse or wallet-sized case. A blood sample between 2–20 μL in volume is obtained from a fingertip puncture and placed on a reagent strip. Older devices required timing and wiping procedures to obtain accurate glucose values. Newer devices, however, employ electrochemical reactions instead of colorimetric reactions and have simplified the process with less user error and more accurate results. Essentially, all the available meters are reliable, with little variability in accuracy and precision when used appropriately. However, patient education in correct use is important, and technique should be checked occasionally. Common causes of erroneous values include insufficient blood on the test strip, touching the sample application area, improper capping of vials (allowing exposure of the reagent strip to moisture), inadequate cleaning of the optical window, and poor operating environmental conditions (such as extremes of light, altitude, humidity, or temperature). Biological variables that could affect accuracy (abnormal hematocrit or triglycerides) and limits of accurate operation differ among units. Machine calibration can be evaluated both with the use of control solutions and by running a sample on the meter and simultaneously sending a sample to the laboratory for comparison. However, capillary whole blood glucose values may be 12% lower than those of venous plasma. Some meters are calibrated to whole blood and others to plasma. In addition, meters requiring smaller (2–5 μL) volume blood samples tend to read lower than meters requiring higher volumes.

Home blood glucose monitoring should be considered mandatory for pregnant patients with diabetes, as well as for all patients who are attempting to achieve near-normalization of blood glucose levels. Target glucose goals must be tailored to the individual. Advanced age, co-morbid medical conditions of cerebral or advanced cardiovascular disease, autonomic neuropathy especially gastroparesis, and inability to sense hypoglycemia are common reasons to raise glucose targets. Glucose targets may change over time, such as during hospitalization when it may be appropriate to raise goals temporarily. The ideal frequency to recommend home glucose monitoring is controversial. For the type 2 patient with near normal glycohemoglobin, sporadic monitoring may be sufficient. However, there is tremendous and immediate feedback to a patient who checks their glucose following a carbohydrate-rich meal or a bout of exercise, helping to direct healthy behaviors. For most patients, monitoring is recommended at preprandially, when there is greatest risk of hypoglycemia, and at a time more easily remembered. However, postprandial monitoring provides valuable information about the extent of glucose excursion and is extremely useful for verifying that the insulin dose administered is correct for the patient trying to perform carbohydrate counting or adjust doses for exercise. Furthermore, postprandial evaluations are recommended during pregnancy. Thus, as in the DCCT, many type 1 individuals striving for near normal glycemia are likely to monitor their glucose about 7× daily, both before and after meals, and occasionally during the night hours. Frequent monitoring has been demonstrated to lower both mean blood glucose and glycohemoglobin levels *(17)*. If patients are not able or willing to perform multiple daily measurements, less frequent home blood glucose determinations can be useful to assess the therapeutic regimen, especially if glucose is sampled at different times of the day on a regular basis throughout the week or month. For either the patient or physician to recognize trends in blood sugars, glucose levels must be charted in an organized manner including information on the time of day, the blood glucose value, the relationship of the measurement to meals, the insulin dose administered, and any unusual physical activity or symptoms. Some meters possess an internal memory, and much of this information can be downloaded into a personal computer. Multiple daily testing does not improve glucose control if the insulin dose remains fixed. In general, for the type 1 patient, dosing of the appropriate insulin should be decreased for the next day after a single unexplained low sugar, and increased after 3–4 d with a pattern of elevated values at a given time of day. Finally, home monitoring is helpful for confirming the clinical diagnosis of hypoglycemia in patients who have equivocal symptoms or hypoglycemic unawareness.

Continuous Blood Glucose Monitoring

The first device to continuously assess glucose has been approved by the Food and Drug Administration (FDA). A small catheter is placed under the skin, and glucose in the interstitial space is assessed at min intervals. Several samples are averaged, and a reading is acquired at 5-min intervals. The catheter generally functions over a 2- to 3-d interval of time prior to requiring replacement. The device does not currently replace home glucose monitoring, as calibration must occur several times daily. Currently, the glucose level is not readily accessible to the patient, but must be downloaded into a computer, at which time the glycemic profiles can be reviewed with the physician for precise medical management. These devices frequently demonstrate previously unrecognized postprandial glucose elevations and severe nocturnal hypoglycemic events, even in patients considered to have optimal management prior to placement of the device *(18)*. Several products are under development, using both minimally invasive and noninvasive measurements, and are likely to be available in the near future. These should have the capacity to demonstrate the direction of movement of glucose to a patient and to have alarms for both hyper- and hypoglycemia. These devices may prove to be lifesaving for the patient with hypoglycemia unawareness. The full range of applications and precautions in use of the extensive glycemic data available and specific limitations of each device will need to be determined.

Urine Glucose Monitoring

Glucose does not pass into the urine until the renal threshold for glucose has been exceeded. Physiologic conditions, such as aging and pregnancy, can raise and lower this threshold, respectively. In most persons, this level is around 180–200 mg/dL . Thus, a negative urine glucose suggests the plasma level has not exceeded this threshold since the time of the last void. The concentration of glucose in the urine if positive, would be a function of both the elevation in plasma glucose and the volume of urine produced. In the setting of home blood glucose meters, this testing has become obsolete, except in the rare patient who is unable to perform the lancing procedure to obtain blood.

Urine Ketone Monitoring

Urine ketones should be measured in patients with type 1 diabetes who have hyperglycemia with glucose levels higher than 250 mg/dL . This test allows physicians and patients to recognize and respond to the development of early diabetic ketoacidosis. It reveals the degree of insulin deficiency, which helps physicians determine how much insulin should be delivered as an additional "booster" to treat hyperglycemia. Booster shots generally consist of 5–25% of a patient's total daily insulin dose, given in the form of regular or short-acting insulin. It is especially important to test for ketones in the setting of hyperglycemia prior to exercise. During exercise, the increased demand for glucose and insulin deficiency can accelerate the metabolic decompensation.

Urine ketone detection systems generally detect the ketone bodies acetoacetic acid and acetone, but not β-hydroxybutyric acid. Freshly voided urine contains about 10× more acetoacetic acid than acetone. Over time, however, acetoacetic acid spontaneously degrades, leaving a greater proportion of acetone. Ketones may be absent from the urine in individuals with uremia. Similarly, urine and serum ketone levels can be falsely low if the ketoacid equilibrium is shifted toward the reduced state (predominantly β-hydroxybutyrate). This occurs when the redox potential of the patient is high, as in severe acidosis. After the initiation of therapy for diabetic ketoacidosis, an apparent worsening of ketone levels can be observed as the redox potential of the patient shifts, due to the clearing of β-hydroxybutyrate through conversion to acetoacetate and acetone, which are measured by the standard assays. Like urine glucose levels, urine ketone levels represent the metabolic status of the patient since the time of the last void. Circulating plasma ketones are cleared through the kidneys and within a short time after serum levels have cleared, urine ketones will become negative, making this a rapid and inexpensive way to monitor the resolution of diabetic ketoacidosis at the bedside.

Other causes of ketoaciduria include alcoholic ketoacidosis, starvation (which is accelerated in late pregnancy and lactation), severely hypocaloric diets, and fasting ketosis. In alcoholic ketoacidosis, there is an underlying nutritional deficiency and an exaggerated response to fasting. Unlike diabetic ketoacidosis, this condition often resolves with the administration of glucose alone and can be differentiated on the basis of history and, sometimes, positive blood alcohol levels. In starvation and pregnancy, hyperglycemia and glycosuria are usually absent. In fasting, urine ketones are rarely above trace levels and total serum ketones rarely exceed 4–6 mmol/L *(19)*.

PROTEIN GLYCATION

Glycohemoglobin

Measurements of glycated hemoglobin (Hb) are of major clinical value for objective monitoring of glucose control in patients with diabetes and have been correlated with long-term complications of diabetes and with fetal outcome in pregnant patients with diabetes. Unfortunately, glycated Hb measurements cannot discriminate IGT or mild diabetes from normal glucose tolerance and are inadequate as a screening test in either the general population or in the diagnosis of gestational diabetes because of the high rate of false negative results. Glycated Hb measurements only provide an estimate of the average blood glucose level over the preceding 6–8 wk and indicate nothing about the variability of the glucose level (i.e., the patients brittleness) during that period. In addition to validating home glucose monitoring accuracy, these levels frequently motivate patients to care for themselves.

Adult Hb consists of about 97% HbAo ($\alpha_2\beta_2$), 2.5% HbA_2 ($\alpha_2\gamma_2$), and 0.5% HbF ($\alpha_2\delta_2$). There also are several minor species: HbA_{1a}, HbA_{1b}, and HbA_{1c}, which are collectively known as glycated Hb. Glycohemoglobin is formed continuously in erythrocytes as the product of a nonenzymatic reaction between Hb and glucose, first forming the labile Schiff base, or pre-A_{1c}, then the more stable Amadori product. HbA_{1c} specifically refers to the Amadori product of the N-terminal valine of each β-chain of HbA with glucose. HbA_{1a} and HbA_{1b} have the carbohydrate moiety attached to other amino acids. HbA_{1c} makes up about 80% of the glycated HbA1 and is the fraction that best reflects average blood glucose concentrations. Other carbohydrate moieties, such as fructose-1,6-diphosphate and glucose-6-phosphate, can react with the Hb molecules to form other glycated Hbs, such as HbA_{1a1} and HbA_{1a2}, respectively. Glycohemoglobin measurements can serve as a reliable index of average blood glucose concentrations over the preceding 6–8 wk, because of the long half-life of red blood cells.

There are two principle methods to measure glycohemoglobin based on the manner in which the glycated and nonglycated Hbs are separated. One relies on charge separation, such as ion-exchange chromatography, electrophoresis, and high-performance liquid chromatography, and the other relies on structural characteristics of the glycation group on the Hb, such as affinity chromatography or immunoassay *(20)*. Glycated Hb results are both method- and laboratory-specific. HbA_1 results tend to be higher than HbA_{1c} results as a greater amount of glucose is measured. The numerous techniques used in different laboratories make it difficult to compare an individual patient's results between laboratories. Additionally, techniques are associated with different causes of false elevation and suppression. Some conditions that cause error include Hb structural variants, like HbS, HbC, or HbE; Hb synthesis variants, such as β-thalassemia; and/or posttranslational modifications of Hb, such as the Schiff base, carbamylated Hb, or acetylated Hb *(21)*. Any condition that leads to increased red blood cell turnover and shortened exposure to glucose will lead to decreased glycosylated Hb levels by all assay methods. Occult bleeding and blood transfusion are the most common causes of falsely low measurements. Likewise, processes that lengthen red blood cell survival, such as iron deficiency anemias, increase glycohemoglobin measurements in all assays. Carbamylated Hb, which increases with renal failure, is least affected by chromatography or immunoassay techniques. The presence of HbS, which would reduce the relative amount of HbA and, therefore, decrease the measured HbA_{1c} by all methods except affinity chromatography, is another common cause of false suppression. The persistence of HbF, which co-elutes with HbA_{1c} in methods based on charge separation would result in a false elevation.

Fructosamine

When metabolic control is changing rapidly, such as with the initiation of new therapy for hyperglycemia, during a superimposed illness, during the planning period for a pregnancy, or at the time of conception, an index of glycemia reflective of a shorter interval of time is desirable. Serum proteins other than Hb, such as albumin, become glycated in the presence of glucose and can be used as alternatives to HbA_{1c}. Albumin has a half-life of 2 to 3 wk, reflecting glycemic control over this shorter interval. As with glycohemoglobins, several assays are currently available and each has different limitations. Changes in albumin concentration, such as those that occur with alterations in nutritional status, or with liver and kidney disease, can affect fructosamine measurements in all assays. First generation assays used nitroblue tetrazolium colorimetric methods to measure glycated serum proteins, particularly albumin, and became known as fructosamines. These methods are limited by the nonspecific nature of the reaction, such that uric acid, bilirubin, and lipids all cause interference, and assay standardization, when compared to the synthetic deoxymorpholinofructose standard, was not reliable in early versions of this test *(22)*. Second generation assays incorporate uricase to eliminate the interference with uric acid and use nonionic surfactants to eliminate the protein-matrix effects and the interference from lipemia. These assays are standardized against more physiologic glycated polylysine standards *(23)*. Further improvements in assay technique are being developed and should lead to more widespread use of these measurements. Fructosamine levels can now be determined by the patient on a portable meter device, but provide less information than multiple glucose determinations.

Although both fructosamine and glycohemoglobin levels correlate well with outpatient measurements of capillary blood glucose concentrations, there is no absolute correlation between fructosamine and glycohemoglobin, as each value depends on the half-lives of the major proteins measured and the average glycemia for the different intervals preceding the blood collection.

DIAGNOSIS AND MONITORING OF DIABETES RELATED COMPLICATIONS

Retinopathy

Diabetes is the leading cause of blindness and visual disability in the U.S. Progressive changes in the retina have been classified as mild preproliferative diabetic retinopathy (PPDR), with microaneurysms only or occasional blotch hemorrhage or hard exudates; transitional diabetic retinopathy (TDR), with more significant blotch hemorrhages or intraretinal microvascular abnormalities (IRMA), soft exudates, or venous abnormalities; moderate to severe PPDR with three or more transitional lesions present in multiple fields, and proliferative diabetic retinopathy (PDR), characterized by new blood vessels (NBV) on the optic disc, or elsewhere (NVE), fibrous proliferation, and preretinal or vitreous hemorrhage. Fundoscopic photograph standards have been developed and are widely used in staging retinopathy *(24)*. Characteristics of proliferative disease carry a 25% risk of severe visual loss within 2 years *(25)*, which can be prevented by panretinal photocoagulation *(26)*. In type 1 diabetes, PPDR typically develops after 5 yr of disease onset, and is present in virtually all patients by 20 yr. In contrast, 20% of patients with type 2 disease have some form of retinopathy present at the time of diagnosis, likely due to the high frequency of prolonged elevations in glucose prior to clinical diagnosis. Annual dilated fundoscopic examination beginning at 5 yr for the type 1 patient, and at the time of diagnosis for the type 2 patient, remains the recommended procedure to diagnose this microvascular complication. Cataracts and glaucoma are also more frequent in patients with diabetes and should be screened for at the time of opthalmological evaluation. Medical control of glycemia and hypertension are critical to both prevention and management of retinopathy *(27)*. With the development of preproliferative vascular changes, the frequency of inspection should be increased. During rapid improvement in metabolic status, during pregnancy, and with nephropathy, the vessels in the retina are at particular risk, and therefore, more frequent dilated inspection is warranted. The use of fundoscopic photographs as screening procedures is currently under evaluation.

Nephropathy

Diabetes mellitus can affect the structure and function of the kidney in multiple ways, including diffuse or nodular glomerulosclerosis, arterionephorsclerosis, chronic interstitial nephritis, a variety of tubular disorders, and/or papillary necrosis. The term diabetic nephropathy covers all lesions, but primarily refers to the most common diffuse intercapillary glomerular lesion and nodular glomerulosclerosis (Kimmelstiel-Wilson lesion). The earliest measurable defect in diabetes-related renal function is a rise in the glomerular filtration rate (GFR), most readily assessed by a 24-h urine for creatinine clearance. The elevated GFR may become associated with leakage of small amounts of the protein albumin through the basement membrane into the urine. As the filtration rate decreases back to normal, larger amounts of protein may pass into the urine. Plasma renin may be normal or low, and acquired hyporeninemic hypoaldosteronism with hyperkalemia and a mild hyperchloremic metabolic acidosis is common. Typically, end stage renal disease develops within 5–10 yr of the development of overt proteinuria *(28)*. Diabetes accounts nationwide for approx 50% of end stage renal disease and remains the leading cause of dialysis or renal transplant in the U.S. Interestingly, despite poor glycemic control, only one-third to one-half of diabetic patients develop nephropathy, and genetic factors appear to play a permissive or protective role. Parental hypertension or a first-degree family member affected with diabetic nephropathy are the clearest risk factors for this complication.

Urine protein can be measured by dipstick analysis; however this measurement is not specific for albumin excretion, which is present with the glomerular disease. Furthermore, dipstick analysis will not be positive until the urine protein levels are above 250–300 mg protein daily, and if other causes of proteinuria have been excluded, would signify significant diabetic renal disease. Normal albumin excretion ranges from 3–25 mg daily. Proteinuria is considered to exist if the urine excretion is greater than 300 mg/d. The range between normal excretion and that detected by the traditional dipstick method, i.e., 30 and 300 mg daily, is considered to be in the microalbuminuric range. Microalbumin measurements, performed by radioimmunoassay, can now detect much lower levels of albumin, at rates 5 µg/min *(29)*. Microalbuminuria has been shown to predict individuals at high risk of progression to advanced diabetic renal disease *(30,31)*, and elevated levels are now considered to represent an early stage of this complication. Microalbumin should be measured annually on a spot urine sample and is best expressed as a ratio to the urine creatinine. The test is considered abnormal when the urine microalbumin is 20 µg/mg of creatinine. Poor metabolic control and hypertension can both cause small increases in urine microalbumin and may reverse with treatment. It is less clear if these transient changes identify patients at risk of progression. Furthermore, the test must be interpreted cautiously, as there are many other causes of increased microalbumin excretion, including exercise, which may impose a circadian variation to microalbumin excretion *(32)*, urinary tract infection, and a series of drugs/toxic exposures associated with glomerular lesions. The more common drug/toxic exposures include nonsteroidal anti-inflamatory drugs, rifampin, heroin, sulfonamides, allopurinol, and mercury or gold exposure. Evaluation for nondiabetic causes of increased urine protein excretion must be guided by the clinical scenario (Table 4).

Improvements in glycemia reduce the development and/or progression of the renal complications of diabetes (DCCT) and all efforts should be made to optimize glycemia. Hypertension contributes to the progression of nephropathy and likewise demands aggressive medical management. There is some suggestion that angiotensin-converting enzyme (ACE) inhibitors and receptor blockers are superior to other antihypertensive agents, but use may be limited in the patient who has significant hyperkalemia. Patients with microalbuminuria and renal disease are at high risk of cardiovascular events *(33,34)* and should have aggressive management of lipids and additional expectant cardiac management.

Table 4
Candidate Laboratory Evaluation for Occult Causes of Microalbuminuria

Daytime and overnight urine microalbumin.
Urine culture.
Thyroid-stimulating hormone (TSH).
Urea nitrogen and creatinine (Bun/Cr).
Liver function tests (LFT'S).
Hepatitis profiles.
Urine or serum protein electrophoresis.
Complete blood count (CBC) with differential.
Erythrocyte sedimentation rate (ESR).
Rheumatoid factor (RF), antinuclear antibodies (ANA).
Toxic screen.
Renal ultrasound.
Renal flow image.

Neuropathy

The prevalence of neuropathy approaches 50% by 25 yr of diabetes *(35)*. The pathophysiology of neuropathy remains unclear. Possible mechanisms include a decrease in myoinositol. Myoinositol is a cyclic alcohol component of phosphoinositides, which is important to cell membrane structure; is part of the cell signaling mechanism through protein kinase C; and is invloved in the regulation of intracellular calcium. Other mechanisms of neuropathy include an increase in the polyol pathway, whereby excess glucose is enzymatically converted to sorbitol and fructose; a decrease in anaerobic glycolysis; glycoslyation of nerve proteins; abnormal fatty acid metabolism; and/or microvascular damage to nerves. Reduction of hyperglycemia lowers the frequency of this complication *(14)*.

The most classic pattern of nerve involvement is a distal symmetrical polyneuropathy that may involve sensory or motor fibers alone or in combination. Other causes of distal symmetric polyneuropathy must be considered, including the metabolic disturbances of hypothyroidism, uremia, folic acid deficiency, and the porphyrias; toxins or drugs, such as alcohol, lead, mercury, and cisplatinum; infiltrative/inflammatory disorders of amyloidosis, sarcoidosis, and polyarteritis nodosa; leukemias, lymphomas, and paraproteinemias; and connective tissue diseases, such as systemic lupus erythematosus. A reasonable laboratory screening evaluation for other etiologies of distal symmetric polyneuropathy must be guided by the patients history and physical examination, but could include studies listed in Table 5. Light touch and vibratory sensation are often diminished before reflexes become abnormal. Electrodiagnostic tests of nerve conduction velocity can be made to the sensory fibers of the ulnar, median, or peroneal nerves, or motor fibers of the ulnar, median, plantar, or sural nerves. Measure-

Table 5
Candidate Laboratory Evaluation for Occult Causes of Distal Symmetrical Polyneuropathy

Thyroid stimulating hormone (TSH).
Urea nitrogen and creatinine (Bun/Cr).
Complete blood count (CBC) with differential.
Urine or serum protein electrophoresis.
Folic acid.
Erythrocyte sedimentation rate (ESR).

ments are made of the relevant muscle or nerve action potential amplitude or latency at each site of stimulation, and a calculation of segmental conduction velocity is made. Additional nerves may need to be evaluated based on the distribution of clinical symptoms or signs. A series of monofilaments can be used to exert a range of light touch stimuli to the extremity to test sensation. Normal nerve function is documented by the ability to perceive a 3.6-g stimuli. In the patient with intact sensation, screening should occur annually. Loss of sensation of the 9-g filament is consistent with early sensory loss, although the ability to perceive a foot injury remains intact. Examination of the foot should be performed at more frequent intervals at this stage. When sensation of a 10-g stimulus is absent, the patient may no longer sense foot injury. Neuropathic foot ulcerations occur with greatest frequency in this group of patients. The patient should be instructed not to walk barefoot or wear open shoes, to wear socks, and to inspect their feet daily with the assistance of a family member if necessary *(36)*. Nail care should be provided by a podiatrist. Tetanus immunization should be up to date. Athlete's foot and excessive dry skin should be treated.

Focal and multifocal neuropathies can be seen involving cranial nerves. Other nerve syndromes may include mononeuropathy (including the common nerve entrapment seen with Carpal Tunnel Syndrome) or mononeuropathy multiplex, radiculopathy, or plexopathy. Again other underlying neuropathies must be considered in the differential diagnosis, as treatments would differ considerably.

Autonomic nerve dysfunction can be present and may have a variety of manifestations. Cardiovascular autonomic dysfunction may be manifest as orthostatic hypotension secondary to the impairment of the sympathetic-mediated increase in peripheral vascular resistance associated with standing. Exercise intolerance may be present from a decreased ability to augment cardiac output with impaired peripheral vasoconstriction. Cardiac denervation is present with advanced autonomic disease and is characterized by a fixed pulse of 80–90 beats/min, unresponsive to exercise or sleep. Tests of heart rate response to valsalva, deep breathing or change of position, and sweating response to temperature or chemical stimuli, such as acetylcholine or pilocarpine, have been used to identify earlier stages of autonomic neuropathy. Devices to measure the spectral analysis of heart rate variability (HRV) are under investigation. Reduced variability appears to precede the clinical expression of autonomic neuropathies and to carry a negative prognosis *(37)*. However, testing is not performed on a regular basis as there have been no studies to demonstrate that early treatment improves outcomes *(38)*. Abdominal bloating, early satiety, or nausea are associated with diabetic gastropathy. Delayed gastric emptying may underlie labile blood sugars. Diabetic diarrhea may be present with intestinal hypermotility from decreased sympathetic inhibition. Diagnosis may be confirmed with radionucleotide imaging studies, but is frequently made on clinical grounds. Autonomic neuropathy may involve the bladder and be manifest as impaired emptying, frequent infections, or incontinence. Sexual dysfunction, impotence, or retrograde ejaculation, is common in males. Questioning may identify persons who would have both improvements in quality of life with therapy and in whom evaluation of cardiac function and risk management is especially important.

Cardiovascular Disease

Cardiovascular events are the leading cause of mortality in patients with diabetes *(39)*. Diabetes, itself, is a classical risk factor for heart disease. Haffner et al. *(40)* recently demonstrated the full importance of this condition in a study showing the probability of death from coronary heart disease in the diabetic patient with no previous myocardial infarction (MI) is equal to that of a nondiabetic person who has sustained a previous MI. This data is supported by the findings in other large-scale clinical trials *(41)*. Thus, diabetes alone may warrant adherence to the American College of Cardiology guidelines for exercise tolerance testing of patients with known coronary artery disease *(42)*. Patients with diabetes frequently have hypertension and abnormal lipid profiles, which impart additional risk (see chapter 11). Thus, screening for and aggressive management of these co-morbid conditions is essential. Nontraditional risk factors for cardiac events include the presence of microalbuminuria and autonomic neuropathy, and warrant smoking cessation and aggressive control of glycemia, blood pressure, and lipids, with a goal to lower low density lipoprotein (LDL) cholesterol to 100 mg/dL (2.60 mmol/L). Patients with diabetes are more likely to have a significant cardiovascular event in the absence of classical anginal symptoms, thus requiring heightened consideration of screening by the physician. Therefore, graded exercise tolerance testing as a screening procedure should be considered in all patients, especially if over 35 yr; with a duration of type 2 diabetes longer than 10 yr or type 1 diabetes greater than 15 yr, with any additional cardiac risk factor, with evidence of microvascular disease (retinopathy or nephropathy, including microalbuminuria), with other peripheral vascular disease, autonomic neuropathy, and/or in patients interested in initiating a high-impact exercise program to manage weight or glycemia. Information on both maximum exercise capacity, which is in part influenced by left ventricular function at rest and in response to exercise, and exercise-induced ischemia are useful to further stratify cardiovascular risk. Patients with abnormal tests must be considered for increased medical management or imaging procedures for potential revascularization procedures. Guidelines for the frequency of testing remain controversial in the patient for whom preliminary testing is negative. There is mounting evidence that ACE inhibitors or receptor blockers may be cardioprotective even in the absence of hypertension *(43)* and are increasingly being considered with low-dose aspirin *(42)* for prophylactic treatment.

The endothelium plays a pivotal role in vascular function by synthesizing and releasing endothelial-derived relaxing factor (EDRF), which has been demonstrated to be nitric oxide. Nitric oxide has been shown to possess a variety of anti-atherogenic properties, including inhibition of leukocyte adhesion, platelet aggregation, and vascular smooth muscle proliferation. Vascular smooth muscle can also vasodilate from endothelium-independent stimuli such as adenosine, verapamil, or to nitric oxide donors (i.e., nitroprusside). Endothelium-dependent relaxation has been shown to be impaired in patients with types 1 *(44–46)* and 2 diabetes mellitus *(47,48)*. In the majority of these studies, the response to exogenous nitric oxide donors (i.e., endothelial-independent vasodilitation) is not reduced, indicating that the defects in vasodilation are not fixed. Endothelium-dependent vasodilation has been demonstrated to be abnormal in association with other cardiac risk factors, including hypertension, hypercholesterolemia, and smoking. There is a strong correlation between vasodilation in the coronary and brachial arteries *(49,50)*, indicating that endothelial dysfunction is a generalized process that is not confined to the vessels that develop overt clinical atherosclerosis and that noninvasive assessment of vasomotor function is predictive of the response in the coronary circulation. Although assessments of endothelial function are widely used in research studies, they have not been demonstrated to be of clinical use either as screening procedures or to assess response to therapy.

REFERENCES

1. Diabetes in America/National Diabetes Data Group. Bethesda, MD, National Institutes of Health, National Institute of Diabetes and Digestive and Kidney Diseases, 1995.
2. ADA Expert Committee on the Diagnosis and Classification of Diabetes Mellitus. Clinical practice recommendations 2000. Diabetes Care 23 Sup 1:S4-19.
3. World Health Organization. Diabetes mellitus: report of a WHO study group. World Health Organization. Tech. Rep. Ser. 77. 1985. Geneva.
4. McCance DR, Hanson RL, Charles MA, et al. Comparison of testes for glycated haemoglobin and fasting and two hour plasma glucose concentration as diagnositc as diagnostics. BMJ 1994;308:1323–1328.
5. Fuller JH, Shipley MJ, Rose G, Jarrett RJ, Keen H. Coronary-heart-disease risk and impaired glucose tolerance. The Whitehall study. Lancet 1980;1:1373–1376.

6. Engelgau MM, Herman WH, Smith PJ, German RR, Aubert RE. The epidemiology of diabetes and pregnancy in the U.S. Diabetes Care 1995;18:1029–1033.
7. Berkus MD, Langer O. Glucose tolerance test: degree of glucose abnormality correlates with neonatal outcome. Obstet Gynecol 1993;81:344–348.
8. Sermer M, Naylor CD, Farine D, et al. The Toronto Tri-Hospital Gestational Diabetes Project. A preliminary review. Diabetes Care 1998;21 (Suppl 2):B33–B42.
9. Moses RG, Calvert D. Pregnancy outcomes in women without gestational diabetes mellitus related to the maternal glucose level. Is there a continuum of risk? Diabetes Care 1995;18:1527–1533.
10. Ilonen J, Reijonen H, Herva E, et al. Rapid HLA-DQB1 genotyping for four alleles in the assessment of risk for IDDM in the Finnish population. The Childhood Diabetes in Finland (DiMe) Study Group. Diabetes Care 1996;19:795–800.
11. Landin-Olsson M: Precision of the islet-cell antibody assay depends on the pancreas. J.Clin.Lab Anal. 4:289-294, 1990
12. Verge CF, Gianani R, Kawasaki E, et al. Prediction of Type I diabetes in first-degree relatives using a combination of insulin, GAD, and ICA512bdc/IA-2 autoantibodies. Diabetes 1996;45:926–933.
13. Bingley PJ, Bonifacio E, Williams AJ, Genovese S, Bottazzo GF, Gale EA. Prediction of IDDM in the general population: strategies based on combinations of autoantibody markers. Diabetes 1997;46:1701–1710.
14. DCCT Research Group. The effect of intensive treatment of diabetes on the development and progression of long-term complications in insulin-dependent diabetes mellitus. N Engl J Med 1993;329:977–986.
15. DCCT Research Group. Epidemiology of severe hypoglycemia in the diabetes control and complications trial. Am J Med 1991;90:450–459.
16. UK Prospective Diabetes Study (UKPDS) Group. Intensive blood-glucose control with sulphonylureas or insulin compared with conventional treatment and risk of complications in patients with type 2 diabetes (UKPDS 33). Lancet 1998;352:837–853.
17. Schiffrin A, Belmonte M. Multiple daily self-glucose monitoring: its essential role in long-term glucose control in insulin-dependent diabetic patients treated with pump and multiple subcutaneous injections. Diabetes Care 1982;5:479–484.
18. Wilson GS, Aussedat B, Reach G, Klein JC, Ward WK. Minimally-invasive real time glucose measurements [abstract]. *Endocrine Society 82nd Annual Meeting June, Toronto, Canada55,* 2000.
19. Cahill GF Jr, Herrera MG, Morgan AP, et al. Hormone-fuel interrelationships during fasting. J Clin Invest 1966;45:1751–1769.
20. Little RR, Wiedmeyer HM, England JD, Naito HK, Goldstein DE. Interlaboratory comparison of glycohemoglobin results: College of American Pathologists Survey data. Clin Chem 1991;37:1725–1729.
21. Weykamp CW, Penders TJ, Muskiet FA, van der Slik SW. Influence of hemoglobin variants and derivatives on glycohemoglobin determinations, as investigated by 102 laboratories using 16 methods. Clin Chem 1993;39:1717–1723.
22. Vogt BW: Development of an improved fructosamine test. In Workshop Report, Fructosamine. Boehringer Mannheim GmbH, Mannheim, Germany, 1989, p. 21
23. Cefalu WT, Bell-Farrow AD, Petty M, Izlar C, Smith JA. Clinical validation of a second-generation fructosamine assay. Clin Chem 1991;37:1252–1256.
24. Klein R, Klein BE, Moss SE, Davis MD, DeMets DL. The Wisconsin epidemiologic study of diabetic retinopathy. II. Prevalence and risk of diabetic retinopathy when age at diagnosis is less than 30 years. Arch Ophthalmol 1984;102:520–526.
25. The Diabetic Retinopathy Study Research Group. Four risk factors for severe visual loss in diabetic retinopathy. The third report from the Diabetic Retinopathy Study. Arch Ophthalmol 1979;97:654–655.

26. The Diabetic Retinopathy Study Research Group. Preliminary report on effects of photocoagulation therapy. Am J Ophthalmol 1976;81:383–396.
27. Dahl-Jorgensen K, Brinchmann-Hansen O, Hanssen KF, et al. Effect of near normoglycaemia for two years on progression of early diabetic retinopathy, nephropathy, and neuropathy: The Oslo study. Br Med J 1986;293:1195–1199.
28. Castellino P, Tuttle KR, DeFronzo RA. Diabetic neuropathy. Curr Ther Endocrinol Metab 1994;5:426–436.
29. Giampietro O, Miccoli R, Clerico A, et al. Urinary albumin excretion in normal subjects and in diabetic patients measured by a radioimmunoassay: methodological and clinical aspects. Clin Biochem 1988;21:63–68.
30. Parving HH, Oxenboll B, Svendsen PA, Christiansen JS, Andersen AR. Early detection of patients at risk of developing diabetic nephropathy. A longitudinal study of urinary albumin excretion. Acta Endocrinol (Copenh) 1982;100:550–555.
31. Mogensen CE. Microalbuminuria predicts clinical proteinuria and early mortality in maturity-onset diabetes. N Engl J Med. 1984;310:356–360.
32. Hishiki S, Tochikubo O, Miyajima E, Ishii M. Circadian variation of urinary microalbumin excretion and ambulatory blood pressure in patients with essential hypertension. J Hypertens 1998;16:2101–2108.
33. Mogensen CE, Christensen CK: Predicting diabetic nephropathy in insulin-dependent patients. N Engl J Med 1984;311:89–93.
34. Schmitz A, Vaeth M: Microalbuminuria: a major risk factor in non-insulin-dependent diabetes. A 10-year follow-up study of 503 patients. Diabet Med 1988;5:126–134.
35. Pirart J, Lauvaux JP, Rey W. Blood sugar and diabetic complications. N Engl J Med 1978;298:1149.
36. Mayfield JA, Reiber GE, Sanders LJ, Janisse D, Pogach LM: Preventive foot care in people with diabetes. Diabetes Care 1998;21:2161–2177.
37. Pagani M, Malfatto G, Pierini S, et al. Spectral analysis of heart rate variability in the assessment of autonomic diabetic neuropathy. J Auton Nerv Syst 1988;23:143–153.
38. Report and recommendations of the San Antonio conference on diabetic neuropathy. Consensus statement. Diabetes 1988;37:1000–1004.
39. National Diabetes Data Group. Diabetes in America Nat Inst Health 1985;85:1468:
40. Haffner SM, Lehto S, Ronnemaa T, Pyorala K, Laakso M: Mortality from coronary heart disease in subjects with type 2 diabetes and in nondiabetic subjects with and without prior myocardial infarction. N Eng J Med 1998;339:229–234.
41. Hu FB, Stampfer MJ, Solomon C, Willett WC, Manson JE. Diabetes mellitus and mortality from all-causes and coronary heart disease in women: 20 years of follow-up [abstract]. Diabetes 2000;49:E20.
42. Gibboms RJ, Balady GJ, Beasley JW, et al. ACC/AHA Guidelines for Exercise Testing. A report of the American College of Cardiology/American Heart Association Task Force on Practice Guidelines (Committee on Exercise Testing). J Am Coll Cardiol 1997;30:260–311.
43. Heart Outcomes Prevention Evaluation Study Investigators. Effects of ramipril on cardiovascular and microvascular outcomes in people with diabetes mellitus: Results of the HOPE sustudy. Lancet 2000;355:253–259.
44. Johnstone MT, Creager SJ, Scales KM, Cusco JA, Lee BK, Creager MA: Impaired endothelium-dependent vasodilation in patients with insulin-dependent diabetes mellitus. Circulation 1993;88:2510–2516.
45. Calver A, Collier J, Vallance P: Inhibition and stimulation of nitric oxide synthesis in the human forearm arterial bed of patients with insulin-dependent diabetes. J Clin Invest 1992;90:2548-2554.

46. Elliott TG, Cockcroft JR, Groop PH, Viberti GC, Ritter JM: Inhibition of nitric oxide synthesis in forearm vasculature of insulin-dependent diabetic patients: blunted vasoconstriction in patients with microalbuminuria. Clin Sci (Colch) 1993;85:687–693.
47. Williams SB, Cusco JA, Roddy MA, Johnstone MT, Creager MA. Impaired nitric oxide-mediated vasodilation in patients with non- insulin-dependent diabetes mellitus. J Am Coll Cardiol 1996;27:567–574.
48. McVeigh GE, Brennan GM, Johnston GD, et al. Impaired endothelium-dependent and independent vasodilation in patients with type 2 (non-insulin-dependent) diabetes mellitus. Diabetologia 1992;35:771–776.
49. Anderson TJ, Gerhard MD, Meredith IT, et al. Systemic nature of endothelial dysfunction in atherosclerosis. Am J Cardiol 1995;75:71B–74B.
50. Anderson TJ, Uehata A, Gerhard MD, et al. Close relation of endothelial function in the human coronary and peripheral circulations. J Am Coll Cardiol 1995;26:1235–1241.

9 Gestational Diabetes

Where Do We Look For It and How Do We Find It?

Robert E. Ratner, MD

CONTENTS

HOW IS GESTATIONAL DIABETES MELLITUS DEFINED?

The First International Gestational Diabetes Workshop *(1)* in 1980 defined gestational diabetes mellitus (GDM) as carbohydrate intolerance of varying severity with onset or first recognition during pregnancy. This definition provides ambiguity of glucose thresholds and recognizes the ascertainment bias of glucose monitoring during pregnancy. It fully acknowledges that some women defined as GDM actually have preexisting diabetes first diagnosed during pregnancy. The accepted definition provides no insight into the genetics, etiology, natural history or complications of the disorder. In fact, some have suggested that GDM is not a unique disorder at all *(2)*, while others are convinced that it is *(3)*.

Traditional diagnosis of disease was based on increased mortality associated with anatomic and pathologic abnormalities found at postmortem examination. In the case of GDM, early reports described a 68% fetal mortality together with a 60% 1-yr maternal mortality following the index pregnancy *(4)*. Mortality is no longer an acceptable diagnostic criteria, and efforts to improve diagnostic sensitivity to promote intervention and prevent morbidity and mortality have led to the development of biochemical measures as markers of disease. In some cases, biochemical results falling outside two standard deviations from the mean may be defined as abnormal and indicative of disease (e.g., abnormalities of salt

From: *Contemporary Endocrinology: Handbook of Diagnostic Endocrinology*
Edited by: J. E. Hall and L. K. Nieman © Humana Press Inc., Totowa, NJ

and water balance defined as hyper- and hyponatremia). In other cases, biochemical cutoffs may be established by consensus at a level at which morbidity and/or mortality is shown to significantly increase (e.g., National Cholesterol Education Program [NCEP] III Guidelines for hypercholesterolemia).

The biochemical diagnosis of GDM, however, is fraught with problems. Should gestational diabetes be defined purely on a statistical basis with those individuals falling more than two standard deviations above the mean plasma glucose being defined as having the disease? Alternatively, should the disease be defined on the basis of morbidity attendant to the mother, either during the pregnancy or postpartum? Finally, given the unique circumstances of pregnancy, should the disease be diagnosed in the mother on the basis of outcomes occurring to the baby? These positions are complicated by the possibility that morbidity may occur along a continuum of plasma glucose rather than in association with a threshold value. These concerns have served to complicate the definition of gestational diabetes around the world, resulting in regional differences in identification of the disease and further complicating assessment of screening effectiveness, maternal complications, indications for therapy, and assessment of fetal outcomes.

CLINICAL FEATURES

GDM effects both the mother and the offspring. Traditional diagnostic criteria have stood the test of time as a predictor of subsequent diabetes in the mother. The initial observations of O'Sullivan and Mahan *(5)* demonstrated a 50% prevalence of diabetes after 28 yr of follow-up in those in whom pregnancy was complicated by GDM. Perinatal maternal morbidity is likewise reflected in the significantly increased incidence of pregnancy-induced hypertension and preeclampsia *(6)*. With current aggressive glycemic management achieving postprandial euglycemia, the traditional maternal complications of polyhydramnios, preterm labor, abnormalities of labor, and birth trauma are not increased in this population with GDM. The predominant acute effects of GDM occur not to the mother, but to the fetus.

Neonatal morbidity in the offspring of women with GDM has long been recognized. The occurrence of metabolic complications including hypoglycemia, hypocalcemia, macrosomia, and hyperbilirubinemia is excessive *(7)*. Older data, reported a four-fold increased mortality rate in infants of mothers with GDM *(8)*. With improved neonatal care, it is difficult to demonstrate changes in fetal mortality. The effects on the offspring are not limited, however, to the immediate perinatal period. As these offspring of mothers with GDM age, they develop premature insulin resistance, obesity, and a high rate of carbohydrate intolerance *(9)*.

Diagnosing GDM is intended to promote aggressive management of the mother to reduce or eliminate the perinatal, neonatal, and long-term complications in the offspring. The current diagnostic criteria, however, in no way take the neonatal outcome into consideration.

HOW IS GDM DIAGNOSED? A CONTINUING CONTROVERSY

The First International Gestational Diabetes Workshop *(1)*, together with the National Diabetes Data Group (NDDG) *(10)*, the American College of Obstetrics and Gynecology (ACOG) *(11)*, and the subsequent Second *(12)* and Third *(13)* International Gestational Diabetes Workshops accepted the modified criteria originally described by O'Sullivan and Mahan *(5)* in their classic study of 1964. A statistical analysis of glucose response over 3 h to a 100-g oral glucose challenge in 752 healthy pregnant women yielded values representing the mean ±2 standard deviations in the fasting state and at 1, 2, and 3 h. By arbitrarily declaring abnormal carbohydrate handling as glucose levels exceeding two standard deviations above the mean on two or more values, 2.5% of the population was defined has having GDM. This statistical means of defining disease is population-specific, with a prevalence of GDM ranging from 0.5% in Northern England to 12.3% in an inner city American population (predominantly Hispanic and African-American) *(14)*. With a mixed inner city African-American and tertiary care population, the George Washington University Medical Center has a 4% prevalence of GDM in its obstetric practice. In a review of an ethnically diverse cohort of 10,187 women undergoing standardized screening for glucose intolerance in New York City, the overall prevalence was 3.2%. The frequency of GDM was lowest for Whites, followed by African-Americans, Hispanics, Asians, and women classified as belonging to another "racial/ethnic group" *(14)*. In addition to ethnic characteristics effecting prevalence rates of GDM, site of maternal birth also strongly impacts the risk of GDM. Regardless of ethnicity, women born outside of the United States, and yet cared for during the index pregnancy within the United States, have an increased relative risk of developing GDM compared to native born women *(15)*.

The original O'Sullivan-Mahan criteria were based upon whole blood glucose measures performed by the Somogyi-Nelson technique *(5)*. Both the technique and the whole blood measures have been replaced by enzymatic techniques on serum or plasma samples. Thus, the O'Sullivan criteria were modified by the NDDG to use a conversion factor of 1.14 to represent plasma glucose determinations by the glucokinase technique *(10)*. Technical modifications of that conversion were recommended by Carpenter and Coustan as being more representative of the true plasma glucose determination *(16)*. This modification results in a lowering of all glucose criteria in the 3-h oral glucose tolerance test (OGTT) (see Table 1). As such, a larger percentage of women undergoing glucose tolerance testing during pregnancy will meet these modified criteria, thus increasing the sensitivity of the test; however, the effects of these more inclusive criteria on specificity remain in question *(17)*. By using the lower modified criteria, the overall incidence of GDM increased by 56%. Data on the modified criteria presented at the Fourth International Workshop on Gestational Diabetes

Table 1
Historical Evolution of O'Sullivan-Mahan Criteria for the Diagnosis of Gestational Diabetes Mellitus

Oral Glucose Tolerance Test	*O'Sullivan-Mahan criteria (mM [mg/dL] whole blood)*	*National Diabetes Data Group criteria (mM[mg/dL] plasma)*	*Carpenter-Coustan Modification (mM [mg/dL] plasma)*
Fasting	5.00 (90)	5.83 (105)	5.28 (95)
1 h	9.17 (165)	10.56 (190)	10.00 (180)
2 h	8.06 (145)	9.17 (165)	8.61 (155)
3 h	6.94 (125)	8.06 (145)	7.78 (140)

Adapted from ref. *38*.

indicated that infants of women meeting these lower criteria are at risk for perinatal morbidity, including macrosomia, similar to that of those patients identified using NDDG criteria *(18)*. Therefore, the Carpenter and Coustan criteria were adopted for diagnosis. Long-term follow-up of this patient population is not yet available.

Recognition of this recommended change in diagnostic criteria for GDM has been slow in coming. Despite its original presentation in 1997 and publication in 1998 *(18)*, The American Diabetes Association (ADA) failed to incorporate these recommendations into their position statement in 1999 on gestational diabetes *(19)*, but did so in their revision of January 2000 *(20)*. The World Health Organization (WHO) and most European and Asian institutions continue to utilize both a different glycemic challenge and different thresholds for the diagnosis of GDM.

The WHO has endorsed a straightforward single glucose challenge study for the diagnosis of GDM *(21)*. In an effort to maintain consistency with the non-pregnant state, the WHO has recommended a 75-g glucose challenge with assessment of fasting and 2-h post-glucose load plasma glucose determinations. The diagnosis of diabetes would remain consistent with those values established in a nonpregnant state (fasting >140 mg/dL [7.8 mmol/L] and 2-h values >200 mg/dL [11.1 mmol/L]). In addition, the WHO recommended initiation of intervention in pregnancy for all women demonstrating impaired glucose tolerance as defined by a 2-h post-glucose load >140 mg/dL (7.8 mmol), but <200 mg/dL (11.1 mmol). The uniformity of testing and criteria between the pregnant and nonpregnant state introduces a level of simplicity for international application, but fails to recognize the dramatic changes in metabolism and circulating substrates inherent in the pregnant state. As such, application of criteria originally defined in the nonpregnant state to that of pregnancy has been severely criticized *(22)*.

Efforts to reconcile the NDDG criteria with the WHO criteria have been undertaken on several occasions. In a high risk population of Pima Indians, pregnant women underwent both a 100-g 3-h OGTT with assessment by NDDG criteria, as well as the 2-h 75-g OGTT with assessment by WHO criteria *(23)*.

Recognizing the small sample size of 127 subjects, the WHO criteria correctly identified all those individuals meeting NDDG criteria for gestational diabetes (sensitivity 100%) with a specificity of 93%. Thus, in 9 cases, the WHO criteria recognized the women with abnormal carbohydrate tolerance, whereas NDDG criteria assessed them as normal. Moreover, the WHO criteria were somewhat better in predicting adverse fetal outcomes than was the NDDG criteria.

In an effort to assuage worldwide desire for a simple 1-step procedure for diagnosing GDM, the Fourth International Workshop on GDM recognized the 75-g OGTT as an alternative diagnostic test for GDM *(18)*. Because outcomes data are unavailable, the cutoff values were arbitrarily defined based on the mean plus 1.5 standard deviations of the OGTT values in a study of over 3500 patients *(24)*. Despite this disparate glucose challenge, the 2-h value was raised to 155 mg/dL to be more consistent with a 2-h value recommended for the 100-g OGTT and the values previously advocated by the European Association for the Study of Diabetes *(25)*. Thus, both fasting (95 mg/dL, 5.3 mmol/L) and 2-h (155 mg/dL, 8.6 mmol/L) cutoffs are consistent between both the 75-g and 100-g OGTT (see Table 2).

These arbitrary cutoffs presuppose a threshold glucose for the occurrence of both maternal and fetal morbidity. Some, however, have suggested that these effects occur on a continuum of maternal glucose *(22)*.

IS THERE A THRESHOLD GLUCOSE FOR PERINATAL MORBIDITY?

The defined cutoffs of glucose response to a glucose load defined by the ADA, the NDDG, and the WHO all presuppose a threshold phenomenon for glucose effects on perinatal outcome. If one accepts the Pedersen hypothesis (transplacental transfer of maternal glucose with subsequent fetal hyperinsulinemia) as the mechanism of fetal morbidity, then a continuum of glycemic effects on neonatal outcome would be logical *(26)*. Tallerigo et al. examined the neonatal outcome in 249 women with normal OGTT results in the third trimester by the O'Sullivan-Mahan criteria *(27)*. They found that the 2-h plasma glucose concentration after a 100-g OGTT significantly correlated with the infant's birth weight: the higher the 2-h plasma glucose concentration, the greater the incidence of macrosomia, toxemia, and cesarean sections. A significant increase was noted as 2-h plasma glucose concentrations exceeded 140 mg/dL compared with the 165 mg/dL cutoff noted in the traditional O'Sullivan-Mahan criteria. Lindsay et al. found that maternal and fetal morbidity increased in women with only a single abnormal value on OGTT during pregnancy *(28)*. Toxemia was increased in the affected group, with an odds ratio of 2.51; macrosomia and subsequent shoulder dystocia were increased with an odds ratios of 2.18 and 2.97, respectively. In mothers with only a single abnormal value on OGTT, Burkus and Langer found the incidence of infants who were large for gestational age to be twice that of

Table 2
Criteria for Diagnosis of GDM with a 75-g Oral Glucose Load

	WHO21 mg/dL (mmol/l)	*European Association for Study of Diabetes (25) mg/dL (mmol/L)*	*4th International Workshop on GDM[a] (18) mg/dL (mmol/L)*
Fasting	Unfavored		95 (5.3)
1 h			180 (10.0)
2 h	140 (7.8)	162 (9.0)	155 (8.6)

[a]Two or more of the venous plasma concentrations must be met or exceeded for a positive diagnosis. The test should be performed in the morning after a 8–14 h fast an after at least 3 d of unrestricted diet and physical activity.

mothers in whom the OGTT was entirely normal *(29)*. Intervention to maintain normal glycemia during pregnancy reduced this adverse outcome to near normal levels.

In the Bellflower Study of Sacks et al. *(24)* 3500 pregnant women underwent a 75-g OGTT with 3.3% demonstrating fasting glucose 105 mg/dL or 2-h values 200 mg/dL. The remaining subjects had their glucose responses masked to the primary care givers. Neonatal macrosomia was defined as the primary outcome variable, and a positive association was found between maternal glucose values and birth weight percentiles. Even after adjustment for maternal age, race, parity, body mass index, gestational weight gain, and family history of diabetes, the fasting, 1- and 2-h OGTT values had an independent positive relationship with the percentiles for birth weights, with the fasting glucose having the strongest positive association. Receiver–operator characteristic curves for prediction of neonatal macrosomia failed to demonstrate any threshold value for the prediction of macrosomia for either fasting or 2-h post-glucose load determinations. In a separate study associated with the Toronto Tri-Hospital Gestational Diabetes Project, 3637 women without GDM by 100-g oral OGTTs were followed prospectively *(30)*. Even in the absence of gestational diabetes, increasing carbohydrate intolerance was associated with an increased incidence of maternal pre-eclampsia and subsequent cesarean section and the birth of macrosomic infants. In a subsequent multivariate analysis, the odds ratio for macrosomia doubled for every 18-mg/dL increment in the fasting glucose *(31)*. In addition, the rate of cesarean section increased 10% for every 18-mg/dL increment in the 3-h glucose value. The investigators further demonstrated that progressively increasing carbohydrate intolerance, short of defined GDM, was associated with an increasing incidence of unfavorable maternal and fetal outcomes. Thus, the value of defined cutoffs of glycemic response to a glucose challenge remains highly controversial as a means of predicting, and subsequently preventing neonatal morbidity.

Difficulties with the OGTT as a diagnostic modality have been raised regardless of the criteria used. Poor reproducibility of glucose tolerance testing has been documented for 60 yr *(32)*. This issue has been further examined during pregnancy, in which high risk pregnant women underwent two sequential glucose tolerance tests 1 wk apart; 24% were found to have discrepant test results on the two examinations *(33)*. Progression from normal to abnormal values stemming from progressive decompensation could not explain this inconsistency, given that 80% of the discrepant tests reverted from abnormal to normal at the second examination.

Because of the lack of reproducibility of the OGTT, together with the discrepancies in the number of abnormalities and the threshold for defining those abnormalities, much effort has gone into establishing simpler diagnostic criteria for GDM. Glycated proteins are used extensively to follow long-term levels of glycemic control (as reviewed in Chapter 8). Many clinicians had hoped to adapt this simple blood test, which can be obtained without dietary preparation and at any time of day, as a diagnostic test for GDM. Unfortunately, neither A_1C, nor fructosamine (see Chapter 8) is sufficiently sensitive for the identification of women with GDM *(34–36)*. The short duration of maternal hyperglycemia and the critical nature of timely intervention precludes the use of these glycated proteins. In addition, increased turnover of hemoglobin and plasma proteins during pregnancy significantly alters the interpretation of A_1C as compared to the nonpregnant state.

An excellent review of alternative diagnostic testing for GDM was provided by Carr at the Fourth International Workshop on Gestational Diabetes *(37)*. In this review, he examines the available data on random glucose testing and the utilization of reflectance meters for diagnostic evaluation of GDM. Traditional reflectance meters (e.g., Accuchek, Glucometer, etc.) lacked the precision necessary for acceptable sensitivity. Thus, a lower limit of glucose would be necessary in order to identify individuals with GDM, sacrificing specificity. Newer reflectance meters (e.g., One Touch, Hemocue, etc.), which have eliminated the potential for user error, appear to have adequate precision, but lack clinical validation in the setting of gestational diabetes. Thus, random glucose testing and reflectance meters are not recommended for the identification of women at risk for GDM.

WHAT IS THE APPROPRIATE SCREENING TEST FOR GDM?

The performance of an OGTT, whether a 75- or a 100-g challenge, is expensive, time-consuming, and poorly accepted by pregnant women who find both prolonged fasting and ingestion of concentrated sweets difficult to tolerate. Universal testing of pregnant women is therefore not recommended. The best screening test for GDM appears to be the 50-g 1-h glucose challenge test *(38)*. It is now

Table 3
Sensitivity and Specificity of the 50-g, 1-h Glucose Challenge Test

	Venous plasma glucose threshold (mg/dL)		
	130	135	140
Sensitivity (%)	100	98	79
Specificity (%)	78	80	87

Ref. *37*.

recognized that a 50-g oral glucose load can be utilized in either the fasting or the fed state without reducing sensitivity or specificity. Utilizing a screening threshold of 130 mg/dL provides a sensitivity approaching 100%, while maintaining specificity at nearly 80% (see Table 3). Altering the threshold to 140 mg/dL significantly improves the specificity to 87%, but drops the sensitivity to 79%. Alteration of these thresholds for undertaking a subsequent 3-h, 100-g OGTT influences the sensitivity, specificity, and ultimate cost of universal screening. Universal screening of all pregnant women using a threshold value of 130 mg/dL resulting in an almost 100% sensitivity costs $249/case diagnosed. Limiting screening to women over the age of 25, or to younger women with the presence of risk factors, maintains the sensitivity at more than 95%, but with only a $35 reduction in cost/case diagnosed *(37)*.

The Second International Workshop Conference on GDM concluded that all pregnant women should be screened for GDM *(12)*. A 1-h plasma glucose determination in excess of 140 mg/dL (lower by Carpenter-Coustan criteria) constitutes a positive screen and requires the performance of a traditional 100-g OGTT for confirmation of GDM. Selective screening based on clinical and obstetric history has previously been deemed inadequate. However, large studies suggest that the inefficiency of screening is improved by assessing only women at high risk. Naylor et al. evaluated data on over 3000 pregnant women and developed a scoring system to determine risks of GDM *(39)*. Scores are based on age, body mass index, and race. They rationalize that those with low scores need not be evaluated, which allowed 34% of women to avoid the glucose challenge test. They also suggested that those with high scores should have a lower cutoff value on their glucose challenge test. The complex formula for integration of historical, anthropometric, and laboratory assessment support the contention of selective screening; however, it has led others to comment that "despite its scientific merits, busy obstetricians are unlikely to wend their way through this complex diagnostic schema for each pregnant woman. It is ironic that the criteria for excluding women from screening are so hard to discern that universal screening would probably be used as a matter of practical convenience" *(40)*.

Table 4
Low Risk Characteristics[a] that Preclude the Need for Screening for Gestational Diabetes[b]

- Age <25 yr.
- Weight normal before pregnancy.
- Member of an ethnic group with a low prevalence of GDM.
- No history of abnormal glucose tolerance.
- No known diabetes in first-degree relatives.
- No history of poor obstetric outcome.

[a] All characteristics must be met.
[b] Ref. *20*.

Others have sought to examine the loss of sensitivity in identifying women with GDM if selective screening were instituted. In a prospective examination of pregnant women meeting criteria for low risk status, the 75-g OGTT identified 2.8% with GDM *(41)*. Perhaps more telling was the observation that GDM, occurring in patients in a low risk category, were no different from the pregnancy outcomes of other women with GDM, specifically in reference to the frequency of insulin use, amount of insulin, morbidity, cesarean section rates, and frequency of large for gestational age babies. These authors suggested that selective screening, as recommended by Naylor et al. *(39)*, would effectively miss 10% of women with GDM. In a retrospective analysis of over 25,000 deliveries, only 10% of women met the criteria for low risk status as it pertains to screening for GDM. Thus, the effective savings from selective screening would be relatively small *(42)*.

Nonetheless, current guidelines recommend screening women with clinical characteristics consistent with high risk of GDM (marked obesity, personal history of GDM, glycosuria, or a strong family history of diabetes) with glucose testing as soon as feasible following the diagnosis of pregnancy *(18)*. Women of average risk are recommended to undergo screening at 24–28 wk of gestation, with low risk status indicating no need for glucose testing reserved for those relatively few women meeting all of the low risk characteristics described in Table 4.

FUTURE DIRECTIONS

Adequate clinical pathophysiologic and epidemiologic data exist to justify the designation of GDM as a specific disorder with attendant morbidity and mortality. The absence of a gold standard for defining the disease has made screening, diagnosis, and evaluation of therapeutic efficacy problematic.

In an effort to definitively elucidate the relationship between maternal glycemia and neonatal outcomes, the National Institutes of Health and an international study group are initiating the "Hyperglycemia and Adverse Pregnancy Out-

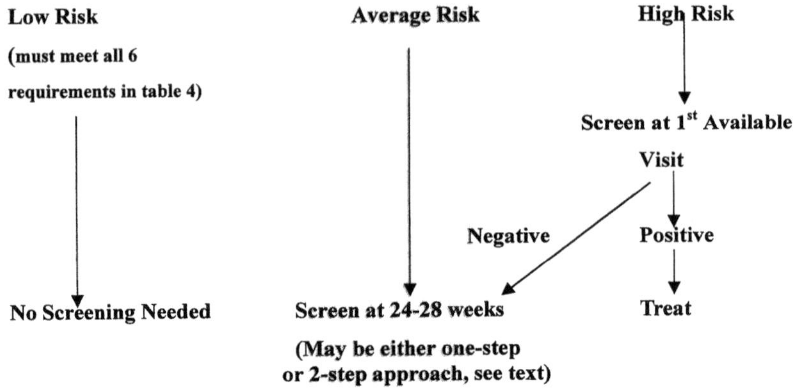

Fig. 1. Recommended screening procedure for gestational diabetes based on risk *(20)*.

comes" (HAPO) Trial. This is intended to be a double blind trial of 25,000 pregnant women recruited over 3 yr in 16 international centers. All women will undergo a 75-g, 2-h OGTT in early third trimester, with results remaining blinded to both patient and primary caregiver, unless the fasting glucose exceeds 105 mg/dL or the 2-h value exceeds 200 mg/dL. Anticipated endpoints include the incidence of cesarean section, large for gestational age infants, and neonatal obesity. It is hoped that this study will clarify whether glucose adversely effects the neonate along the continuum or if a threshold phenomenon can be identified to support diagnostic criteria. With completion of this study, it is hoped that sensible recommendations for screening, diagnosis, and intervention may be provided to clinicians.

SUMMARY

In January 2000, publication of the American Diabetes Association Clinical Practice Recommendations for Gestational Diabetes finally complied with the final recommendations of the Fourth International Workshop on Gestational Diabetes concerning screening and diagnosis *(20)*.

Selective screening is advocated with no screening necessary only in those women meeting all of the low risk characteristics described in Table 4. High risk women require glucose screening at the first clinical contact following diagnosis of pregnancy, with women of average risk being screened at 24–28 wk gestation (see Fig. 1.)

Glucose testing may proceed along either a one step or a two step approach depending upon the preference of the individual center and the risk characteristics of their population. The one-step approach involves the performance of a diagnostic 75-g, OGTT without prior glucose screening. The test should be done in the morning after an overnight fast between 8 and 14 h and after at least 3 d of unrestricted diet (150 g carbohydrate/d) and unlimited physical activity.

The 2-step approach is anticipated for populations with average risk. A 1-h, 50-g oral glucose challenge test may be performed randomly throughout the day, independent of the timing of the last meal. A 1-h glucose threshold 140 mg/dL identifies approx 80% of women with GDM, and the yield is further increased to >90% by using a cutoff of 130 mg/dL. Women meeting the above criteria on the 50-g glucose challenge proceed to a 3-h, 100-g OGTT, following the same preparation described above.

The diagnosis of GDM is made on the basis of either of the OGTT results. Two abnormalities exceeding the limits defined by Carpenter and Coustan on the 100-g OGTT or a single abnormality exceeding the limits on the 75-g OGTT confirm the diagnosis of GDM.

REFERENCES

1. Summary and recommendations, First International Workshop-Conference on Gestational Diabetes. Diabetes Care 1980;3:499–501.
2. Harris MI. Gestational diabetes may represent discovery of pre-existing glucose intolerance. Diabetes Care 1988;11:402–411.
3. Hod M, Rabinerson D, Peled Y. Gestational diabetes: is it a clinical entity? Diabetes Reviews 1995;3:602–613.
4. Hadden DR. A historical perspective on gestational diabetes. Diabetes Care 1998;21 (Suppl 2):B3–B4.
5. O'Sullivan JB, Mahan CM. Criteria for the oral glucose tolerance test in pregnancy. Diabetes 1964;13:278–285.
6. Goldman M, Kitzmiller JL, Abrams B, et al. Obstetric complications with GDM: Effect of maternal weight. Diabetes 1991;40(Suppl 2):79–82.
7. Hod M, Merlob P, Friedman S, et al. Gestational Diabetes Mellitus a survey of perinatal complications in the 1980's. Diabetes 1991;40(Suppl 2):74–78.
8. O'Sullivan JB, Charles D, Mahan CM, et al. Gestational diabetes and perinatal mortality rate. Am J Obstet Gynecol 1973;116:901–904.
9. Pettitt DJ, Bennett PH, Saad MF, et al. Abnormal glucose tolerance during pregnancy in Pima Indian women: long-term effects on offspring. Diabetes 1991;40 (Suppl 2):126–130.
10. National Diabetes Data Group. Classification and diagnosis of diabetes mellitus and other categories of glucose intolerance. Diabetes 1979;18:1039–1057.
11. American College of Obstetricians and Gynecologists. Diabetes in pregnancy. Washington, D.C., ACOG, 1994 (Technical Bulletin No. 200).
12. Freinkel N (ed.). Proceedings of the second international workshop-conference on gestational diabetes mellitus. Diabetes 1985;34(Suppl 2):123–127.
13. Metzger BE (ed.). Proceedings of the third international workshop-conference on gestational diabetes mellitus. Diabetes 1991;40(Suppl 2):197–201.
14. Berkowitz GS, Lapinski RH, Wein R, Lee D. Racial/ethnicity and other risk factors for gestational diabetes. Am J Epidemiol 1992;135:965–973.
15. Kieffer EC, Martin JA, Herman WH. Impact of maternal nativity on the prevalence of diabetes during pregnancy among U.S. ethnic groups. Diabetes Care 1999;22:729–735.
16. Carpenter MW, Coustan DR. Criteria for screening tests for gestational diabetes. Am J Obstet Gynecol 1982;144:768–773.

17. Magee MS, Walden CE, Benedetti TJ, Knopp RH. Influence of diagnostic criteria on the incidence of gestational diabetes and perinatal morbidity. JAMA 1993;269:609–615.
18. Metzger BE, Coustan DR, The Organizing Committee. Summary and recommendations of the Fourth International Workshop Conference on gestational diabetes mellitus. Diabetes Care 1998;21(Suppl. 2):B161–B167.
19. American Diabetes Association. Position statement: gestational diabetes mellitus. Diabetes Care 1999;22(Suppl 1):S74–S76.
20. American Diabetes Association. Position Statement: Gestational diabetes mellitus. Diabetes Care 2002;25(Suppl 1):594–596.
21. World Health Organization. Diabetes mellitus: report of a WHO study group. Geneva, World Health Organization, 1985 (Tech Report Series No. 727).
22. Coustan DR. Diagnosis of gestational diabetes: are new criteria needed? Diabetes Reviews 1995;3:614–620.
23. Pettitt DJ, Bennett PH, Hanson RL, Narayan KMV, Knowler WC. Comparison of World Health Organization and National Diabetes Data Group procedures to detect abnormalities of glucose tolerance during pregnancy. Diabetes Care 1994;17:1264–1268.
24. Sacks DA, Greenspoon JS, Abu-Fadil S, Henry HM, Wolde-Tsadik G, Yao JFF. Toward universal criteria for gestational diabetes: the 75-gram glucose tolerance test in pregnancy. Am J Obstet Gynecol 1995;172:607–614.
25. LindT, Phillips PR, the DPSG of the EASD. Influence of pregnancy on the 75 g OGTT: a prospective multicenter study. Diabetes 1991;40(Suppl 2):8–13.
26. Pedersen J. The Pregnant Diabetic and Her Newborn. Williams & Wilkins Co., Baltimore, 1977. pp 211–220.
27. Tallarigo L, Giampietro O, Penno G, et al. Relation of glucose tolerance test to complications of pregnancy in nondiabetic women. N Engl J Med 1986;315:989–992.
28. Lindsay MK, Graves W, Klein L. The relationship of one abnormal glucose tolerance test value in pregnancy complications. Obstet Gynecol 1988;73:103–106.
29. Berkus MD, Langer O. Glucose tolerance test: degree of glucose abnormality correlates with neonatal outcome. Obstet Gynecol 1993;81:344–348.
30. Sermer M, Naylor CD, Gare DJ, et al. Impact of increasing carbohydrate intolerance on maternal-fetal outcomes in 3637 women without gestational diabetes. Am J Obstet Gynecol 1995;173:146–156.
31. Sermer M, Naylor CD, Farine D, et al. The Toronto tri-hospital gestational diabetes project. Diabetes Care 1998;21(Suppl 2):B33–B42.
32. Freeman H, Looney JM, Hoskins RG. Spontaneous variability of oral glucose tolerance. J Clin Endocrinol 1942;2:431–434.
33. Catalano PM, Avallone D, Drago NM, Amini SV. Reproducibility of the oral glucose tolerance test in pregnant women. Am J Obstet Gynecol 1193;169:874–881.
34. Hod M, Orvieto R, Friedman S, et al. Glycated proteins in gestational diabetes mellitus. Isr J Med Sci 1990;26:638–644.
35. Huter O, Drexel H, Brezinka C, et al. Low sensitivity of serum fructosamine as a screening parameter for gestational diabetes mellitus. Gynecol Obstet Invest 1992;34:20–23.
36. Aziz NL, Abdelwahab S, Moussa M, Georgy M. Maternal fructosamine and glycosylated hemoglobin in the prediction of gestational glucose intolerance. Clin Exp Obstet Gynecol 1992;19:235–241.
37. Carr SR. Screening for gestational diabetes mellitus: a perspective in 1998. Diabetes Care 1998;21(Suppl 2):B14–B18.
38. Carpenter MW. Rationale and performance of tests for gestational diabetes. Clin Obstet Gynecol 1991;34:544–557.
39. Naylor CD, Sermer S, Chen E, Farine D. Selective screening for gestational diabetes mellitus. N Engl J Med 1997;337:1591–1596.

40. Greene MF. Screening for gestational diabetes mellitus. N Engl J Med 1997;337:1625–1626.
41. Moses RG, Moses J, Davis WS. Gestational diabetes: Do lean young caucasian women need to be tested? Diabetes Care 1998;21:1803–1806.
42. Williams CB, Iqbal S, Zawacki CM, Yu D, Brown MB, Herman WH. Effect of selective screening for gestational diabetes. Diabetes Care 1999;22:418–421.

10 Hypoglycemic Disorders

F. John Service, MD, PhD

Contents

INTRODUCTION

Low concentrations of blood glucose were recognized as a concomitant of some disease states in the nineteenth century *(1)*. However, it was not until insulin became available for the treatment of diabetes mellitus in the early 1920s that symptoms similar to those arising from overtreatment of diabetes mellitus were recognized in nondiabetic persons. This observation led to the postulation of a new disease entity called hyperinsulinism *(2)*. Support for the existence of hyperinsulinism was provided from the identification of a malignant pancreatic islet cell tumor in 1926 in a patient who had episodes of severe hypoglycemia *(3)*. Postmortem extracts of tissue metastatic to the liver from this patient caused marked hypoglycemia when injected into rabbits. The first surgical cure of hyperinsulinism was reported by Howland et al. *(4)* in 1929, following successful removal of a benign insulinoma from a hypoglycemic patient. Consequent to the development of a radioimmunoassay for insulin *(5)*, hyperinsulinism was confirmed as the pathophysiologic basis for hypoglycemia caused by insulinoma. Elucidation of the biochemistry of glucose metabolism and hormonal control of glucose counterregulation has permitted identification of other non-insulin-mediated causes of hypoglycemia.

CLASSIFICATION

A classification based on fasting and reactive hypoglycemia should be abandoned, because it does not facilitate selection of appropriate diagnostic maneuvers or expedite identification of the correct underlying disorder. The term

From: *Contemporary Endocrinology: Handbook of Diagnostic Endocrinology*
Edited by: J. E. Hall and L. K. Nieman © Humana Press Inc., Totowa, NJ

reactive hypoglycemia is only a descriptor, it describes the timing of hypoglycemia without any implication regarding etiology. Like fever, it is an indicator of an abnormality without indication of cause.

A more useful approach for the practitioner is a classification based on clinical characteristics (Table 1 and Fig. 1) *(6)*. Persons who appear healthy *(7–26)* have different hypoglycemic disorders from persons who are ill *(27)*. Hospitalized patients are at additional risk for hypoglycemia, often from iatrogenic factors *(59,60)*. The potential for mediation by drugs in the generation of a low serum glucose exists in any patient with hypoglycemia. Episodes of hypoglycemia may result from accidental drug ingestion in healthy persons (e.g., ethanol in children) *(7)*, the mistaken dispensing of a sulfonylurea for the intended drug *(21,22)*, or the idiosyncratic action of a drug used for the treatment of an ill patient *(27–32)*. The occurrence of hypoglycemia in a patient with an illness known to be associated with the risk for low serum glucose requires little if any investigation of its cause, only a recognition of the association of the disease with the risk for hypoglycemia.

Patients may have a history of neuroglycopenic spells or may be observed during a hypoglycemic episode. Asymptomatic patients may have artifactual hypoglycemia due to leukemia *(61)* or severe hemolysis *(62)* or may have adapted to lifelong hypoglycemia caused by glycogen storage disease *(63)*.

The healthy-appearing adult patient with a history of episodes of neuroglycopenia usually has a hyperinsulinemic hypoglycemic disorder.

Insulinoma may occur at any age, is more frequent in women, and has an estimated incidence of 1 case/250,000 patient years *(11)*. Multiple endocrine neoplasia (MEN) 1 syndrome, multiplicity, or malignancy occur in less than 10%. Recurrence rate is less than 10% without MEN 1 and 20% with MEN 1. Treatment is surgical removal. Long-term survival after removal of a benign insulinoma is normal *(11)*.

Factitial hypoglycemia, whether from sulfonylurea *(16)* or insulin use *(15)* is probably more common than reported. It may occur as self-injury, suicide, homicide, or child abuse. Perpetrators are more frequently women in a health-related occupation or who have diabetes. Treatment is discontinuation of the drug. Insulin autoimmune hypoglycemia is extraordinarily rare, reported mostly, but not exclusively, in Asians of all ages without gender preference *(19)*. There may be a history of antecedent autoimmune disease or use of drugs containing sulfhydril. Insulin antibody titers are high. Spontaneous remission may occur in Asians, but is less likely in Caucasians. There is no known effective treatment. Non-insulin pancreatogenous hypoglycemia syndrome (NIPHS) is a newly described hypoglycemic entity characterized by male predominance, neuroglycopenia occurring postprandially, negative 72-h fast, negative radiologic localization studies, but positive calcium stimulation test, amelioration of symptoms by gradient-guided partial pancreatectomy, and presence of islet hyperplasia and nesidioblastosis in resected pancreata *(13,14)*.

Table 1
Clinical Classification of Hypoglycemic Disorders

Patient appears healthy		
A.	No coexistent disease	
	Drugs:	Ethanol *(7)*
		Salicylates *(8)*
		Quinine *(9)*
		Haloperidol *(10)*
	Insulinoma *(9)*	
	Islet hyperplasia/nesidioblastosis:	
		Persistent hyperinsulinemic hypoglycemia of infancy *(12)*
		Non-insulinoma pancreatogenous hypoglycemia syndrome *(13,14)*
	Insulin factitial hypoglycemia *(15)*	
	Sulfonylurea factitial hypoglycemia *(16)*	
	Severe exercise *(17)*	
	Ketotic hypoglycemia *(18)*	
	Insulin autoimmune hypoglycemia *(19)*	
B.	Compensated coexistent disease	
	Drugs:	Dispensing error *(21,22)*
		Disopyramide *(23)*
		β-Adrenergic blocking agents *(24)*
		Unripe ackee fruit and undernutrition *(25,26)*
Patient appears ill		
A.	Drugs:	Pentamidine and pneumocystis pneumonia *(27)*
		Sulfamethoxazole and trimethoprim and renal failure *(28)*
		Propoxyphene and renal failure *(29)*
		Quinine and cerebral malaria *(30)*
		Quinine and malaria *(31)*
		Topical salicylates and renal failure *(32)*
B.	Predisposing illness:	
		Small for gestational age infant *(33)*
		Beckwith-Wiedemann syndrome *(34)*
		Erythroblastosis fetalis *(35)*
		Infant of diabetic mother *(36)*
		Glycogen storage disease *(37)*
		Defects in amino acid and fatty acid metabolism *(38)*
		Reye's syndrome *(39)*
		Cyanotic congenital heart disease *(40)*
		Hypopituitarism *(41)*
		Isolated growth hormone deficiency *(42)*
		Isolated adrenocorticotrophic hormone (ACTH) deficiency *(43)*
		Addison's disease *(41)*
		Galactosemia *(44)*

(continued)

Table 1
Clinical Classification of Hypoglycemic Disorders *(continued)*

Hereditary fructose intolerance *(45)*
Carnitine deficiency *(46)*
Defective type 1 glucose transporter in the brain *(47)*
Spinal muscular atrophy *(48)*
Acquired severe liver disease *(49)*
Nonislet cell tumor hypoglycemia *(50)*
Sepsis *(51)*
Renal failure *(52)*
Congestive heart failure *(53)*
Lactic acidosis *(54)*
Starvation *(55)*
Anorexia nervosa *(56)*
Post-operative removal of pheochromocytoma *(57)*
Insulin receptor antibody hypoglycemia *(58)*
C. Hospitalized patient:
Diseases predisposing to hypoglycemia
Total parenteral nutrition and insulin therapy *(59)*
Questran interference with glucocorticoid absorption *(60)*
Shock *(59)*

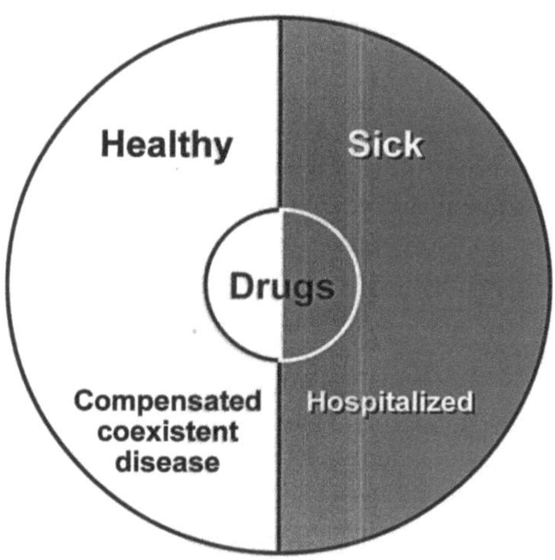

Fig. 1. A clinical approach to hypoglycemic disorders separates patients into those who appear healthy and those who are sick. Among the former are those without and those with a compensated coexistent disease. Medications may be the cause of hypoglycemia in the former through accidental ingestion, e.g., ethanol in children or in the latter, by a dispensing error, e.g., sulfonylurea for the intended drug. Sick persons may have an illness that predisposes to hypoglycemia or experience drug-illness interaction leading to hypoglycemia. Hypoglycemia in hospitalized patients can often be ascribed to iatrogenic factors.

The mechanisms of hypoglycemia among patients whose low glucose is mediated by drugs or a predisposing illness are varied—insulin- or non-insulin-mediated hypoglycemia or unknown. Not all patients with a disease, which has a proclivity to generate hypoglycemia, actually experience low blood glucose. Why some patients and not others experience hypoglycemia is unknown.

DIAGNOSTIC EVALUATION

A healthy-appearing patient with no coexisting disease who has a history of neuroglycopenic spells requires an approach quite different from that taken for a patient with concurrent illness or a hospitalized patient with acute hypoglycemia.

The Healthy-Appearing Patient

SERUM GLUCOSE LEVELS

Because symptoms of hypoglycemia are nonspecific, it is necessary to verify a low serum glucose level at the time that spontaneous symptoms occur and demonstrate that symptoms are relieved through correction of the low glucose level ("Whipple's triad") *(64)*.

A normal serum glucose level, reliably obtained during the occurrence of spontaneous symptoms, eliminates the possibility of a hypoglycemic disorder, and no further evaluation is required. Glucose measurements made by the patient with a reflectance meter during the occurrence of spontaneous symptoms are likely to provide false information. Patients are usually not experienced in this technique. The measurements are obtained under adverse circumstances (i.e., while the patient is symptomatic), and the method may not even provide an accurate measurement of glucose levels in the hypoglycemic range *(65)*. However, reliably measured capillary glucose levels in the normal range values should virtually eliminate the possibility of hypoglycemia as the cause of symptoms. Normoglycemia during symptoms cannot be ascribed to spontaneous recovery of glycemia from prior hypoglycemia, and the reverse is the actual phenomenon: symptoms ease before euglycemia is achieved.

Often, the measurement of serum glucose level is not feasible when spontaneous symptoms occur during activities of ordinary life. Under such circumstances, a judgement by a physician whether to proceed with further evaluation depends on a detailed history. A history of neuroglycopenic symptoms or a confirmed low (<50 mg/dL) serum glucose level warrants further testing.

THE PROLONGED (72-H) FAST

The prolonged (72-h) fast is the classic diagnostic test for hypoglycemia. It should be conducted following standardized procedures. A suggested protocol is shown in Table 2. The fast may be conducted for different purposes: to establish that hypoglycemia is the basis for the patient's symptoms, or to establish the

Table 2
Protocol for Prolonged Supervised Fast

1. Date the onset of the fast as of the last ingestion of calories. Discontinue all nonessential medications.
2. Allow the patient to drink calorie-free and caffeine-free beverages.
3. Ensure that the patient is active during waking h.
4. Measure serum glucose, insulin, C-peptide, and, if an assay is available, proinsulin in the same specimen: repeat measurements every 6 h until the serum glucose is <60 mg/dL, when the interval should then be reduced to every 1 to 2 h.
5. End the fast when the serum glucose is <45 mg/dL and the patient has symptoms and/or signs of hypoglycemia or <55 mg/dL if Whipple's triad is not the goal.
6. At the end of the fast, measure serum glucose, insulin, C-peptide, proinsulin, β-OH, and sulfonylurea in the same specimen; then inject 1 mg of glucagon IV and measure serum glucose after 10, 20, and 30 min. Then feed the patient.

Reprinted from ref. *39* with the permission of the publisher.

mechanism for the hypoglycemia. In the former, Whipple's triad must be demonstrated. In the latter, the sole purpose is to measure β-cell polypeptides and serum sulfonylurea since Whipple's triad had been previously documented. In the latter case, the fast can be terminated when serum glucose 55 mg/dL (even better, 50 mg/dL), because β-cell polypeptides can be expected to be suppressed at this serum glucose level and sulfonylurea absent from the serum (unless that drug is mediating the hypoglycemia) (Fig. 2). In patients who have neither symptoms nor signs of hypoglycemia and in those without severely depressed serum glucose concentrations (>40 mg/dL), the fast should be terminated at 72 h. Fasting should be terminated prior to 72 h when a patient has both symptoms of hypoglycemia and a serum glucose level in the hypoglycemic range or in the event that demonstration of Whipple's triad is not the goal when serum glucose is 55 mg/dL. Truncation of the 72-h fast at 48 h as recommended by some is ill advised *(66)*.

The decision to end the fast may not be easy to make when Whipple's triad is the goal. Because of possible delays in the availability of the results of serum glucose testing, the bedside reflectance meter may have to serve as a guide to glucose levels. Some patients have slightly depressed glycemic levels without symptoms or signs of hypoglycemia. Other patients may reproduce during fasting the symptoms they experienced in ordinary life, but may have serum glucose levels that are sometimes in and sometimes above the hypoglycemic range. In such instances, the attribution of symptoms to hypoglycemia is difficult, especially if all additional measurements made during fasting are normal. To complicate matters, young, lean, healthy women and, to a lesser degree, some men,

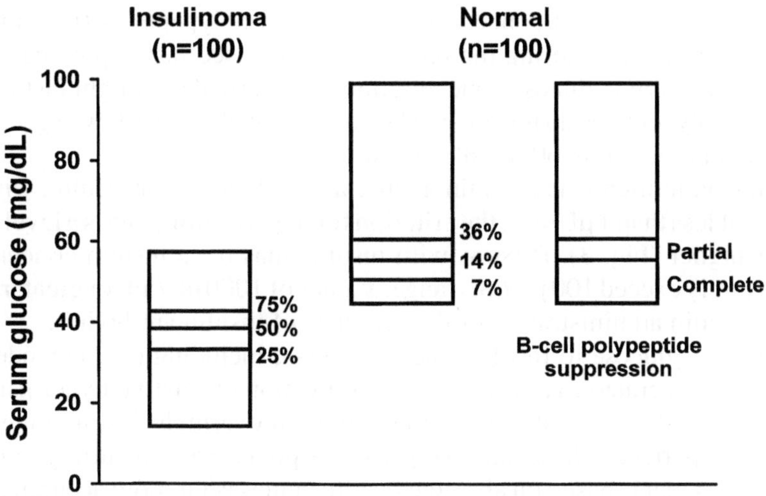

Fig. 2. Serum glucose concentrations at the termination of the prolonged (72 h) fast (72 h in normals and Whipple's triad in patients with insulinoma) show considerable overlap. Among 100 recently operated patients with insulinoma, median serum glucose was 37 mg/dL, 75% 42 mg/dL, 25% 33 mg/dL, with highest value of 57 mg/dL. In contrast, among 100 normal subjects who recently underwent the prolonged fast, 36% had terminal serum glucose 60 mg/dL, 14% 55 mg/dL and 7% 50 mg/dL, with 2 patients having values as low as 44 mg/dL. Suppression of β-cell polypeptides (insulin, C-peptide, and proinsulin) may be observed when the serum glucose is 60 mg/dL. When the serum glucose is 55 mg/dL, all three β-cell polypeptides were uniformly suppressed below diagnostic criteria for hyperinsulinemia.

may have serum glucose levels in the range of 40 mg/dL or even lower during prolonged (but never overnight) fasting *(67)*. Careful examination and testing for subtle signs or symptoms of hypoglycemia should be conducted repeatedly when the patient's serum glucose level is near or in the hypoglycemic range. To end fasting solely on the basis of a low serum glucose level, in the absence of symptoms or signs of hypoglycemia, jeopardizes the possibility of discriminating between normal persons and those with hypoglycemia not mediated by insulin.

On the other hand, concluding that a fast is negative on the basis of the absence of symptoms and/or signs is an equally egregious error. It is essential to monitor patients closely during the fast and be vigilant for subtle signs of neuroglycopenia. We have encountered patients who were unnecessarily fasted for the full 72-h period, when earlier in the fast serum glucose was low but evidence for neuroglycopenia was not appreciated.

In one large study, the prolonged (72-h) fast was terminated within 12 h in 33%, within 24 h in 65%, and within 48 h in 93% of patients with insulinoma *(68)*. No patient with a negative fast at 72 h became positive by extending the fast to 96 h.

The interpretation of concentrations of β-cell polypeptides (insulin, C peptide, and proinsulin) during the prolonged supervised fast is predicated on the concomitant serum glucose concentration. The normal overnight fasting ranges for these polypeptides do not apply when the serum glucose is low, e.g., 50 mg/dL or lower and probably 60 mg/dL or lower.

Using an immunochemiluminometric assay (ICMA) for insulin, with a sensitivity of less than 1 μU/mL, the criterion for hyperinsulinemia is a level of 3 μU/mL or higher (Fig. 3). Persons with insulinomas have insulin concentrations which rarely exceed 100 μU/mL range. Values of 1000 μU/mL or greater suggest recent insulin administration or the presence of insulin antibodies.

Ratios of glucose to insulin, and vice versa, including the "amended ratio" have been generated to assist in the identification of relative hyperinsulinemia when the insulin concentration is in the normal overnight fasting range. In the author's experience, these ratios (Fig. 3) have poor diagnostic utility. A diagnostic criterion that is based on absolute insulin values is far more accurate. Criteria for hyperinsulinemia using C-peptide and proinsulin (each measured by ICMA) are levels of 200 pmol/L *(68)* or greater and 5 pmol/L or greater, respectively *(6)* (Fig. 3). The molar ratio of insulin to C-peptide is the same for patients with insulinomas and healthy individuals (approx 0.2) *(69)*. Although a ratio >1.0 for the diagnosis of insulin factitial hypoglycemia has been suggested *(70)*, the insulin concentration is usually high, and C-peptide concentration is undetectable or very low, making a ratio superfluous. Proinsulin concentration mirrors that of C-peptide *(71)*.

Because of the antiketogenic effect of insulin, plasma (β-Hydroxy) β-OH butyrate is measured at the end of the fast. Patients with insulin-mediated hypoglycemia have concentrations of <2.7 mmol/L, whereas others (normal individuals or those with non-insulin-mediated hypoglycemia) have higher levels (Fig. 3) *(72)*. Because insulin is glycogenic and antiglycogenolytic, the response of serum glucose to glucagon, 1 mg injected intravenously at the end of the fast can be useful (Fig. 4) *(72)*. Patients with insulin-mediated hypoglycemia have a maximum increment of 25 mg/dL or more above the terminal fasting serum glucose, whereas, others (normal individuals or those with non-insulin-mediated hypoglycemia) have lower increments (Fig. 3). Both insulin surrogates (β-OH butyrate and glucose response to intravenous glucagon) are applicable when the serum glucose is 60 mg/dL or lower at the end of the fast. When the serum glucose exceeds 60 mg/dL at the end of the fast, knowledge of β-cell polypeptides and insulin surrogates is unnecessary, as the fast is negative by virtue of the serum glucose level. The criteria for hyperinsulinemia apply both in the fasting and postprandial states.

Measurement of first- and second-generation sulfonylureas and meglitinides in the serum at the end of the fast is an essential component of the prolonged

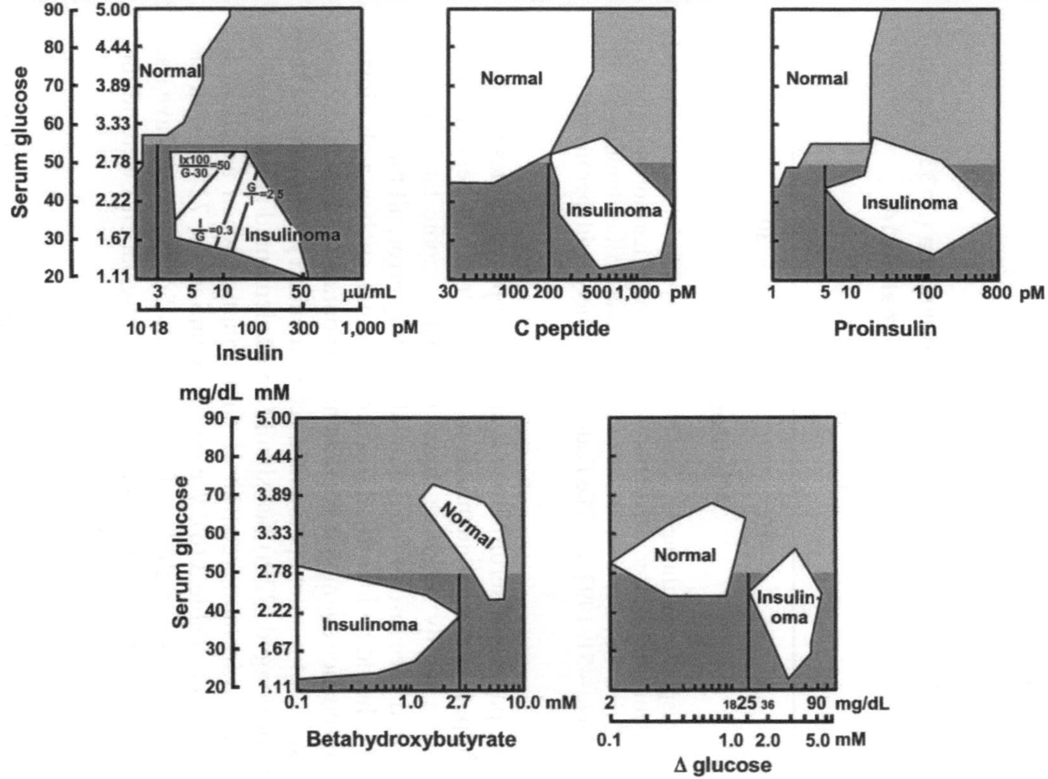

Fig. 3. Limits of serum insulin, C-peptide, proinsulin, and β-OH levels and changes in serum glucose levels in response to intravenous glucagon, according to serum glucose levels at the end of a 72-h fast in normal persons and when the features of Whipple's triad were noted in patients with histologically-confirmed insulinomas. Shaded areas represent serum glucose levels 50 mg/dL (2.8 mmol/L). Vertical lines represent diagnostic criteria for insulinoma: insulin, 3 μU/mL (18 pmol/L); C-peptide, 200 pmol/L; proinsulin, 5 pmol/L; β-OH, 2.7 mmol/L; and change in glucose level (from preglucagon concentrations to peak after), 25 mg/dL. The lack of diagnostic utility of various ratio of insulin and glucose: glucose/insulin = 2.5, insulin/glucose = 0.3, and insulin ×100/glucose-30 = 50 is apparent from their distribution within the insulinoma range.

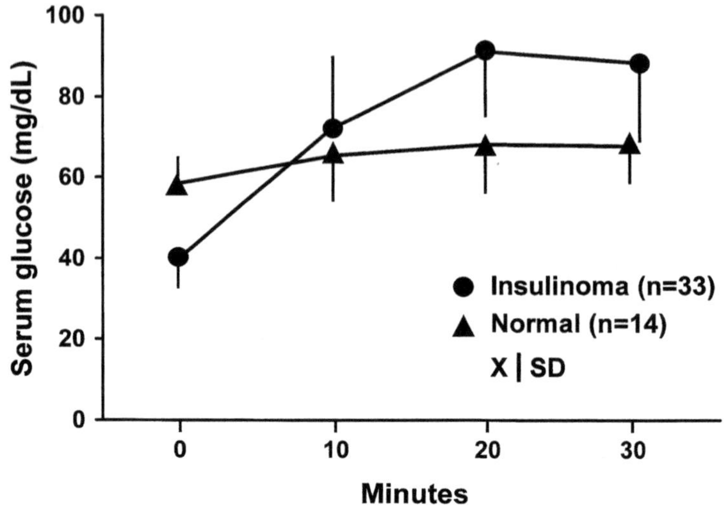

Fig. 4. Serum glucose responses to glucagon, 1 mg intravenously administered at the end of the prolonged fast (0 min) are greater in patients with insulinoma than normal subjects. From O'Brien T, O'Brien PC, Service FJ: Insulin surrogates in insulinoma. J Clin Endocrinol Metab 77:448-451, 1993; (c) The Endocrine Society; with permission.

supervised fast. The pattern of serum glucose and β-cell polypeptides in sulfonylurea-induced hypoglycemia is identical to that observed in persons with insulinoma. We use a highly sensitive liquid chromatographic tandem mass spectrography method. Because of the potential for drug error, all medications taken by the patient should be identified by a professional, such as a physician or pharmacist. In the chance event that a patient has a spontaneous hypoglycemic episode in the presence of medical personnel, recommended procedures for the termination of the prolonged (72-h) fast should be implemented at that time.

A suggested diagnostic interpretation of data obtained when a patient is hypoglycemic is shown in Table 3 *(6)*. We routinely initiate the 72-h fast in the outpatient setting after an overnight fast. Forty percent of our patients have had positive fasts by the end of the business day; the remaining patients were admitted for completion of the 72-h fast *(68)*.

Mixed Meal Test

For persons with a history of neuroglycopenic, symptoms within 5 h of food ingestion, a mixed meal test may be conducted. Unfortunately, there are no standards for the interpretation of this procedure. Patients should eat a meal that is similar to that which has led to symptoms during ordinary life activities. The test is considered to be positive should the patient experience neuroglycopenic symptoms when a concomitant serum glucose is low, for example, 50 mg/dL or

Table 3

Diagnostic Interpretation of the Results of a Prolonged (72-h) Fast[a]

Diagnostic interpretation or signs	*Symptoms*	*Glucose[b] (mg/dL)*	*Insulin[c] (µU/mL)*	*C-Peptide[c,d] (pmol/L)*	*Proinsulin[c,e] (pmol/L)*	*b-OH-butyrate (mmol/L)*	*Change in glucose[f] (mg/dL)*	*Sulfonylurea in Serum*
Normal	No	40	<3[g]	<200	<5	>2.7	<25	No
Insulinoma	Yes	45	3[h]	200	5	2.7	25	No
Factitious hypoglycemia from insulin	Yes	45	3[i]	<200	<5	2.7	25	No
Sulfonylurea-induced hypoglycemia	Yes	45	3	200	5	2.7	25	Yes
Hypoglycemia mediated by insulinlike growth factor	Yes	45	3	<200	<5	2.7	25	No
Non-insulin-mediated hypoglycemia	Yes	45	<3	<200	<5	>2.7	<25	No
Inadvertent feeding during the fast	No	45	<3	<200	<5	2.7	25	No
Nonhypoglycemic disorder	Yes	40	<3	<200	<5	>2.7	<25	No

[a] Measurements are made at the point the decision is made to end the fast.

[b] Sequential serum glucose measurements in the hypoglycemic range fluctuate. Serum glucose levels 45 mg/dL at the time a decision is made to end the fast may rise to as much as 56 mg/dL when the fast is actually ended approx 1 h later. Serum glucose levels may be as low as 40 mg/dL during prolonged fasting in normal women.

[c] In normal subjects serum insulin, C-peptide, and proinsulin levels may be higher if the serum glucose level is >60 mg/dL.

[d] Measured by the immunochemiluminometric technique (lower limit of detection, 33 pmol/L).

[e] Measured by the immunochemiluminometric technique (lower limit of detection, 0.2 pmol/L).

[f] In response to intravenous glucagon (peak value minus value at end of fast).

[g] Measured by immunochemiluminometric technique (lower limit of detection, 0.1 µU/mL).

[h] Ratios of insulin to glucose are of no diagnostic value in patients with insulinomas.

[i] Serum insulin levels may be very high (>100 µU/mL or even approx 1000 µU/mL) in factitious hypoglycemia from insulin.

From Service FJ: Hypoglycemic disorders. N Engl J Med 332:1144-1152, 1995; with permission.

lower. There are no standards for the interpretation of levels of β-cell polypeptides measured during this test. However, considering the short half-life of insulin, its level should be suppressed after 5 half-lives (approx 30 min), after peak insulinemia if the serum glucose is low. A positive mixed meal test, in and of itself, does not provide a diagnosis, only biochemical confirmation of the history. Because patients with insulinoma may have neuroglycopenic symptoms after meals, and in some instances only after meals, all patients with a positive mixed meal test should undergo a prolonged (72-h) fast. In those patients with a positive mixed meal test and/or a history of neuroglycopenia postprandially confirmed biochemically and a negative prolonged (72-h) fast, the possibility of non-insulinoma pancreatogenous hypoglycemia syndrome should be considered. These patients should undergo the selective arterial calcium stimulation test. For patients with negative responses to this procedure, other mechanisms to explain the postprandial hypoglycemia should be explored. Glucagon levels should be measured during the mixed meal test to ensure that there was an increase in response to the low serum glucose. Nuclear gastric emptying studies to detect accelerated transit as a cause of postprandial hypoglycemia should be considered, and if found, prokinetic gastrointestinal hormones should be measured. This investigative area of a positive mixed meal test and negative 72-h fast and no evidence for β-cell hyperfunction is somewhat murky and difficult clinically. In the evaluation of such patients, neuroglycopenia, regardless of when it happens, requires intensive evaluation usually carried out through dynamic diagnostic tests. The 5-h oral glucose tolerance test should never be used as a diagnostic test for hypoglycemia, because a substantial percentage of healthy persons may have a serum glucose nadir 50 mg/dL or lower *(73–75)*.

The C-Peptide Suppression Test

The C-peptide suppression test *(76)* may be used to provide additional diagnostic information, especially if data from the prolonged (72-h) fast are not conclusive. This test can also be used as a screening test. When the likelihood of a hypoglycemic disorder is not high, a normal result on this test may preclude the need for a 72-h fast. The C-peptide suppression test is based on the observation that insulin secretion (as measured by levels of C-peptide) is suppressed during hypoglycemia to a lesser degree in persons with insulinomas than in normal persons. Interpretation of the C-peptide suppression test requires normative data appropriately adjusted for the patient's body mass index and age (Fig. 5 and Table 4) *(77)*.

At one point, there was optimism that the C-peptide suppression test might replace the prolonged (72-h) fast as the preferred diagnostic test for persons with neuroglycopenia. The C-peptide test has the advantage of being brief (2 h) and not requiring hospitalization. As experience increased, however, this expectation became less sanguine. There are no sensitivity and specificity data regarding

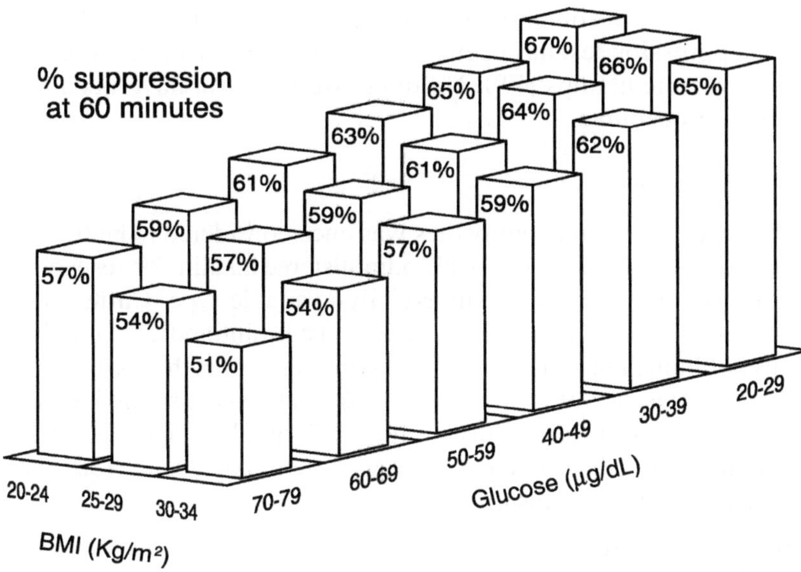

Fig. 5. Normative data for the interpretation of the results of the C-peptide suppression test. Data derived from a study of 101 normal subjects in whom hypoglycemia was induced by the administration of insulin (0.125 U/kg body weight over a period of 60 min). In each body-mass-age subgroup, 95% of the subjects had a level of C-peptide suppression at 60 min that was greater than the value shown. Body mass index (BMI) was calculated as the weight in kilograms divided by the square of the height in meters. From Service FJ, Hypoglycemic Disorder: NEJM 332:1144–1152, 1995.

Table 4
C-peptide Suppression Test

		5th Percentile for percent decrease of C-peptide		
Time	*Age,*		*BMI[a] (kg/m²)*	
60 min	*yr*	*20–24*	*25–29*	*30–34*
	20–29	67	66	65
	30–39	65	64	62
	40–49	63	61	59
	50–59	61	59	57
	60–69	59	57	54
	70–79	57	54	51

[a]BMI, body mass index. An abnormal test is less suppression than shown in the table, e.g., for a person age 55 yr with a BMI of 25–29 kg/m^2. C-peptide suppression (60-min value minus basal value divided by basal value) <59% would be abnormal, but a value 59% would be normal.

the C-peptide test in comparison with the prolonged supervised fast. The C-peptide suppression test has been modified as hyperinsulinemic euglycemic or hypoglycemic clamps *(78)*. No diagnostic criteria have been generated from these procedures.

INSULIN ANTIBODIES

The detection of insulin antibodies was once considered to be firm evidence of factitious hypoglycemia due to self-administered insulin *(79)*, especially when animal insulin was the only commercially available type. Currently, patients with this disorder usually have no detectable insulin antibodies, possibly because of the use of human insulin, which is less antigenic than the form derived from animals. The presence of insulin antibodies has been considered to be the *sine qua non* for a diagnosis of insulin autoimmune hypoglycemia *(19)*, but low titers of antibodies may be detected in persons without hypoglycemia *(80)* and, in rare instance, in patients with insulinomas *(81)*.

GLYCATED HEMOGLOBIN

Glycated hemoglobin concentrations (affinity chromatography) are statistically significantly lower in patients with insulinomas than in control subjects. However, there is too much overlap to provide a diagnostic criterion *(82)* (Fig. 6). Nevertheless, a value 4.1% uniformly was associated with insulinoma, but only 25% of patients with insulioma had values in that range.

IMAGING STUDIES

There has been a consensus among endocrinologists that the diagnosis of a hypoglycemic disorder should be made biochemically. Should the data point to a pancreatic lesion, localization procedures are then undertaken. The success in localization often depends on local skill and experience. Ultrasound is heavily operator-dependent; computed tomography (CT) is technologically dependent, i.e., best results with triple phase technique. Octreoscan has been generally disappointing. Transhepatic portal venous sampling for insulin has been abandoned by major centers. Merging of localization and diagnostic maneuvers has occurred with the development of the selective arterial calcium stimulation test *(83,84)*. Although conducted in the vascular radiology suite and requiring access to various intra-abdominal vessels (e.g., hepatic vein, splenic artery, gastroduodenal artery, and superior mesenteric artery), the test may be viewed as a dynamic biochemical test. A twofold to threefold step up in insulin concentration in response to calcium injection into one or more of the arteries noted above suggests that the region of the pancreas served by that artery harbors abnormal β-cells, either insulinoma or hyperplasia/nesidioblastosis. This may be the dynamic test of choice for the evaluation of hypoglycemia in the patient with chronic renal failure.

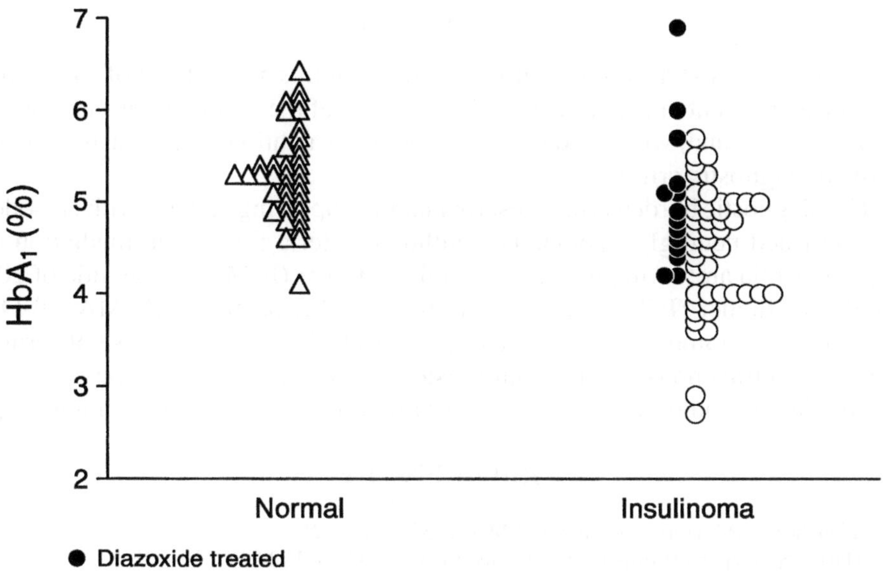

Fig. 6. Glycated hemoglobin measured by boronate affinity chromatography (normal range 4–7%) is significantly lower in patients with insulinoma whether treated with diazoxide than in normal controls. However, there is considerable overlap between the two groups. Nevertheless, no normal subject and 25% of insulinoma patients had glycated hemoglobin values 4.1%. From Hassoun et al., Endocr Pract 4:181–183, 1998.

The Ill-Appearing Patient

In persons with coexisting disease, it may be sufficient to recognize the underlying disease and its association with hypoglycemia and to take action to minimize recurrences of hypoglycemia (Table 1). Confirmation of the suspected mechanism of the hypoglycemia may be sought, such as low insulin and C-peptide levels in ethanol hypoglycemia, elevated insulin-like growth factor II levels in non-β-cell tumor hypoglycemia, low levels of cortisol in adrenal insufficiency, and blunted serum glucose responses to intravenous glucagon in hypoglycemias due to abnormal liver function (e.g., glycogen storage disease, sepsis, and congestive heart failure).

Hospitalized patients are often severely ill persons with multisystem disease. They are at risk for iatrogenic hypoglycemias (insulin added to total parenteral nutrition), as well as for any hypoglycemia that may be produced by the underlying disease. In determining the cause of hypoglycemia in a hospitalized, seriously ill patient, a diligent examination of the record may be more profitable than examination of the patient.

CONCLUSION

The diagnosis of a hypoglycemic disorder requires a high level of suspicion, careful assessment of the patient for the presence of mediating drugs or a predisposing illness, and, where indicated, methodic evaluation on the basis of well-defined diagnostic criteria.

The diagnostic burden is heaviest for healthy appearing persons with episodes of confirmed neuroglycopenia. The author's criteria for insulin mediation of hypoglycemia are: serum insulin 3 μU/mL or higher (ICMA), C-peptide of 200 pmol/L or higher (ICMA), proinsulin of 5 pmol/L or higher (ICMA), β-OH butyrate of 2.7 mmol/L or lower, and generous (25 mg/dL) response of serum glucose to intravenous glucagon administered when the patient is hypoglycemic. Sulfonylurea should be sought in the serum of any hypoglycemic patient.

REFERENCES

1. Wauchope GM. Hypoglycemia. Q J Med 1933;2:117–125.
2. Harris S. Hyperinsulinism and dysinsulinism. JAMA 1924;83:729–733.
3. Wilder RM, Allan RN, Power MH, et al. Carcinoma of the islands of the pancreas: hyperinsulinism and hypoglycemia. JAMA 1927;89:348–355.
4. Howland G, Campbell WR, Maltby EJ, et al. Dysinsulinism: convulsions and coma due to islet cell tumor of pancreas, with operation and cure. JAMA 1929;93:674.
5. Yalow RS, Berson SA. Immunoassay of endogenous plasma insulin in man. J Clin Invest 1960;39:1157.
6. Service FJ: Hypoglycemic Disorders. N Engl J Med 1995;332:1144–1152.
7. Madison LL. Ethanol-induced hypoglycemia. Adv Metab Disord 1968;3:85–109.
8. Hecht A, Goldner MG. Reappraisal of the hypoglycemic action of acetyl-salicylate. Metabolism 1959;8:418–428.
9. Limburg PJ, Katz H, Grant CS, et al. Quinine-induced hypoglycemia. Ann Intern Med 1993;119:218.
10. Kojak G Jr, Barry MJ Jr, Gastineau CF. Severe hypoglycemic reaction with haloperidol: report of a case. Am J Psychiatry 1969;126:573–576.
11. Service FJ, McMahon MM, O'Brien PC, et al. Functioning insulinoma—incidence, recurrence, and long-term survival of patients: a 60-year study. Mayo Clin Proc 1991;66:711–719.
12. Thomas PM, Cote GJ. Persistent hyperinsulinemic hypoglycemia of infancy. In: Arnold, A, ed. Endocrine Neoplasms. Kluwer Academic Publishers, Norwell, MA, 1997, pp. 348–363.
13. Service FJ, Natt N, Thompson GB, et al. Noninsulinoma pancreatogenous hypoglycemia: a novel syndrome of hyperinsulinemic hypoglycemia in adults independent of mutations in Kir6.2 and SUR1 genes. J Clin Endocrinol Metab 1999;84:1582–1589.
14. Thompson GB, Service FJ, Andrews JC, et al. Noninsulinoma pancreatogenous hypoglycemia syndrome: an update in 10 surgically treated patients. Surgery 2000;128:937–945.
15. Service FJ. Factitial hypoglycemia. Endocrinologist 1992;2:173–176.
16. Natt N, Service FJ. The highway to insulinoma: road signs and hazards. Endocrinologist 1997;7:89–96.
17. Felig P, Cherif A, Minagawa A, et al. Hypoglycemia during prolonged exercise in normal men. N Engl J Med 1982;306:895–900.
18. Kogut MD, Blaskovics M, Donnell GN. Idiopathic hypoglycemia: a study of twenty-six children. J Pediatr 1969;74:853–871.

19. Archambeaud-Mouveroux F, Huc MC, Nadalon S, Fournier MP, Conivet B. Autoimmune insulin syndrome. Biomed Pharmacother 1989;43:581–586.
20. Ahlquist DA, Nelson RL, Callaway CW. Pseudoinsulinoma syndrome from inadvertent tolazamide ingestion. Ann Intern Med 1980;93:281–282.
21. Miller DR, Orson J, Watson D. UpJohn, down glucose. N Engl J Med 1977;297:339.
22. Sketris I, Wheeler D, York S. Hypoglycemic coma induced by inadvertent administration of glyburide. Drug Intell Clin Pharm 1984;18:142–143.
23. Nappi JM, Dhanani S, Lovejoy JR, et al. Severe hypoglycemia associated with disopyramide. West J Med 1983;138:95–97.
24. Nelson RL. Drug induced hypoglycemias. In: Service FJ, ed. Hypoglycemic Disorders: Pathogenesis, Diagnosis and Treatment. G.K. Hall, Boston, 1983, pp. 97–109.
25. Billington D, Osmundsen H, Sherratt H. Mechanisms of the metabolic disturbances caused by hypoglycin and by pent-4-enoic acid: in vitro studies. Biochem Pharmacol 1978;27:2879–2890.
26. Morbidity and Mortality Weekly Report. Toxic hypoglycemic syndrome—Jamaica, 1989-1991. MMWR 1992;41:53–55.
27. Bouchard PH, Sai P, Reach G, et al. Diabetes mellitus following pentamidine-induced hypoglycemia in humans. Diabetes 1982;31:40–45.
28. Arem R, Garber AJ, Field JB. Sulfonamide-induced hypoglycemia in chronic renal failure. Arch Intern Med 1983;143:827–829.
29. Almirall J, Montoliu J, Torras A. Propoxyphene-induced hypoglycemia in a patient with chronic renal failure. Nephron 1989;53:273–275.
30. White NJ, Warrell DA, Chanthavanich P, et al. Severe hypoglycemia and hyperinsulinemia in falciparum malaria. N Engl J Med 1983;309:61–66.
31. Phillips RE, Looareesuwan S, White NJ, et al. Hypoglycaemia and antimalarial drugs: quinine and release of insulin. BMJ 1986;292:1319–1321.
32. Raschke R, Arnold-Capell PA, Richeson R, et al. Refractory hypoglycemia secondary to topical salicylate intoxication. Arch Intern Med 1991;151:591–593.
33. Collins JE, Leonard JV, Teale D, et al. Hyperinsulinaemic hypoglycaemia in small for dates babies. Arch Dis Child 1990;65:1118–1120.
34. Cohen MM Jr, Gorlin RJ, Feingold M, et al. The Beckwith-Weidemann syndrome: seven new cases. Am J Dis Child 1971;122:515–519.
35. Barrett CT, Oliver TK Jr. Hypoglycemia and hyperinsulinism in infants with erythroblastosis fetalis. N Engl J Med 1968;278:1260–1263.
36. Pedersen J, Bojsen-Møller B, Poulsen J. Blood sugar in newborn infants of diabetic mothers. Acta Endocrinol 1954;15:33–52.
37. Talente GM, Coleman RA, Alter C, et al. Glycogen storage disease in adults. Ann Intern Med 1994;120:218–226.
38. Søvik O. Inborn errors of amino acid and fatty acid metabolism with hypoglycemia as a major clinical manifestation. Acta Paediatr Scand 1989;78:161–170.
39. Glasgow AM, Cotton RB, Dhiensiri K. Reye syndrome. III. The hypoglycemia. Am J Dis Child 1973;125:809–811.
40. Benzing G III, Schubert W, Sug G, et al. Simultaneous hypoglycemia and acute congestive heart failure. Circulation 1969;40:209–216.
41. Zimmerman BR. Hypoglycemia from hepatic, renal and endocrine disorders. In: Service FJ, ed. Hypoglycemia: Pathogenesis, Diagnosis, and Treatment. G.K. Hall, Boston, 1983.
42. Merimee TJ, Felig P, Marliss E, et al. Glucose and lipid homeostasis in the absence of human growth hormone. J Clin Invest 1971;50:574–582.
43. Ooi TC, Holdaway IM, Donald RA. Isolated ACTH deficiency confirmed by ACTH radioimmunoassay. J Endocrinol Invest 1980;3:45–49.
44. Segal S. Disorders of galactose metabolism. In: Stanbury JB, Wyngaarden JB, Frederickson DS, et al. eds. The Metabolic Basis of Inherited Disease, ed. 5. McGraw Hill, New York. 1983, pp. 167–191.

45. Froesch ER. Essential fructosuria and hereditary fructose intolerance. In Stanbury JB, Wyngaarden JB, Frederickson DS, et al. eds. The Metabolic Basis of Inherited Disease. McGraw-Hill, New York, 1978, pp. 121–136.
46. Treem WR, Stanley CA, Finegold DN, et al. Primary carnitine deficiency due to a failure of carnitine transport in kidney, muscle, and fibroblasts. N Engl J Med 1988;319:1331–1336.
47. De Vivo DC, Trifiletti RR, Jacobson RI, et al. Defective glucose transport across the blood-brain barrier as a cause of persistent hypoglycorrhachia, seizures, and developmental delay. N Engl J Med 1991;325:703–709.
48. Bruce AK, Jacobsen E, Dossing H, Kondrup J. Hypoglycaemia in spinal muscular atrophy. Lancet 1995;346:609.
49. Felig P, Brown WV, Levine RA, et al. Glucose homeostasis in viral hepatitis. N Engl J Med 1970;283:1436–1440.
50. Daughaday WH. Hypoglycemia in patients with non-islet cell tumors. Endocrinol Metab Clin North Am 1989;18:91–101.
51. Miller SI, Wallace RJ Jr, Musher DM, et al. Hypoglycemia as a manifestation of sepsis. Am J Med 1980;68:649–654.
52. Garber AJ, Bier DM, Cryer PE, et al. Hypoglycemia in compensated chronic renal insufficiency: substrate limitation of gluconeogenesis. Diabetes 1974;23:982–986.
53. Block MB, Gambetta M, Resnekov L. Spontaneous hypoglycaemia in congestive heart-failure. Lancet 1972;2:736–738.
54. Heinig RE, Clarke EF, Waterhouse C. Lactic acidosis and liver disease. Arch Intern Med 1979;139:1229–1232.
55. Heard CRC. The effect of protein-energy malnutrition on blood glucose homeostasis. World Rev Nutr Diet 1978;30:107–147.
56. Rich LM, Caine MR, Findling JW, et al. Hypoglycemic coma in anorexia nervosa: case report and review of the literature. Arch Intern Med 1990;150:894–895.
57. Levin H, Heifetz M. Phaeochromocytoma and severe protracted postoperative hypoglycaemia. Can J Anaesth 1990;37:477–478.
58. Service FJ. Hypoglycemia including hypoglycemia in neonates and children. In: DeGroot LJ, ed. Endocrinology, 3rd ed. W.B. Saunders, Philadelphia, 1995, pp. 1605–1623.
59. Fischer KF, Lees JA, Newman JH. Hypoglycemia in hospitalized patients: causes and outcomes. N Engl J Med 1986;315:1245–1250.
60. Johansson C, Adamsson U, Stierner U, et al. Interaction by cholestyramine on the uptake of hydrocortisone in the gastrointestinal tract. Acta Med Scand 1978;204:509–512.
61. Goodenow TJ, Malarkey WB. Leukocytosis and artifactual hypoglycemia. JAMA 1977;237:1961–1962.
62. Macaron CI, Kadri A, Macaron Z. Nucleated red blood cells and artifactual hypoglycemia. Diabetes Care 1981;4:113–115.
63. Service FJ, Veneziale CM, Nelson RA, et al. Combined deficiency of glucose-6-phosphate and fructose-1,6-diphosphate: studies of glucagon secretion and fuel utilization. Am J Med 1978;64:698–706.
64. Whipple AE. The surgical therapy of hyperinsulinism. J Int Chir 1938;3:237–276.
65. American Diabetes Association. Consensus statement on self-monitoring of blood glucose. Diabetes Care 1987;10:95–99.
66. Hirshberg B, Livi A, Bartlett DL, et al. Forty-eight-h fast: the diagnostic test for insulinoma. J Clin Endocrinol Metab 2000;85:3222–3226.
67. Merimee TJ, Fineberg SE. Homeostasis during fasting II. Hormone substrate differences between men and women. J Clin Endocrinol Metab 1973;37:698–702.
68. Service FJ, Natt N. Clinical perspective: the prolonged fast. J Clin Endocrinol Metab 2000;85:3973–3974.

69. Service FJ, O'Brien PC, McMahon MM, Kao PC. C-peptide during the prolonged fast in insulinoma. J Clin Endocrinol Metab 1993;76:655–659.
70. Lebowitz MR, Blumenthal SA. The molar ratio of insulin to C-peptide. An aid to the diagnosis of hypoglycemia due to surreptitious (or inadvertent) insulin administration. Arch Intern Med 1993;153:650–655.
71. Kao PC, Taylor RL, Service FJ. Proinsulin by immunochemiluminometric assay for the diagnosis of insulinoma. J Clin Endocrinol Metab 1994;78:1046–1051.
72. O'Brien T, O'Brien PC, Service FJ. Insulin surrogates in insulinoma. J Clin Endocrinol Metab 1993;77:448–451.
73. Andreani D, Marks V, LeFebvre PJ, eds. Hypoglycemia. Vol. 38 of Serono symposia publications. Raven Press, New York, 1987:312.
74. Hogan MJ, Service FJ, Sharbrough FW, et al. Oral glucose tolerance test compared with a mixed meal in the diagnosis of reactive hypoglycemia; a caveat on stimulation. Mayo Clin Proc 1983;58:491–496.
75. Lev-Ran A, Anderson RW. The diagnosis of postprandial hypoglycemia. Diabetes 1981;30:996–999.
76. Service FJ, Horwitz DL, Rubenstein AH, et al. C-peptide suppression test for insulinoma. J Lab Clin Med 1977;90:180–186.
77. Service FJ, O'Brien PC, Kao PC, Young WF Jr. C-peptide suppression test: effects of gender, age and body mass index: implications for the diagnosis of insulinoma. J Clin Endocrinol Metab 1992;74:204–210.
78. Yki-Jarvinen H, Pelkonen R, Koivisto A. Failure to suppress C-peptide secretion by euglycemic hyperinsulinemia: a new diagnostic test for insulinoma? Clin Endocrinol 1985;23:461–466.
79. Service FJ, Palumbo PJ. Factitial hypoglycemia: three cases diagnosed on the basis of insulin antibodies. Arch Intern Med 1974;134:336–340.
80. Takei M. Insulin autoantibodies produced by methimazole treatment in patients with Graves' disease. J Tokyo Wom Med Coll 1980;50:54–68.
81. Fushimi H, Tsukuda S, Hanafusa T, et al. A case of insulin autoimmune syndrome associated with small insulinomas and rheumatoid arthritis. Endocrinol Jpn 1980;27:679–687.
82. Hassoun AAK, Service FJ, O'Brien PC. Glycated hemoglobin in insulinoma. Endocrine Practice 1998;(4)4:181–183.
83. Doppman JL, Miller DL, Chang R, et al. Insulinomas: localization with selective intra-arterial injection of calcium. Radiology 1991;178:237–241. [Erratum, Radiology 1993;187:880.]
84. Oshea D, Rohrer-Thens W, Lynn JA, et al: Localization of insulinomas by selective ultra-arterial calcium injection. J Clin Endocrinol Metab 1996;81:1623–1627.

11 The Evaluation of Dyslipidemia and Obesity

William T. Donahoo, MD, Elizabeth Stephens, MD, and Robert H. Eckel, MD

CONTENTS

LIPIDS

Fasting Lipid Panel

Lipids, including cholesterol triglyceride (TG) and phospholipids, are essential components of life functioning in membranes, as second messengers, and as a major source of energy. Their physical properties (i.e., their lipophilicity or hydrophobicity) are in part what suit them for this role. However, due to this hydrophobicity, lipids are not soluble in the aqueous environment of the plasma. Therefore, lipids must be carried in lipoprotein particles that allow for the hydrophobic components to be protected from the hydrophilic plasma. In addition, the lipoprotein particles contain surface proteins that target them for metabolism or uptake. Figure 1 is an overview of the metabolism of lipoprotein particles (see ref. *1* for a review of lipoprotein metabolism). There are two general pathways of lipid metabolism, one involving chylomicrons absorbed from the intestine and the other starting with very low density lipoprotein (VLDL) from the liver. In the first or exogenous pathway, chylomicrons, which are large (75–1200 nm) TG-rich (>80% TG and <10% cholesterol) particles, are produced through intestinal absorption of lipids. Chylomicrons include apolipo-proteins B48, C1, C2, C3, and E. They are catabolized by lipoprotein lipase in peripheral tissues yielding fatty acids for the tissues and forming chylomicron remnant lipoproteins, which are taken up by the liver. In the second (endogenous) pathway, the liver produces VLDL particles that are also large (30–80 nm) and TG rich (approx 50% TG and 20% cholesterol). VLDL contains apolipoproteins

From: *Contemporary Endocrinology: Handbook of Diagnostic Endocrinology*
Edited by: J. E. Hall and L. K. Nieman

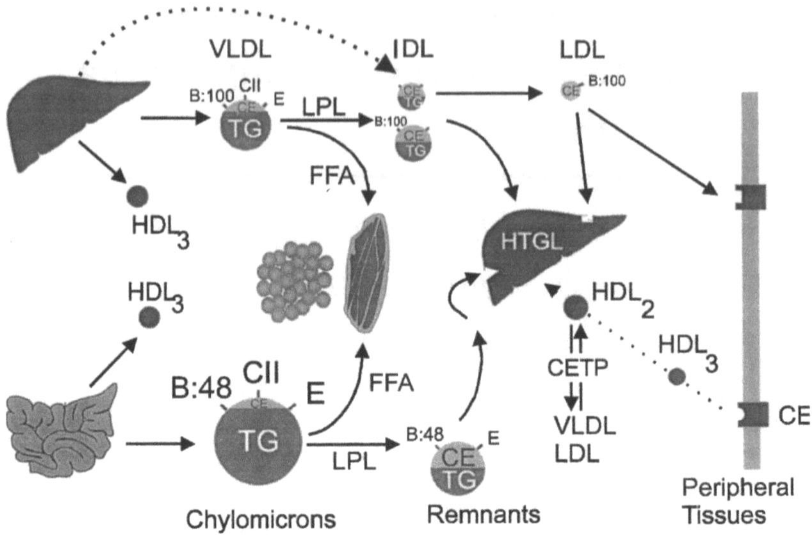

Fig. 1. Lipoprotein metabolism

B100, C1, C2, C3, and E. VLDL are also acted upon by lipoprotein lipase forming free fatty acids for peripheral tissues and VLDL remnants. Intermediate density lipoproteins (IDL) are also produced by the liver but are limited in concentration, are somewhat smaller (25–35 nm), and contain less TG and more cholesterol (approx 30% TG and approx 30% cholesterol). IDL have the same apolipoproteins as VLDL. VLDL remnants and IDL are further catabolized to form LDL, a small (18–25 nm) cholesterol-rich (<10% TG, approx 45% cholesterol) particle, which is the major cholesterol carrier in the blood. The only apolipoprotein in LDL is apoB100. LDL is taken up by the liver and peripheral tissues through a receptor-mediated mechanism. However, LDL can also be oxidized and taken up by macrophages in the vascular wall, initiating the cascade leading to an atherosclerotic plaque.

A final lipoprotein pathway is that of high density lipoprotein (HDL). HDL is secreted as a discoid particle by the liver and small intestine. Nascent HDL picks up free cholesterol secreted from cells via the ABC A1 cassette to become HDL_3, which is small (5–12 nm) and contains primarily cholesterol (<10% TG and approx 30% cholesterol). HDL always contains apolipoprotein A1, but, variably, can contain apolipoproteins A2, C1, C2, C3, and E as well. Through cholesterol ester transfer protein, HDL_3 acquires cholesterol from the peripheral tissues forming HDL_2. HDL_2 then returns to the liver, likely providing a means for "reverse cholesterol transport" back to the liver and presumably imparting the protective effects of HDL.

Epidemiological data have shown a correlation between increased cholesterol and increased risk of cardiovascular disease (CVD) *(2)*. Additionally, several well-designed studies have shown decreases in both cardiovascular morbidity and total mortality with lowering of LDL-cholesterol (LDL-C) by diet and medications *(3–9)*. Therefore, a working knowledge of how to assess cholesterol abnormalities is essential in clinical medicine due to the proven benefit of treating such abnormalities.

Current recommendations for screening and treatment of lipid disorders are based on National Cholesterol Education Program (NCEP) guidelines. Presently, it is recommended that adults 20 yr old have a fasting lipid panel obtained every 5 yr. Case finding may be considered more frequently in those with a history of vascular disease, pancreatitis, renal disease, or liver disease. Treatment is based on a goal LDL-C, and this varies by risk for CVD.

Current cardiovascular risk factors (exclusive of LDL-C) that modify LDL goals are:

1. Age (male 45 yr, female >55 yr).
2. Family history (coronary heart disease [CHD] in male first degree relative 55 yr or female first degree relative 65 yr).
3. Current cigarette smoking.
4. Hypertension (HTN) (blood pressure [BP] 140/90 or on antihypertensive medications).
5. Low HDL-cholesterol (HDL-C) (40 mg/dL) (Note: HDL-C 60 mg/dL is a negative risk factor).

In order to eliminate postprandial lipoproteins, the duration of the fast prior to drawing a fasting lipoprotein analysis should be 9–12 h *(10)*. The analysis of the fasting lipid panel begins with the measurement of total cholesterol by an enzymatic method *(11)*. Then, apoB containing lipoproteins (non-HDL-C) are precipitated by a variety of means including Mg^{+2}, phosphotungstate, or heparin-Mn^{+2} *(12)*. Finally, cholesterol (now only HDL-C) is measured again using the same method described above. Alternatively, HDL-C can be measured following ultracentrifugal separation *(12)*.

Total TG are measured in whole plasma. This is usually done using a multistep process that first hydrolyzes TG to free fatty acids and glycerol, then the glycerol is measured using several additional steps *(13)*. The addition of a lipase is the method presently most often used to hydrolyze TG into free fatty acids and glycerol. However, at least 14 other methods have been developed for the measurements of TG. These methods differ in the means of hydrolysis of fatty acids from glycerol or in the steps used to measure glycerol *(14)*.

Several assumptions are inherent in the measurement of a lipid panel. First, it is assumed that cholesterol is carried in fasting plasma by only three particles: VLDL-C, LDL-C, and HDL-C. However when TG are very elevated (>1000 mg/dL), some cholesterol is carried by chylomicrons, which are nearly always present *(15)*. Additionally, chylomicrons can even be present in fasted patients

Table 1
Goal LDL-C Based on Non-LDL Cardiovascular Risk Factors

Number of risk factors	*Goal LDL-C*
0–1	160 mg/dL
2 and 10-yr risk <20% [a]	130 mg/dL
CHD, other atherosclerotic disease, diabetes, or a 10-yr risk >20%[a]	100 mg/dL

[a]See Table 2 for calculation of 10-yr risk.

with TG >400 mg/dL, thus invalidating the assumptions described above *(16)*. Finally, when TG are <400 mg/dL, the mass ratio of TG to VLDL-C is 5:1 (or 2.2:1 on a molar basis), so that VLDL-C can be calculated by dividing the serum TG by 5. This is the basis for the Friedewald formula *(17)*, whereby LDL-C is calculated (e.g., LDL-C = total cholesterol –(TG/5)–HDL-C). Thus, this formula only holds when the TG are <400 mg/dL.

However, there are data to suggest that a calculated LDL-C may not adequately reflect the measured LDL-C in some patient groups, including type 2 diabetes mellitus *(18)*, type 1 diabetes *(19)*, and alcoholics with liver disease *(20)*. These are all conditions in which IDL might be present, even in fasting serum with TG <400 mg/dL. Indeed, there is a direct relation between the amount of IDL and the error in calculating LDL-C by the Friedewald formula *(21)*.

LDL-C calculation is usually adequate for initial risk assessment using NCEP guidelines *(10)*. Figure 2 is a description of the evaluation of dyslipidemia using NCEP guidelines, but also incorporating additional laboratory testing when appropriate. The initial evaluation using the left 2 branch points on Fig. 2 follow NCEP guidelines.

The current goal LDL-C is based on the number of risk factors above (see Table 1). Those with coronary artery disease, other clinical forms of atherosclerotic disease (peripheral arterial disease, abdominal aortic aneurysm, symptomatic carotid artery disease), diabetes, or multiple risk factors that confer a 10-yr risk for CHD >20% are at the highest risk, and should be treated to an LDL-C 100 mg/dL

To determine if someone has a 10-yr risk for CHD >20%, a point scoring system derived from the Framingham cohort is used. This calculation only needs to be done if there are no other high risk diseases present (which would automatically set the LDL-C goal at <100 mg/dL), and if there are 2 risk factors described above. This calculation can be done using a handheld PDA. A program using the Palm OS can be downloaded free from the National Institutes of Health (NIH) or using Table 2.

Table 2
Estimated 10-yr Risk Based on Framingham Point Scores

Age

Age (yr)	*Points male*	*Points female*
20–34	–9	–7
35–39	–4	–3
40–44	0	0
45–49	3	3
50–54	6	6
55–59	8	8
60–64	10	10
65–69	11	12
70–74	12	14
75–79	13	16

Total cholesterol

TC	*Sex*	*20–39 yr*	*40–49 yr*	*50–59 yr*	*60–69 yr*	*70–79 yr*
<160	Both	0	0	0	0	0
160–199	Male	4	3	2	1	0
160–199	Female	4	3	2	1	1
200–239	Male	7	5	3	1	0
200–239	Female	8	6	4	2	1
240–279	Male	9	6	4	2	1
240–279	Female	11	8	5	3	2
280	Male	11	8	5	3	1
280	Female	13	10	7	4	2

Tobacco use

Smoker	*Sex*	*20–39 yr*	*40–49 yr*	*50–59 yr*	*60–69 yr*	*70–79 yr*
No	Both	0	0	0	0	0
Yes	Male	8	5	3	1	1
Yes	Female	9	7	4	2	1

HDL-C

HDL (mg/dL)	*Points*
60	–1
50–59	0
40–49	1
<40	2

Systolic blood pressure

Systolic BP (mmHg)	*Sex*	*Untreated*	*Treated*
<120	Both	0	0
120–129	Male	0	1
120–129	Female	1	3
130–139	Male	1	2
130–139	Female	2	4
140–159	Male	1	2
140-159	Female	3	5
160	Male	2	3
160	Female	4	6

(continued)

Table 2
Estimated 10-yr Risk Based on Framingham Point Scores *(continued)*

	10-yr Risk point summary	
Point total	*% Risk male*	*% Risk female*
0	1	<1
1	1	<1
2	1	<1
3	1	<1
4	1	<1
5	2	<1
6	2	<1
7	3	<1
8	4	<1
9	5	1
10	6	1
11	8	1
12	10	1
13	12	2
14	16	2
15	20	3
16	25	4
17	30	5
18	30	6
19	30	8
20	30	11
21	30	14
22	30	17
23	30	22
24	30	27
25	30	30

Those with two or more risk factors and a 10-yr risk for CHD >20% should be treated to an LDL-C <100 mg/dL. Those with two or more risk factors, a 10-yr risk for CHD <20%, and no known CVD should be treated to an LDL-C 130 mg/dL. And, those with no known CVD and <2 risk factors should have an LDL-C <160 mg/dL.

Evaluation Beyond the Fasting Lipid Panel

The fasting lipid panel often is all that is needed to risk-stratify patients, determine cardiovascular risk, and decide if therapy is needed. However, there are cases where additional information is required to help in diagnosis and treatment decisions. The right 2 branch points of Fig. 2 illustrate where additional lipid testing may be indicated. Fig. 2 is designed based on experience in an adult lipid practice, but is generalizable to any adult primary care practice. This flow diagram assumes that secondary causes of hyperlipidemia (medications, diabetes mellitus, hypothyroidism, hepatic disease, and renal disease) have been ruled out or treated

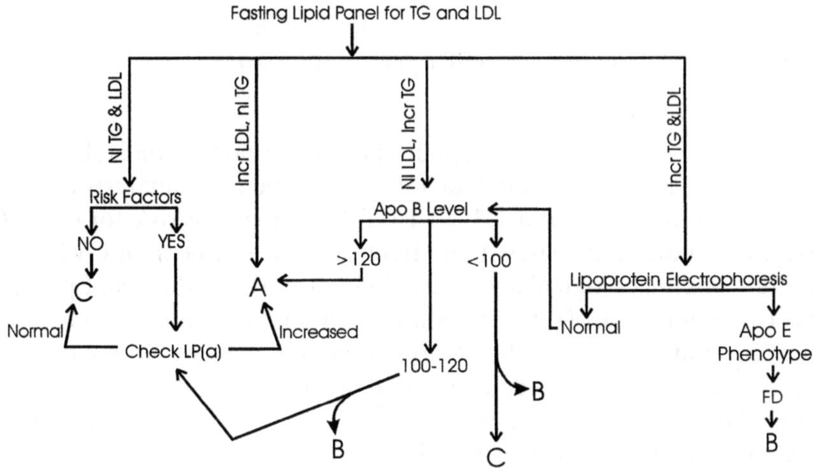

Fig. 2. The figure represents a flow diagram to aid in the assessment of lipoprotein disorders. A fasting lipid panel is used to determine the need for additional work-up. Following the diagram down the left-most arm, when both LDL and TG are normal, an assessment of risk factors is undertaken (see text and Table 2). If risk factors are present, then obtaining a Lp(a) is the next step to further risk-stratify the patient. In the 2nd arm from the left, when LDL alone is increased, then treatment should proceed in accordance with NCEP-Adult Treatment Panel (ATP) II guidelines. In the third arm from the left, when LDL is normal but TG are elevated (but <400 mg/dL, see text), then an apoB will assist in determining if atherogenic particles are present, which would necessitate a different treatment course. In the right-most arm, when elevations in both LDL and TG occur, an evaluation for FD is indicated starting with a lipoprotein electrophoresis and continuing with apoE phenotyping if indicated. Each pathway ends with a treatment recommendation. **(A)** Dietary therapy to decrease dietary fat and cholesterol (American Heart Association Step 1 or Step 2 diet) with progression to drug therapy targeted toward lowering of apoB containing particles (LDL and VLDL). **(B)** Lifestyle therapy to decrease dietary fat, increase activity, and limit ethanol intake, with progression to drug therapy targeted toward lowering of TG (i.e., decreasing VLDL production and/or increasing VLDL and chylomicron catabolism). **(C)** Encouragement of lifestyle modification and routine follow-up of lipids every 2–5 yr.

adequately. These recommendations obviously go beyond the NCEP guidelines, but given the impact of atherosclerotic coronary or vascular disease (CVD) on society and the proven benefit of lipid lowering therapy on morbidity and mortality, such additional evaluation and guidance in therapy can be justified. In Fig. 2, the fasting TG and LDL-C levels dictate which path is followed. For definition, "normal" values are LDL-C <130 mg/dL and TG <150 mg/dL. Although these values are somewhat arbitrary, they are consistent with NCEP guidelines and provide a basis from which to begin analysis. When LDL-C and TG are normal but additional traditional (single) risk factors are present, further lipid evaluation with lipoprotein(a) might be appropriate (see below). If no risk factors are present, routine follow-up yearly or every other year is appropriate.

Lipoprotein(a) Levels

There is extensive evidence to support the use of lipoprotein(a) [Lp(a)] as an additional lipid cardiovascular risk factor *(22)*. In one meta-analysis of 14 studies, elevated Lp(a) imparted a 1.3- to 1.4-fold increase in risk for CVD *(22)*. However, no studies have shown an effect of altering Lp(a) on CVD, in part because few pharmacological agents can lower Lp(a). In addition, Lp(a) levels do not correlate with risk of CVD in some populations, including African-American men *(23)* and the elderly *(24)*. Thus, although the measurement of Lp(a) is not a part of current NCEP guidelines, Lp(a) levels can be used clinically to help determine if therapy (or more aggressive therapy, i.e., further decreases in LDL-C or increases in HDL-C) is warranted.

Lp(a) is a lipoprotein that is covalently attached to the apolipoprotein B component of LDL *(25)*. It has the structure of multiple repeats of a kringle motif *(26)*. Lp(a) likely has a normal physiological role in clotting and wound healing. However, there are numerous ways in which Lp(a) may be playing a role in atherogenesis including: induction of adhesion molecules, induction of monocyte chemotaxis, enhancement of LDL atherogenicity, prothrombosis, and impaired vasodilation *(27)*.

Unfortunately, there are many issues in the measurement of Lp(a). First, there is a variable number of one of the kringle repeats, thus the value can be either overestimated or underestimated when Lp(a) is analyzed by radioimmunoassay *(28)*. Second, the determination of Lp(a) by techniques that involve monoclonal antibodies often lack accuracy if the Lp(a) has been modified by oxidation or removal of carbohydrates *(28)*. Third, although Lp(a) cholesterol levels can be determined, it is not known clinically if the risk from Lp(a) is due to the particle number [and thus proportional to the Lp(a) cholesterol] or to the mass of the Lp(a) itself.

A final method to assess elevations in Lp(a) is by lipoprotein electrophoresis (see the section on Lipoprotein Electrophoresis below). The presence of a sinking pre-β-band often indicates an elevated Lp(a) and has been correlated with increased CVD *(29)*. However, the use of electrophoresis lacks the sensitivity and specificity normally required of such a test *(30)*. Nonetheless, in the almost 1500 patients in our Lipid Clinic, in whom both an Lp(a) value and a lipoprotein electrophoresis were obtained, those with the presence of a sinking pre-β-band had significantly higher Lp(a) levels than those without such a band (25 mg/dL vs 58 mg/dL, $p = 2 \times 10^{-30}$) (Eckel et al. personal observation). In summary, sufficient information exists that Lp(a) is a risk factor for CVD in most populations (except elderly and African-American men) and thus should be considered in the establishment of LDL-C and HDL-C goals.

Apolipoprotein B Levels

In addition to the total amount of cholesterol in LDL and VLDL, there is sufficient evidence that the number of particles present imparts a risk. There is only one apolipoprotein B (apoB) per lipoprotein particle. Lipoproteins that include apoB are VLDL, LDL, IDL, Lp(a), chylomicrons and remnants. In the fasting state, when only VLDL and LDL are present (see discussion above under Fasting Lipid Panel section for exceptions), the amount of apoB correlates well with the number of LDL and VLDL particles. Several studies have shown that elevated apoB levels have an independent correlation with increased risk for CVD *(31–34)*.

ApoB is particularly helpful when TG are elevated and LDL-C is normal. In such patients, there could either be predominately large VLDL-like particles (similar to familial hypertriglyceridemia), where there is low risk for CVD, or predominately smaller LDL particles, where there is a more significant risk for CVD. In the former patients, apoB will be lower (i.e., <100 mg/dL), whereas in the latter, apoB will be elevated (>120 mg/dL). Thus, those with elevated apoB would benefit from LDL and VLDL lowering, while it is questionable if the benefit of treatment directed at apoB (i.e., statins) in those with a low apoB would be worthwhile. This approach has some support from the literature. In an analysis of the Third National Health and Nutrition Examination Survey (NHANES III) database, it was found that in people with LDL-C <130 mg/dL apoB is helpful only when TG are elevated *(35)*. Specifically, less than 2% of people with TG <200 mg/dL had an elevated apoB, whereas almost 30% of people with TG between 200–400 mg/dL had an elevated apoB *(36)*. Additionally, in the Quebec Cardiovascular Study, men who had an elevated apoB had a 3-fold increased risk of CVD *(31)*.

The benefits of using apoB levels in clinical assessment are limited by the lack of standardization with respect to measurements and reference material. ApoB is measured by a variety of methods including: electroimmunoassay, radioimmunoassay (RIA), enzyme-linked immunosorbent assay (ELISA), radial immunodiffusion, immunoturbidimetric assay, and immunonephelometric assay *(36)*. Most currently approved methods use an immunoturbidimetric assay. The coefficient of variance with measurements of apoB can be as high as 30% *(36)*. Additionally, the development of apoB standards has proven to be a challenge. Purified lipid-free apoB has self-self interactions and, thus, is inappropriate for use as a standard, and there are matrix interactions when the standards are lyophilized *(36)*. However, with respect to reference material, a liquid stabilized material has been developed that appears suitable and that has been endorsed for use by the World Health Organization (WHO) *(37)*. The Food and Drug Administration (FDA)'s National Committee For Clinical Laboratory Standards (NCCLS) is currently developing standards for the measurement of apoB. Overall, apoB is a useful measurement for risk assessment in the setting of a normal

LDL-C (i.e., <130 mg/dL) and elevated TG (>200 mg/dL) *(38)*. However, the differences in methodology of laboratories limit the generalizability of this measurement. Finally, most assays do not distinguish between apoB 100 (from LDL, Lp(a), and VLDL particles) and apoB-48 (from chylomicrons). Thus, apoB measurements should not be performed when TG are above 400 mg/dL, because under this circumstance, when chylomicrons may be present, there will be a (variable) contribution of apoB-48 to the measurement, thus making it clinically less interpretable.

Lipoprotein Electrophoresis

The importance of LDL-C to CVD was shown in the laboratory by gel electrophoresis before other measures were available for the determination of LDL-C *(39)*. The present role of separating the major lipoprotein classes by electrophoresis is not used to estimate LDL-C, but rather to identify abnormalities in the distribution of lipoproteins that may distinguish disturbances in IDL and remnant metabolism (i.e., familial dysbetalipoproteinemia (FD) or broad-β disease) from increases in VLDL and LDL *(40)*. In addition, the presence of a sinking pre-β-band by lipoprotein electrophoresis correlates with an Lp(a) as described above.

The purpose for specifically diagnosing FD is threefold. First, people with FD often respond significantly to lifestyle alterations. Second, the preferred pharmacological agents are those that alter VLDL metabolism more than LDL metabolism (i.e., fibric acid derivatives rather than a statins). Thus, knowledge of the diagnosis will help guide therapy. Third, FD is an autosomal recessive genetically inherited disease (unlike most other inherited diseases of lipoprotein metabolism, which are autosomal dominant), and therefore, the knowledge of the diagnosis will help with genetic counseling *(41)*.

Electrophoresis of fasting plasma separates VLDL or pre-β-lipoproteins, LDL or beta-lipoproteins, and HDL or α-lipoproteins *(42)*. Lipoprotein electrophoresis is performed in the following manner: The plasma or serum is ultracentrifuged to separate the VLDL from the LDL and HDL fractions. The tube is then sliced at the interface (density of 1.006), and the fractions are transferred quantitatively to other tubes. The top fraction contains only VLDL, so when cholesterol is measured in the top fraction (known as the β-quant), a true determination of VLDL-C is obtained that bypasses the problems of the Friedewald formula described above. Each fraction is then analyzed by electrophoresis on agarose gel. The lipid bands on the gel are finally visualized by staining with fat red 7B.

When FD is present, there is inadequate clearance of the IDL and remnants, and thus, there is a band between the VLDL and LDL bands (i.e., a beta-VLDL or broad-β-band). As the fasting plasma in patients with FD characteristically has approximately equivalent elevations in both cholesterol and TG, a lipoprotein electrophoresis is recommended only when there is an increase in both LDL-C and TG. Additional information received from the above analysis (the β-quant) allows for the calculation of a VLDL-C to TG ratio. A VLDL-C to TG ratio of >0.3 is suggestive of FD, with a VLDL-C to TG ratio of >0.4 being diagnostic *(43)*. The specific cutoff of LDL-C and TG to maximize the sensitivity and specificity have yet to be determined, but using an LDL-C above 160 mg/dL with TG >200 mg/dL will certainly maximize the sensitivity (although likely at the expense of some specificity). A complete analysis of our database is currently underway, but using the criteria described above in >800 lipoprotein electrophoreses, the yield for FD (as diagnosed by a broad-β-band and apoE phenotyping [see below]) has been about 8%. In a patient with suspected FD, if a broad-β-band is present, the work-up should continue with the assessment of apoE phenotyping.

ApoE Phenotyping

When the lipoprotein electrophoresis reveals a broad-β-band, the diagnosis of FD must be entertained. The next step in the evaluation is apoE genotyping. Apolipoprotein E comes in 3 possible phenotypes, E-2, E-3, and E-4 *(41)*. The E-2/E-2 or E-2/- phenotype (usually in the setting of another etiology for a disturbance in VLDL metabolism, such as diabetes) results in FD and abnormal clearance of remnant particles.

In most laboratories, the apoE polymorphism is determined by isoelectric focusing of serum *(44)*. The apoE isoform bands are detected by Coomassie blue staining *(45)* or by antibodies against human apoE *(46,47)*. There is also an assay to genotypically separate the three isoforms using a specific restriction enzyme, DNA probes, and polymerase chain reaction technology *(48)*.

Lipoprotein Subfractionation

There are data to suggest that not only are the LDL particles atherogenic, but that specific subfractions of LDL have even greater athrogenicity than others *(49)*. Several methods have, therefore, been developed to help differentiate subclasses of particles and help further define cardiovascular risk in patients. These methods include density gradient centrifugation, gradient gel electrophoresis (GGE), liquid chromatography, and proton nuclear magnetic resonance (NMR) spectroscopy. However, the use of these methods at present remains largely a research tool, and their applicability in the clinical setting is still being defined. Thus, determination of particle size is not present in the flow diagram, but has been considered by some to be a partial risk factor to use when other data are equivocal. Several methods used to separate lipoprotein subfractions will be briefly described.

GGE is different than simple lipoprotein electrophoresis described above, in that it better separates particles by both size and electrophoretic charge. The method is accomplished by injecting plasma onto a 2–16% gradient gel, running this over an electrophoretic field, and then visualizing the separated particles with a stain (Sudan black) *(50)*. With GGE, a separation into several LDL peaks can be obtained *(50)*. The typical approach used with GGE is to determine an overall phenotypic pattern of A (less dense LDL and thus less atherogenic) or B (more dense LDL and thus more atherogenic) *(49)*.

High-performance liquid chromatography (HPLC) is another means to separate out lipoprotein subfractions. With HPLC, a sample of plasma is injected onto a column that separates particles based on their size *(51)*. The separated fractions are then collected and can be assayed for cholesterol, TG, or apoproteins. Although the separation of the subfractions of LDL by HPLC is not as complete as with GGE, the dominant LDL fraction (and any changes with therapies) can be determined with HPLC. Additionally, HPLC allows the opportunity for further analysis of the fractions for cholesterol, TG, or apolipoproteins.

The newest method to separate lipoprotein subfractions is by proton NMR spectroscopy. NMR has the advantage that it is much easier and less labor-intensive to perform *(52)*. Additionally, good agreement between NMR and GGE has been shown *(53)*. Specific description of the methods behind NMR spectroscopy of lipoproteins is beyond the scope of this text, therefore, for further information see the review by Otvos et al. *(52)*. Clinically, particle distribution by NMR has been correlated with CVD *(54,55)*. However, at present, few sites have the hardware, software, and technical expertise to appropriately run lipid samples by NMR.

Additional Analysis When Pure Elevations in LDL-C Are Present

In patients with marked elevations of LDL-C (e.g., LDL-C >250 mg/dL) and in whom secondary causes have been ruled out and the other lipid values (TG and HDL-C) are normal, the diagnosis of heterozygous familial hypercholesterolemia (FH), autosomal recessive hypercholesterolemia, β-sitosterolemia, or heterozygous familial defective apolipoprotein-B (FDB) should be entertained. It is worthwhile making this diagnosis for several reasons. Patients homogyzous for FH or FDB do not respond well to standard pharmacotherapy, and it is important to have the diagnosis for genetic counseling. Patients with β-sitosterolemia have an increased intestinal absorption of phytosterols (plant sterols) and shellfish sterols, and thus are treated by dietary intervention.

FH can be diagnosed by measurement of LDL receptor activity on cultured skin fibroblasts *(56)*. Additionally, FH or FDB can be diagnosed by DNA haplotype analysis *(57)*. Other methods are also available to diagnose FDB, including heteroduplex analysis, single-strand conformation polymorphism, and denaturing gradient gel electrophoresis *(58)*. Obviously, these are highly specialized methods performed in a few specialized laboratories.

OBESITY

The purpose for assessing excess weight is threefold. First, mortality risk increases with increasing body fat *(59–61)*, and thus, overweight and obesity is determined as a means to evaluate a patient's overall mortality risk. Second, numerous diseases are caused or worsened by overweight or obesity. These include diabetes, dyslipidemia and CVD, hypertension, menstrual irregularities and polycystic ovarian syndrome, osteoarthritis, some cancers, obstructive sleep apnea, and gout *(62)*. And third, determining the degree of excess body fat will help in assessing the risk of, appropriate screening for, and adequate treatment of these diseases. Methods for the determination of obesity and body composition are described below. For a review of the evaluation and treatment of overweight and obesity, the reader is referred to the National Institutes of Health guidelines *(62)* or the Canadian Task Force *(63)*.

Height and Weight

The beginning of the assessment of obesity is simply weight and height. As with lipids, where the fasting lipid panel was often the end to assessment of lipid disorders, height and weight are often all that is needed to adequately assess obesity. It is interesting to note that life insurance companies have had data linking increased weight to mortality for almost a century *(64,65)*. From this actuarial data, the Metropolitan Life Insurance Company developed height–weight tables to determine ideal body weight *(64)*. However, the tables are cumbersome and have adjustments for frame size that are of questionable importance. The recommended test for the determination of obesity has become the body mass index (BMI). Of note, the BMI correlates very highly ($r^2 = 0.992–0.999$) with the Metropolitan Life tables *(67)*, but yields a single number that is much easier to interpret and act upon.

The BMI (or Quetelet index) is calculated as the weight in kg divided by the square of the height in m (i.e., kg/m^2). Those with a BMI <18.5 kg/m^2 are classified as underweight, a BMI between 18.5–24.9 kg/m^2 normal, a BMI between 25–29.9 kg/m^2 overweight, and a BMI >30 kg/m^2 obese, and a BMI >40 kg/m^2 extreme obesity *(62)*.

BMI has been shown to correlate with other measures of body fat. BMI explains between 25–55% of the variance in percent body fat *(68–71)*. However BMI predicts between 60–85% of the variance in fat weight *(68,70)*. Using the criteria of obesity being >20% body fat in men and >25% body fat in women, BMI has a sensitivity between 13–55%, but a specificity of 92–100% *(70,72,73)*. In the diagnosis of those with extreme obesity (those who are at extreme risk from their obesity and in whom surgical therapy may be an appropriate option, as defined as body fat >45%), a BMI of >45 kg/m^2 has a sensitivity of 55% with a specificity of 82% *(67)*.

Despite this relatively poor sensitivity, increased BMI correlates well with increased risk of medical complications, including increased risk of overall mortality *(59–61)*. Additionally, the chance of having cardiovascular risk factors, including hypertension, dyslipidemia, and diabetes, all increase with increasing BMI *(74,75)*. Even without risk factors at baseline, an increased BMI is associated with increased risk of CVD *(76,77)*.

Looking at mortality data such as that from the Nurses Health *(77)* or the Cancer Prevention Studies *(60,61)*, the reasoning behind the BMI cutoff points becomes evident. Although there is a slight increase in the relative risk of death between a BMI of 20–25 kg/m^2, the risk increases more between 25–30 kg/m^2, and rises even more dramatically above a BMI of 30 kg/m^2. Therefore, the NIH and WHO have defined normal weight as a BMI <25 kg/m^2, overweight as a BMI between 25–30 kg/m^2, and obesity as a BMI >30 kg/m^2.

Body Composition

The health risks associated with obesity are primarily due to excess fat. Currently, there are a number of differing techniques available to assess body composition which can be grouped broadly into three categories: anthropomorphic methods, two-compartment model methods, and multicompartment model methods. Each has certain advantages and disadvantages, differences in accuracy and precision, and issues in practicality that will be discussed below.

Anthropometric Methods

Anthropometric methods include weight and height measures (BMI, see above), circumferences (see below), and skinfold measurements. While these techniques are limited in their ability to estimate abdominal or visceral body fat, they do correlate with risk factors for diabetes and CVD and are advocated as proxy measures for public health initiatives *(78)*. Importantly, these methods are easy to perform in the clinical setting and do not require extensive equipment or testing.

Skinfold Thickness

Measurement of skinfold thickness is one anthropometric technique used to estimate the amount of body fat. With this method, specially designed calipers are used to measure subcutaneous fat in specific locations, most commonly the triceps, biceps, subscapular and suprailiac regions. Because 70–90%of total adipose tissue is subcutaneous, skin fold thickness can be used to grade or predict total body fat *(79)*. These values can then be compared to grouped values or norms, or can be incorporated into specific equations that can predict body density, total body fat mass, or percent body fat. When proper measurement technique is applied these equations can predict body fat with errors between 3.5–5% *(80)*. Problems with this technique include variability between procedure performed and caliper type used, variability between observers, and difficulty with obese patients being too large for the caliper.

Multicompartmental Models

To increase the accuracy of measuring body composition, multicompartmental models have been developed. The two-compartment model for the evaluation of body composition is based on the presumption that the body is composed of two components: fat mass (FM) and fat-free mass (FFM). With these methods, the composition of FFM is presumed to be constant among individuals in terms of density, levels of potassium, and total body water, which has been observed in older autopsy series *(81)*. With these assumptions, the described parameters are evaluated and incorporated into equations to determine separate measures of body composition. Examples of two-compartment model techniques include underwater weighing, bioelectrical impedance, assessment of total body water, and assessment of total body potassium.

Underwater Weighing

Underwater weighing is a procedure to determine body density based on the Archimedian principle that a solid object submerged in water is subject to a buoyant force that is equal to the weight of the water displaced by the object or the loss in weight of the object when it is weighed while submerged in the water *(82)*. Thus, body density can be calculated by dividing body mass by vol, with vol determined by the amount of water displaced by an individual, or by the difference between water weight and air weight, after making corrections for the vol of air in the lungs and the gut. Once density is determined, equations can be used to estimate the corresponding degree of body fat. Prior to the development of multicompartmental model techniques, this procedure was considered by some to be the gold standard for the determination of body composition and was frequently utilized for the determination of body composition in research studies. However, while reproducible and fairly easy to perform, this procedure is often difficult for patients to tolerate due to the required submersion, respiratory problems associated with obesity, and the tendency for obese subjects to float and therefore require weight belts in order to be submerged.

Bioelectric Impedence Analysis

Bioelectric impedence analysis (BIA) utilizes the conductance of current by tissues, specifically the electrolytes in body water to estimate the amounts of FM and FFM. The amount of current conducted depends on the quantity of water present and is, therefore, proportional to total body water, which is only present in FFM not adipocytes. Most commonly, a high-frequency low amplitude electric current is administered (typically 50 kHz), with the change in voltage due to resistance measured between a proximal and distal electrode. Prediction equations can then be used to convert the measured impedance into an estimate of body composition from previous comparisons with isotope dilution studies *(78)*. Traditionally, the electrodes had been placed on the right ankle and hand, although newer machines allow individuals to stand on two metal plates while the machine measures impedance from foot to foot. Portable BIA devices are now available, making it a more attractive and practical alternative for the evaluation of body composition. However, the specific prediction equation utilized and hydration status of the patient, which may be elevated in the obese, can significantly impact the accuracy of this tool. A final limitation to BIA is due to differences in cross-sectional area. The current is most affected by those parts of the body that have the highest resistance (e.g., the limbs); however, these segments do not contribute nearly as much to the overall FM and FFM. Therefore, smaller differences in conductance through the limbs can have a major (albeit not accurate) impact on body composition by BIA *(83)*.

Isotope Dilution

With the assumption that fat does not contain water and that FFM has an established proportion of water, total body water can be measured to estimate FFM. This is done by isotope dilution methods, in which a dose of tracer is administered (water labeled with an isotope of hydrogen such as deuterium, $^{2}H_{2}0$, or oxygen, $H_{2}{}^{18}0$), followed by equilibration during which time the isotope is exchanged with other nonlabeled molecules and subsequently excreted and measured. Overall, this is a fairly simple procedure, with the isotope being administered either orally or intravenously, and measuring the levels in either saliva, urine, or plasma. The precision of measurements of total body water is 1 to 2% *(84)*. Concerns with this technique includes the question of whether obese individuals may have increased levels of hydration of fat-free tissue as mentioned above; in addition, the presence of edema, which is common in the obese, adds to the difficulty of estimating the hydration status of the FFM.

^{40}K

Potassium is found exclusively in FFM. A naturally occurring isotope of potassium, ^{40}K, can be measured by whole body counters to estimate levels of total body potassium in individuals. Measurement of this isotope requires that the patient remain in a small space for approx 40–90 min since repeated scans are frequently required. Values measured can then be incorporated into equations, in which a constant relationship between total body potassium and FFM are assumed. A major limitation to this technique is the shielding of γ-counts emitted in the obese due to the excessive fat. Also, lower levels of potassium in the FFM of the obese have been observed, thus biasing measurements in this population. Finally, there is limited availability of the equipment needed for these measurements, as most instruments are located in research centers.

Each of these two-compartment methods has drawbacks as described above. Overall though, as a group, these methodologies are primarily limited by the assumption made regarding the consistent composition of FFM, which in further studies has been shown to be more variable than previously believed, particularly between obese and lean *(85–87)*. These measures are also confounded in those undergoing weight loss, with unpredictable shifts in both body water and potassium levels. Concerns regarding the accuracy of the two-compartment model for the determination of body composition have led to the development of models that more precisely evaluate the multiple components of FFM. Examples of multicompartment models include dual energy X-ray absorptiometry (DEXA), and imaging techniques (such at computed tomography [CT] or magnetic resonance imaging [MRI]) as described below.

DEXA

The ability to measure components of the FFM, such as bone, is exemplified by DEXA, a technique that was originally developed for the measurement of bone mineral content. However, it was also noted that the attenuation data could provide information on the fat/lean composition of soft tissue as a byproduct of the bone mineral measurements *(88)*. In the procedure, soft tissue composition is measured in a whole body scan, which takes between 5–20 min to complete. The scan utilizes two low-dose X-rays scanning at different energies, typically 70 and 140 kev, which is roughly equivalent to the background radiation received in one day. A detector system measures the intensity of the beam on the other side of the individual, with beam attenuation depending on the amount of bone, fat, and lean tissue present.

The primary advantage to using DEXA technology for the determination of body composition is the excellent precision of measurement and theoretical capacity to detect small changes in body composition *(89)*. In addition, while the machine for evaluation is very expensive, it is now more commonly available, due to the increased diagnosis and treatment of osteoporosis. Problems with the DEXA in the evaluation of obese patients predominantly relate to difficulty with measurement, given the small scanning area (approx 190 × 60 cm), and the possibility of soft tissue falling outside of the scanning area. A similar problem exists with the evaluation of regional body composition due to difficulty with positioning. In these circumstances, some authors recommend multiplying body weight by percent fat estimates on half-body scans to estimate whole fat and FFM, which will provide information in those with little anatomical asymmetry *(82)*.

Computed Tomography and Magnetic Resonance Imaging

Imaging techniques such as CT and MRI also provide information on body composition either by organ, tissue, or region, and are currently considered the most accurate method available. CT provides information about fat stores by utilizing radiation, whereas MRI uses magnetic pulses in which signal intensity is determined by the concentration and relaxation properties of water and fat in the tissues being studied *(78)*. With both imaging techniques, it is possible to measure total body composition, although currently, the reported reliability of estimates from MRI is somewhat less than CT. This is changing, however, as new imaging techniques and software become available. The obvious advantage of these techniques is their accuracy, minimal risk (although CT does use ionizing radiation), short scanning times, and current wide availability of these machines. Disadvantages include higher cost and difficulty with claustrophobic or severely obese individuals with studies generally being limited to those with BMI <35 kg/m^2. These last two methods are described in more detail below.

Adipose Tissue Distribution

There is much data to suggest that more than simply the amount of adipose tissue present, but rather the location of the adipose tissue is what is resulting in the metabolic disturbances associated with obesity. Specifically, intra-abdominal or visceral adipose tissue (VAT) is a better predictor than BMI for risk of diabetes *(90,91)*, HTN *(91)*, and stroke *(92)*. However, the problem in using VAT as an indicator for risk of obesity-related diseases is that it is not easily measured directly. In cadavers, the use of MRI to determine the total adipose tissue present in the visceral bed correlates very well with the amount obtained from dissection *(93)*. Similarly, the total amount of VAT can be accurately determined by CT *(94,95)*. When compared, the absolute mass obtained by CT and MRI may be slightly different, although they both yield similar ranking of increased VAT among a population *(96)*. Additionally, a single MRI or CT slice at the L2-L3 intervetebral disc level is highly predictive of VAT, with the advantages of being safer and cheaper *(97,98)*. It has been proposed that the cutoff between normal and abnormal be at 130 cm^2 of adipose tissue at the L2-L3 level *(99)*. Unfortunately from a clinical standpoint, CT and MRI are not appropriate screening tools due to the risk of radiation and the cost. Thus, other measures have been developed as markers for VAT, notably waist circumference (WC) and sagital diameter.

Waist Circumference

WC is performed with the patient standing at the level half way between the top of the iliac crests and the bottom of the ribs. It should be done at the end of a normal expiration. It has been recommended by the NIH that an abnormal WC is >40 inches (102 cm) in men and >35 inches (88 cm) in women *(62)*. Using these cutoffs, the likelihood of having any cardiovascular risk increases 2.5- to 4-fold in those with an elevated compared to normal WC *(100)*.

In postmortem evaluation of the correlation with VAT, WC was able to explain 61% of the variance in VAT (compared to 37% by BMI and 43% by waist-to-hip [WHR] ratio) *(99)*. In studies using MRI or CT to determine VAT, WC accounts for between 44–79% of the variance in VAT *(102–104)*. Using the cutoff of 130 cm^2 of adipose tissue area, a WC 100 cm has a sensitivity of 83%, however this is at the expense of a 38% false positive rate *(103)*.

WC correlates with disease in many studies, and WC correlates better than BMI or WHR ratio. WC is a better predictor for the development of type 2 diabetes than is BMI or WHR *(105)*. Additionally, changes in WC with weight loss correlate well with changes in VAT, whereas there was no such correlation between change in VAT and WHR *(103)*. Third, it has been shown that with increased WC, there is a concomitant increase in both objective health-related consequences (e.g., type 2 diabetes and cardiovascular risk factors) and impairment in the activities of daily living *(106,107)*. Finally, WC is an independent predictor of fasting insulin levels and is an even better predictor than body fat in women *(108)*.

There are potential problems with the use of WC, the foremost being that the correlation of WC with VAT is generally better in women than men and varies with race *(104)*. Additionally, the relatively high false positive rate described above would misclassify individuals with a low VAT as abnormal. However, both the NIH and the WHO feel that the increased risk with increasing VAT and the ability to estimate this with WC is an important tool in the assessment of obesity.

Waist-to-Hip and Waist-to-Height Ratios

The question arises as to the utility of ratios in measuring VAT, namely WHR and waist-to-height ratios. Numerous studies have shown WHR to be much less precise (compared to WC alone) in its correlation with VAT *(101,103,104,109–111)*. Some have suggested that height plays a role in the increased mortality with obesity *(112)* and, thus, have recommended the use of WC-to-height ratios *(113)*. However, there are several other studies which do not support the use of WC-to-height ratios *(114–116)*. There are several reasons why the ratios are not as good of a measure as WC alone: (i) two different measures are needed, which increases the error; (*ii*) a change in body fat may not be reflected by a change in the ratio; (*iii*) ratios are more difficult to interpret than a single number; and (*iv*) (with respect to WHR) WC measures visceral organs and abdominal fat, whereas hip circumference measures muscle mass, fat mass, and skeletal frame size, and thus, WHR includes components that are of lower interest with respect to VAT *(117)*.

Sagittal Diameter

A method similar to WC used to estimate VAT is sagittal diameter. Sagittal diameter is measured in the supine position and is usually defined as the largest anterioposterior diameter *(118)*. Several studies have shown sagittal diameter to correlate with VAT in a degree similar to WC (explaining 40–77% of the variance) *(104,109,116,118)*. Like WC, there are some gender and race differences with sagittal diameter that need further evaluation *(104)*. Additionally, no definite criteria have been established to differentiate a "normal" from an "abnormal" sagittal diameter, thus limiting its usefulness clinically. Thus, although sagittal diameter may be as useful clinically as WC, more data are needed on its ability to correlate with disease and its generalizability before it can be adopted as a routine clinical tool.

In summary, although sophisticated research techniques are available to precisely and accurately characterize body composition and differences in fat distribution, two simple measures will give a clinically meaningful evaluation of obesity: BMI and WC. These can be done in virtually any setting and provide a means to identify people at risk, select those appropriate for intervention, evaluate the effects of interventions, and exclude those inappropriate for intervention. Although the criteria for the differentiation between normal and abnormal were chosen differently for BMI (BMI >30 kg/m^2 being the point where the relative health risk increases) and WC (WC 40 inches for men and 35 inches for women correlates with 130 cm^2 of adipose tissue which is a critical amount), they both provide important clinical information.

Energy Homeostasis

Once the diagnosis of obesity has been established, the next step is to evaluate for the cause of obesity. The etiology of obesity is a positive excess in energy balance in the genetic setting where surplus calories are efficiently stored. Thus, the evaluation of obesity entails an examination of energy intake and expenditure. There are secondary causes of obesity, which help enable weight gain or make weight loss more difficult. Concern for any endocrine secondary causes of obesity or alterations in body composition (e.g., Cushing's syndrome, hypothyroidism, hypoandrogenism, polycystic ovarian syndrome, insulinoma, or growth hormone deficiency) should be evaluated as described elsewhere. However, it is rare that such a cause will be found.

The evaluation of energy intake in the free-living patient is done through the use of dietary recall, dietary history, or food frequency questionnaires. For a complete review of methods to determine energy intake, see the review by Buzzard *(119)*. The dietitian is much more experienced in obtaining an analysis of dietary intake and recommending the appropriate dietary adjustments and, thus, should play a major role in this assessment. However, by being able to assess the patient's dietary intake, the physician can help guide dietary changes and also help in the avoidance of any dietary pitfalls. Additionally, by showing such interest, the physician conveys to the patient the importance of diet in the management of obesity.

The assessment of intake by the physician in the office is probably best done using a 24-h recall method. The patient is asked to recount all food that was eaten in the last 24 h, so that the physician can obtain an appreciation of meal timing, skipped meals, and a gross estimate of dietary fat intake. A dietary history is similar but covers a longer period of time than the food frequency questionnaires, which are used to assess one aspect of the diet (e.g., fat intake). Any assessment of dietary intake should be used with extreme caution, especially in the obese, as these assessments often underestimate the true caloric intake *(120)*. Nonetheless, the role of nutrition assessment described above justifies their use despite the limitations in accuracy.

Similar to the assessment of intake, the assessment of energy expenditure is also fraught with difficulties. Energy expenditure is divided into three components: (*i*) resting metabolic rate (RMR); (*ii*) thermic effect of food (TEF); and (*iii*) activity-related energy expenditure (AEE). The basal metabolic rate accounts for about two-thirds of the total daily energy expenditure, and the lean body mass accounts for approx 75% of the variance in RMR. With weight gain there is an increase in lean mass as well as FM, so the RMR increases with increased weight and decreases with weight loss *(121)*. The TEF is about 10% of the total energy daily expenditure (TDEE), and varies with macronutrients (carbohydrates use about 8% of their available energy for digestion, whereas fat only uses about 2%) *(122)*. Nonetheless, there is no significant variation with obesity. The AREE accounts for the remaining daily energy expenditure. Although several research methods are available to measure energy expenditure (including direct or indirect calorimetry and doubly labeled water) none of these have yet been shown to have a clinical utility *(122)*. Clinically, several equations have been developed to determine energy expenditure. The most frequently used equation is the Harris-Benedict equation, although other appropriate alternatives include the Food and Agriculture Organization of WHO equation and Schofield equation. The Harris-Benedict equation for women and men are :

$$\text{Women's basal energy expenditure} = 655.1 + 9.56 \times \text{weight (in kg)} + 1.85 \times \text{height (in cm)} - 4.68 \times \text{age (in yr)}.$$

$$\text{Men's basal energy expenditure} = 66.47 + 13.75 \times \text{weight (in kg)} + 5 \times \text{height (in cm)} - 6.76 \times \text{age (in yr)}.$$

In normal individuals, the Harris-Benedict equation has a precision of approx ±14% *(123)*, however it has been shown to overestimate energy expenditure in several populations *(124,125)*. Despite the limitations of these equations, they can play a role in the overall clinical assessment of energy expenditure.

In summary, highly sensitive techniques have yet to be developed to measure energy homeostasis in a free-living population and in a way that is clinically meaningful. The assessment of energy balance by the physician, despite the crude level at which it is done, imparts to the patient a higher level of appreciation of the dietary and exercise components of weight management. Through a 24-h dietary recall and a 1-wk exercise history or calculation of energy requirements from an equation, the physician completes the assessment of obesity and can begin to make treatment recommendations.

REFERENCES

1. Havel RJ. Structure and metabolism of plasma lipoproteins. In: Scriver CR, Beaudet A, Sly WS, Valle D, eds. The Metabolic and Molecular Basis of Inherited Disease, 7th ed. McGraw Hill, New York, 1995:1841–1852.
2. LaRosa JC, Hunninghake D, Bush D, et al. The cholesterol facts. A summary of the evidence relating dietary fats, serum cholesterol, and coronary heart disease. A joint statement by the American Heart Association and the National Heart, Lung, and Blood Institute. The Task Force on Cholesterol Issues, American Heart Association. Circulation 1990;81:1721–1733.

3. Anonymous. Randomised trial of cholesterol lowering in 4444 patients with coronary heart disease: the Scandinavian Simvastatin Survival Study (4S). Lancet 1994;344:1383–1389.
4. Shepherd J, Cobbe SM, Ford I, et al. Prevention of coronary heart disease with pravastatin in men with hypercholesterolemia. West of Scotland Coronary Prevention Study Group. N Engl J Med 1995;333:1301–1307.
5. Sacks FM, Pfeffer MA, Moye LA, et al. The effect of pravastatin on coronary events after myocardial infarction in patients with average cholesterol levels. Cholesterol and Recurrent Events Trial investigators. N Engl J Med 1996;335:1001–1009.
6. Anonymous. Prevention of cardiovascular events and death with pravastatin in patients with coronary heart disease and a broad range of initial cholesterol levels. The Long-Term Intervention with Pravastatin in Ischaemic Disease (LIPID) Study Group. N Engl J Med 1998;339:1349–1357.
7. Downs JR, Clearfield M, Weis S, et al. Primary prevention of acute coronary events with lovastatin in men and women with average cholesterol levels: results of AFCAPS/TexCAPS. Air Force/Texas Coronary Atherosclerosis Prevention Study. JAMA 1998;279:1615–1622.
8. Anonymous. The Lipid Research Clinics Coronary Primary Prevention Trial results. II. The relationship of reduction in incidence of coronary heart disease to cholesterol lowering. JAMA 1984;251:365–374.
9. Ornish D, Scherwitz LW, Billings JH, et al. Intensive lifestyle changes for reversal of coronary heart disease JAMA 1998;280:2001–2007.
10. Anonymous. Summary of the second report of the National Cholesterol Education Program (NCEP) Expert Panel on Detection, Evaluation, and Treatment of High Blood Cholesterol in Adults (Adult Treatment Panel III). JAMA 2001;285:2846.
11. Allain CC, Poon LS, Chan CS, Richmond W, Fu PC. Enzymatic determination of total serum cholesterol. Clin Chem 1974;20:470–475.
12. Lopes-Virella MF, Stone P, Ellis S, Colwell JA. Cholesterol determination in high-density lipoproteins separated by three different methods. Clin Chem 1997;23:882–884.
13. Bucolo G, David H. Quantitative determination of serum TGs by the use of enzymes. Clin Chem 1973;19:476–482.
14. Klotzsch SG, McNamara JR. Triglyceride measurements: a review of methods and interferences. Clin Chem 1990;36:1605–1613.
15. Brunzell JD, Bierman EL. Chylomicronemia syndrome. Interaction of genetic and acquired hyperTGmia. Med Clin North Am 1982;66:455–468.
16. Brunzell JD, Hazzard WR, Porte DJ, Bierman EL. Evidence for a common, saturable, TG removal mechanism for chylomicrons and very low density lipoproteins in man. J Clin Invest 1973;52:1578–1585.
17. Friedewald WT, Levy RI, Fredrickson DS. Estimation of the concentration of low-density lipoprotein cholesterol in plasma, without use of the preparative ultracentrifuge. Clin Chem 1972;18:499–502.
18. Rubies-Prat J, Reverter JL, Senti M, et al. Calculated low-density lipoprotein cholesterol should not be used for management of lipoprotein abnormalities in patients with diabetes mellitus. Diabetes Care 1993;16:1081–1086.
19. Kazi-Aoul T, Benmiloud M. The Friedewald formula: another restriction? Clin Chem 1987;33:1301.
20. Matas C, Cabre M, La Ville A, et al. Limitations of the Friedewald formula for estimating low-density lipoprotein cholesterol in alcoholics with liver disease. Clin Chem 1994;40:404–406.
21. Senti M, Pedro-Botet J, Nogues X, Rubies-Prat J. Influence of intermediate-density lipoproteins on the accuracy of the Friedewald formula. Clin Chem 1991;37:1394–1397.
22. Craig WY, Neveux LM, Palomaki GE, Cleveland MM, Haddow JE. Lipoprotein(a) as a risk factor for ischemic heart disease: metaanalysis of prospective studies. Clin Chem 1998;44:2301–2306.

23. Schreiner PJ, Heiss G, Tyroler HA, Morrisett JD, Davis CE, Smith R. Race and gender differences in the association of Lp(a) with carotid artery wall thickness. The Atherosclerosis Risk in Communities (ARIC) Study. Arterioscler Thromb Vasc Biol 1996;16:471–478.
24. Baggio G, Donazzan S, Monti D, Mari D, Martini S, Gabelli C, et al. Lipoprotein(a) and lipoprotein profile in healthy centenarians: a reappraisal of vascular risk factors. FASEB J 1998;12:433–437.
25. Berg K. A new serum type system in man. Acta Pathol Microbiol Scand 1963;59:369.
26. Marcovina SM, Koschinsky ML. Lipoprotein(a) as a risk factor for coronary artery disease. Am J Cardiol 1998;82:57U–66U.
27. Hobbs HH, White AL. Lipoprotein(a): intrigues and insights. Curr Opin Lipidol 1999;10:225–236.
28. Marcovina SM, Albers JJ, Gabel B, Koschinsky ML, Gaur VP. Effect of the number of apolipoprotein(a) kringle 4 domains on immunochemical measurements of lipoprotein(a). Clin Chem 1995;41:246–255.
29. Bostom AG, Cupples LA, Jenner JL, et al. Elevated plasma lipoprotein(a) and coronary heart disease in men aged 55 years and younger. A prospective study. JAMA 1996;276:544–548.
30. Nguyen TT, Ellefson RD, Hodge DO, Bailey KR, Kottke TE, Abu-Lebdeh HS. Predictive value of electrophoretically detected lipoprotein(a) for coronary heart disease and cerebrovascular disease in a community-based cohort of 9936 men and women. Circulation 1997;96:1390–1397.
31. Lamarche B, Tchernof A, Mauriege P, et al. Fasting insulin and apolipoprotein B levels and low-density lipoprotein particle size as risk factors for ischemic heart disease. JAMA 1998;279:1955–1961.
32. Lamarche B, Moorjani S, Lupien PJ, et al. Apolipoprotein A-I and B levels and the risk of ischemic heart disease during a five-year follow-up of men in the Quebec cardiovascular study. Circulation 1996;94:273–278.
33. Sniderman A, Shapiro S, Marpole D, Skinner B, Teng B, Kwiterovich POJ. Association of coronary atherosclerosis with hyperapobetalipoproteinemia [increased protein but normal cholesterol levels in human plasma low density (beta) lipoproteins]. Proc Natl Acad Sci USA 1980;77:604–608.
34. Brunzell JD, Sniderman AD, Albers JJ, Kwiterovich POJ. Apoproteins B and A-I and coronary artery disease in humans. Arteriosclerosis 1984;4:79–83.
35. Bachorik PS, Lovejoy KL, Carroll MD, Johnson CL. Apolipoprotein B and AI distributions in the United States, 1988-1991: results of the National Health and Nutrition Examination Survey III (NHANES III). Clin Chem 1997;43:2364–2378.
36. Albers JJ, Marcovina SM. Standardization of apolipoprotein B and A-I measurements. Clin Chem 1989;35:1357–1361.
37. Marcovina SM, Albers JJ, Kennedy H, Mei JV, Henderson LO, Hannon WH. International Federation of Clinical Chemistry standardization project for measurements of apolipoproteins A-I and B. IV. Comparability of apolipoprotein B values by use of International Reference Material. Clin Chem 1994;40:586-592, 1994.
38. Eckel RH. Familial combined hyperlipidemia and insulin resistance - Distant relatives linked by intra-abdominal fat? Arterioscler Thromb Vasc Biol 2001;21:469–470.
39. Ose L, Kalager T, Grundt IK. Serum beta-lipoprotein subfractions in polyacrylamide gel electrophoresis associated with coronary heart disease. Scand J Clin Lab Invest 1976;36:75–79.
40. Zhao SP, Smelt AH, Leuven JA, Vroom TF, van der Laarse A, van 't Hooft FM. Changes of lipoprotein profile in familial dysbetalipoproteinemia with gemfibrozil. Am J Med 1994;96:49E-E56.
41. Mahley RW, Rall SC Jr. Type III hyperlipoproteinemia. In: Scriver CR, Beaudet AL, Sly WS, Valle D, eds. The Metabolic and Molecular Basis of Inherited Diseases. 7th ed. McGraw Hill, New York, 1995, pp. 1953–1980.

42. Frings CS, Foster LB, Cohen PS. Electrophoretic separation of serum lipoproteins in polyacrylamide gel. Clin Chem 1971;17:111–114.
43. Warnick GR, Knopp RH, Fitzpatrick V, Branson L. Estimating low-density lipoprotein cholesterol by the Friedewald equation is adequate for classifying patients on the basis of nationally recommended cutpoints. Clin Chem 1990;36:15–19.
44. Hill JS, Pritchard PH. Improved phenotyping of apolipoprotein E: application to population frequency distribution. Clin Chem 1990;36:1871–1874.
45. Warnick GR, Mayfield C, Albers JJ, Hazzard WR. Gel isoelectric focusing method for specific diagnosis of familial hyperlipoproteinemia type 3. Clin Chem 1979;25:279–284.
46. Kamboh MI, Ferrell RE, Kottke B. Genetic studies of human apolipoproteins. V. A novel rapid procedure to screen apolipoprotein E polymorphism. J Lipid Res 1988;29:1535–1543.
47. Havekes LM, de Knijff P, Beisiegel U, Havinga J, Smit M, Klasen E. A rapid micromethod for apolipoprotein E phenotyping directly in serum. J Lipid Res 1987;28:455–463.
48. Hixson JE, Vernier DT. Restriction isotyping of human apolipoprotein E by gene amplification and cleavage with HhaI. J Lipid Res 1990;31:545–548.
49. Austin MA, Breslow JL, Hennekens CH, Buring JE, Willett WC, Krauss RM. Low-density lipoprotein subclass patterns and risk of myocardial infarction. JAMA 1988;260:1917–1921.
50. Campos H, Blijlevens E, McNamara JR, Ordovas JM, Posner BM, Wilson PW, et al. LDL particle size distribution. Results from the Framingham Offspring Study. Arterioscler Thromb 1992;12:1410–1419.
51. Okazaki M, Ohno Y, Hara I. High-performance aqueous gel permeation chromatography of human serum lipoproteins. J Chromatogr 1980;221:257–264.
52. Otvos JD, Jeyarajah EJ, Bennett DW. Quantification of plasma lipoproteins by proton nuclear magnetic resonance spectroscopy. Clin Chem 1991;37:377–386.
53. Otvos JD, Jeyarajah EJ, Bennett DW, Krauss RM. Development of a proton nuclear magnetic resonance spectroscopic method for determining plasma lipoprotein concentrations and subspecies distributions from a single, rapid measurement. Clin Chem 1992;38:1632–1638.
54. Bathen TF, Engan T, Krane J. Principal component analysis of proton nuclear magnetic resonance spectra of lipoprotein fractions from patients with coronary heart disease and healthy subjects. Scand J Clin Lab Invest 1999;59:349–360.
55. Freedman DS, Otvos JD, Jeyarajah EJ, Barboriak JJ, Anderson AJ, Walker JA. Relation of lipoprotein subclasses as measured by proton nuclear magnetic resonance spectroscopy to coronary artery disease. Arterioscler Thromb Vasc Biol 1998;18:1046–1053.
56. Spengel FA, Harders-Spengel KM, Keller CF, Wieczorek A, Wolfram G, Zollner N. Use of fibroblast culture to diagnose and genotype familial hypercholesterolaemia. Ann Nutr Metab 1982;26:240–247.
57. Schuster H, Keller C, Wolfram G, Zollner N. Diagnosis of familial hypercholesterolemia using DNA haplotype analysis in three large families with two hyperlipidemic parents. Ann Nutr Metab 1992;36:79–86.
58. Henderson BG, Wenham PR, Ashby JP, Blundell G. Detecting familial defective apolipoprotein B-100: three molecular scanning methods compared. Clin Chem 1997;43:1630–1634.
59. Garrison RJ, Castelli WP. Weight and thirty-year mortality of men in the Framingham Study. Ann Intern Med 1985;103:1006–1009.
60. Stevens J, Cai J, Pamuk ER, Williamson DF, Thun MJ, Wood JL. The effect of age on the association between body-mass index and mortality. N Engl J Med 1998;338:1–7.
61. Calle EE, Thun MJ, Petrelli JM, Rodriguez C, Heath CWJ. Body-mass index and mortality in a prospective cohort of U.S. adults. N Engl J Med 1999;341:1097–1105.

62. National Institutes of Health Obesity Task Force. The evaluation and treatment of overweight and obesity. Obesity Res 1998;6(Suppl 2):51S–209S.
63. Douketis JD, Feightner JW, Attia J, Feldman WF. Periodic health examination, 1999 update: 1. Detection, prevention and treatment of obesity. Canadian Task Force on Preventive Health Care. Can Med Assoc J 1999;160:513–525.
64. The Association of Life Insurance Medical Directors and the Actuarial Society of America. Medico-Actuarial Mortality Investigation. New York: The Association of Life Insurance Medical Directors and the Actuarial Society of America, 1913.
65. Bray GA. Life insurance and overweight. Obesity Res 1995;3:97–99.
66. Metropolitan Life Insurance Company. New weight standards for men and women. Met Life Stat Bull 1959;40:1.
67. Gray DS, Fujioka K. Use of relative weight and body mass index for the determination of adiposity. J Clin Epidemiol 1991;44:545–550.
68. Himes JH, Bouchard C, Pheley AM. Lack of correspondence among measures identifying the obese. Am J Prev Med 1991;7:107–111.
69. Israel RG, Pories WJ, O'Brien KF, McCammon MR. Sensitivity and specificity of current methods for classifying morbid obesity. Diabetes Res Clin Pract 1990;10(Suppl 1):S145–S147.
70. Smalley KJ, Knerr AN, Kendrick ZV, Colliver JA, Owen OE. Reassessment of body mass indices. Am J Clin Nutr 1990;52:405–408.
71. Roubenoff R, Dallal GE, Wilson PW. Predicting body fatness: the body mass index vs estimation by bioelectrical impedance. Am J Public Health 1995;85:726–728.
72. Hortobagyi T, Israel RG, O'Brien KF. Sensitivity and specificity of the Quetelet index to assess obesity in men and women. Eur J Clin Nutr 1994;48:369–375.
73. Curtin F, Morabia A, Pichard C, Slosman DO. Body mass index compared to dual-energy x-ray absorptiometry: evidence for a spectrum bias. J Clin Epidemiol 1997;50:837–843.
74. Thompson D, Edelsberg J, Colditz GA, Bird AP, Oster G. Lifetime health and economic consequences of obesity. Arch Intern Med 1999;159:2177–2183.
75. Huang Z, Willett WC, Manson JE, et al. Body weight, weight change, and risk for hypertension in women. Ann Intern Med 1998;128:81–88.
76. Hubert HB, Feinleib M, McNamara PM, Castelli WP. Obesity as an independent risk factor for cardiovascular disease: a 26-year follow-up of participants in the Framingham Heart Study. Circulation 1983;67:968–977.
77. Manson JE, Willett WC, Stampfer MJ, Colditz GA, Hunter DJ, Hankinson SE, et al. Body weight and mortality among women. N Engl J Med 1995;333:677–685.
78. Jebb SA. Measuring body composition. In: Kopelman PG, Stock MJ, eds. Clinical Obesity. Blackwell Science, London, 1998, pp. 18–49.
79. Roche AF, Baumgartner RN, Guo S. Anthropometry: classical and modern approaches. In: Whitehead RG, Prete PE, eds. New Techniques in Nutritional Research. Academic Press, New York, 1991, pp. 242–260.
80. Lohman TG. Advances in body composition analysis. Human Kinetics Publishers, Champaign, IL, 1992, pp. 37–56.
81. Widdowson E, Dickerson J. Chemical composition of the body. In: Comar C, Bronner F, eds. Mineral Metabolism. Academic Press, New York, 1964, pp. 2–210.
82. Heymsfield SB, Allison DB, Wang ZM, Baumgartner RN, Ross R. Evaluation of total and regional body composition. In: Bray GA, Bouchard C, James WPT, eds. Handbook of Obesity. Marcel Dekker, New York, 1998, pp. 41–77.
83. NIH Technonogy Assessment Conference. (http://text.nlm.nih.gov/nih/ta/www/15.html) Bioelectrical Impedance Analysis in Body Composition Measurement. NIH Technonogy Assessment Conference. 1994.
84. Coward WA, Parkinson SA, Murgatroyd P. Body composition measurements for nutrition research. Nutr Res Rev 1988;1:115–124.

85. Colt EW, Wang J, Stallone F, Van Itallie TB, Pierson RNJ. A possible low intracellular potassium in obesity. Am J Clin Nutr 1981;34:367–372.
86. Morgan DB, Burkinshaw L. Estimation of non-fat body tissues from measurements of skinfold thickness, total body potassium and total body nitrogen. Clin Sci 1983;65:407–414.
87. Deurenberg P, Leenen R, Van der Kooy K, Hautvast JG. In obese subjects the body fat percentage calculated with Siri's formula is an overestimation. Eur J Clin Nutr 1989;43:569–575.
88. Nord RH, Payne RK. Body composition by dual-energy X-ray absorptiometry. Asia Pac J Clin Nutr 1995;4:167–171.
89. Tothill P, Avenell A, Reid DM. Precision and accuracy of measurements of whole-body bone mineral: comparisons between hologic, lunar and norland dual-energy X-ray absorptiometers. Br J Radiol 1994;67:1210–1217.
90. Carey VJ, Walters EE, Colditz GA, et al. Body fat distribution and risk of non-insulin-dependent diabetes mellitus in women. The Nurses' Health Study. Am J Epidemiol 1997;145:614–619.
91. Okosun IS, Cooper RS, Rotimi CN, Osotimehin B, Forrester T. Association of waist circumference with risk of hypertension and type 2 diabetes in Nigerians, Jamaicans, and African-Americans. Diabetes Care 1998;21:1836–1842.

12 Hyper- and Hypocalcemia

Benjamin Z. Leder, MD
and Joel S. Finkelstein, MD

CONTENTS

INTRODUCTION

Abnormalities in circulating levels of calcium are commonly encountered by the internist and endocrinologist. Ninety-nine percent of the body's calcium is found in bone, with the remaining fraction in either the extracellular or intracellular compartments of all other tissues. Approximately half of the circulating blood calcium is bound to serum proteins, but it is the nonbound fraction (or ionized calcium) that is tightly controlled by the calcium homeostatic hormones. The role of calcium in many cellular functions, including the excitation of nerves and muscle and the contraction of muscle (including the myocardium), directly relates to the symptoms of both its excess and insufficiency in the circulation. Because of the physiologic importance of maintaining the blood calcium concentration in a tight range, the feedback loop that controls calcium homeostasis is highly sensitive (Fig. 1). The two main calcium regulatory hormones are parathyroid hormone (PTH) and 1,25$(OH)_2$ vitamin D. Calcitonin's role in human physiology is less clear. Similarly, the role, if any, of PTH-related protein (the peptide responsible for humoral hypercalcemia of malignancy) in normal physiology has not yet been elucidated.

PTH is a peptide hormone secreted by the chief cells of the parathyroid gland and regulates the blood calcium concentration on a minute-to-minute basis. Circulating PTH levels are regulated by the serum calcium level, which affects secretion, and 1,25$(OH)_2$ vitamin D, which inhibits transcription of the PTH

From: *Contemporary Endocrinology: Handbook of Diagnostic Endocrinology*
Edited by: J. E. Hall and L. K. Nieman © Humana Press Inc., Totowa, NJ

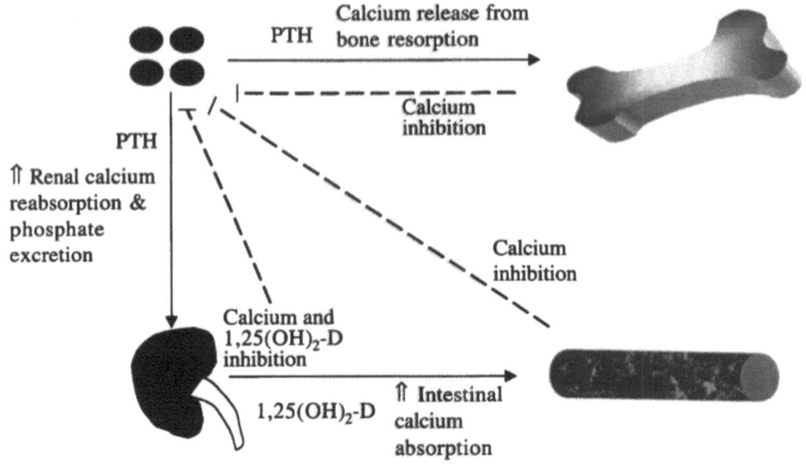

Fig. 1. The hormonal regulation of calcium homeostasis by PTH and 1,25-$(OH)_2$ vitamin D.

gene. The parathyroid cell's responsiveness to calcium levels is mediated through the calcium sensor, which is a member of the G-protein-coupled receptor family. Mutations in the gene for this receptor are associated with various abnormalities in calcium homeostasis *(1)*. PTH is secreted both as the intact molecule (84 amino acids in length) and as carboxyl terminal fragments. The intact hormone is metabolized in the liver and kidney, while the carboxyl terminal fragments are metabolized exclusively in the kidney *(2)*. Before the introduction of immunological assays, which distinguished between PTH and its fragments (two-site assays), this pattern of metabolism made the evaluation of patients with renal insufficiency especially difficult.

The primary sites of action of PTH are the kidney and the bone and are mediated by the PTH receptor. In the kidney, PTH promotes calcium reabsorption and inhibits phosphate reabsorption. In the bone, PTH stimulates bone resorption by indirectly activating osteoclasts (via the stimulation of osteoblasts) and by stimulating differentiation of osteoclast precursors *(3,4)*. These effects on the bone and kidney raise blood calcium concentrations and thus inhibit PTH release as per the classic endocrine feedback loop.

Vitamin D is a steroid compound formed in the body when precursor molecules are exposed to ultraviolet light. Dietary sources of vitamin D include fortified dairy products, egg yolk, and some plants. Vitamin D is not biologically active until it is 25-hydroxylated in the liver and 1α-hydroxylated in the kidney. The 1α-hydroxylation is the regulated enzymatic step, and PTH and hypophosphatemia are the major stimulators of this reaction. While 1,25$(OH)_2$ vitamin D is the main biologically active metabolite, 25-OH vitamin D, which is 1/100 to

1/1000 less potent, can have biologic activity at pharmacological concentrations. The physiologically important actions of $1,25(OH)_2$ vitamin D are mediated via its interaction with the nuclear vitamin D receptor and its subsequent effects on gene transcription. The primary target organ of vitamin D is the gut, but vitamin D has effects on the parathyroid glands and the bone as well. Vitamin D facilitates intestinal calcium absorption through its effects on the transcellular route of calcium transport from the lumen through the enterocyte. Thus, vitamin D is necessary for the body to maintain calcium homeostasis by allowing dietary intake of calcium to replenish the obligate losses of calcium occurring through intestinal and urinary secretion. Other properties of vitamin D include its ability to inhibit PTH excretion by the parathyroid and its role in the regulation of the transcription of bone matrix proteins *(2)*.

In this chapter, we discuss both hyper- and hypocalcemia. The regulatory mechanisms and integral hormones described above not only provide a framework to understand the pathophysiology of these conditions, but also provide a background to form a logical approach to their diagnosis.

HYPERCALCEMIA

Hypercalcemia is a common disorder, as its prevalence has been reported to be between 1.1–3.9% in normal populations and between 0.2–2.9% in hospitalized patients *(5)*. In almost all instances, the elevation in measured calcium is due to true increases in the serum ionized calcium concentration but, rarely can be caused by elevations in binding protein levels (pseudohypercalcemia). Despite the many causes of hypercalcemia, in the vast majority of cases (>90%) the underlying disorder is either hyperparathyroidism or malignancy. The former is the most prevalent etiology among outpatients and the latter, among inpatients *(6)*. Hypercalcemia is rarely seen in occult malignancy. Thus, in asymptomatic patients, the hypercalcemia is usually caused by hyperparathyroidism.

Symptoms of hypercalcemia are often nonspecific. Central nervous system symptoms include weakness, fatigue, mental disturbance, depression, psychomotor retardation, and, if severe, coma and death. Gastrointestinal symptoms include anorexia, nausea, and constipation. In the kidney, hypercalcemia can produce nephrogenic diabetes insipidus and lead to polyuria. When both serum calcium and phosphate levels are elevated (as in vitamin D toxicity), soft tissue calcifications can occur. While there is great patient to patient variability, the symptoms of hypercalcemia are generally related to both the degree of hypercalcemia and the rate at which the calcium elevations have developed.

Etiology and Pathogenesis

The causes of hypercalcemia can be classified by their underlying etiology (Table 1). In some cases, multiple mechanisms may contribute.

Table 1
Causes of Hypercalcemia

Parathyroid-related	*Vitamin D-related*	*Malignancy-related*	*Other causes*
Primary hyperparathyroidism: adenoma, hyperplasia (MEN)	Vitamin D intoxication	PTHrP producing: squamous cell tumors (lung and head/neck most common) kidney, breast.	Milk-Alkali syndrome
Tertiary hyperparathyroidism	Granulomatous Disease: sarcoidosis tuberculosis inflammatory bowel disease	Osteolytic metastases: multiple myeloma, breast	Immobilization
Familial hypocalciuric hypercalcemia		PTH-producing (rare)	Vitamin A intoxication
Lithium		Other humoral factors: lymphoma, leukemia multiple myeloma	Aluminum intoxication
			Hyperthyroidism
			Thiazide use
			Adrenal insufficiency
			Phenochromocytoma
			Theophylline toxicity

Primary Hyperparathyroidism

Primary hyperthyroidism is caused by excess PTH secretion from either an autonomous adenoma in a parathyroid gland (or glands) or by generalized parathyroid hyperplasia. In these abnormal glands, the set point for PTH suppression by calcium is shifted, and the resultant increase in calcium is not sufficient to suppress PTH levels normally. The peak incidence of primary hyperparathyroidism is in the fifth and sixth decade of life, and it rarely occurs prior to adolescence. Between 1983 and 1992, the overall incidence rate in both urban and rural populations was approx 21/100,000 person-yr with a female-to-male ratio of 2–3:1 *(7)*. In 80–85% of patients with primary hyperparathyroidism, the underlying cause is a single adenoma *(8,9)*. Most of the remaining patients have parathyroid hyperplasia. Hyperplasia is more common in younger patients and is often associated with the syndromes of multiple endocrine neoplasia (MEN) type I and IIa *(10)*. Parathyroid carcinoma is rare and is the cause of primary hyperparathyroidism in only 0.1–1.0 % of cases *(10,11)*.

There are several heritable syndromes associated with primary hyperparathyroidism. MEN I (also called Wermer's Syndrome) is associated with parathyroid hyperplasia, pancreatic islet cell tumors, and anterior pituitary adenomas. In over 90% of patients with MEN I, hyperparathyroidism is the first clinical manifestation. MEN I is an autosomal dominant disorder caused by defects in the *MEN I* gene encoding a 610-amino acid protein called "MENIN" *(12)*. Of the mutations identified, most are loss of function mutations consistent with MENIN's proposed role as a tumor suppression gene.

MEN IIa (also called Sipple's Syndrome) consists of medullary thyroid cancer, pheochromocytoma, and primary hyperparathyroidism. In contrast to MEN I, hyperparathyroidism occurs in only 15–30% of patients with MEN II. Like MEN I, MEN II is inherited in an autosomal dominant fashion. Mutations in the *c-ret* proto-oncogene have been found in most patients with MEN II *(13)*.

In nonfamilial hyperparathyroidism, most parathyroid adenomas result from the clonal expansion of a single somatic cell. Tumor-specific genetic defects have been characterized in a minority of sporadic parathyroid adenomas including: (*i*) a pericentric inversion on chromosome 11, resulting in a relocation of *PRAD 1* (parathyroid adenoma 1 or cyclin D1) proto-oncogene next to the 5'-PTH gene-promoter *(14,15)*; (*ii*) loss of heterozygosity in the *MENI* gene *(16)*; and (*iii*) deletions in the retinoblastoma (*RB*) gene (particularly in parathyroid carcinomas) *(17)*.

The clinical manifestations of primary hyperparathyroidism are related to both the level of hypercalcemia and the elevation of PTH. Because of routine blood screening, approx 80% of patients with primary hyperparathyroidism are diagnosed while asymptomatic. The classic bone abnormality associated with the primary hyperparathyroidism, osteitis fibrosa cystica, is now rarely seen. Similarly, local destructive bone lesions (Brown tumors) are also vanishingly rare. Cortical bone osteopenia with relative preservation of trabecular bone, however, is a commonly encountered abnormality in patients with primary hyperparathyroidism, but this pattern is not universal. Some patients will be globally osteopenic, while others will have normal bone density *(2)*.

The renal manifestations of primary hyperparathyroidism have also changed. Nephrocalcinosis (bilateral calcification of the renal parenchyma) once common, is now rarely seen. Nephrolithiasis, once thought to be nearly universal, is now reported in only 5–25% of these patients, though more subtle abnormalities in renal function (such as mild reduction in glomerular filtration rate [GFR] and renal tubular defects) are seen more frequently *(11)*.

Neuropsychiatric manifestations of hyperparathyroidism include depression, cognitive impairment, anxiety, and personality changes. Whether there is a clear cause and effect relationship with primary hyperparathyroidism, however, has not been determined *(18)*.

Rarely, patients with primary hyperparathyroidism may present with life threatening severe hypercalcemia or "parathyroid crises," which is a surgical emergency. Patients with hyperparathyroidism and a neck mass are at increased risk for parathyroid carcinoma, as palpable neck masses are not a manifestation of adenoma or hyperplasia.

Hypercalcemia of Malignancy

Hypercalcemia of malignancy is the second most common cause of hypercalcemia and is the most common cause among hospital inpatients. Many tumors have been associated with hypercalcemia. In general, these can be stratified into those that produce PTH-related protein (PTHrP) or other humoral factors and those that cause hypercalcemia by local bony invasion. At times, the hypercalcemia can result from both mechanisms (Table 1).

Humoral Hypercalcemia of Malignancy. It had long been theorized that a PTH-like humoral factor was the cause of the hypercalcemia in patients with cancer, but no obvious skeletal metastases. The identification of PTHrP and the elucidation of its role in the humoral hypercalcemia of malignancy, however, did not occur until relatively recently *(19)*. PTHrP is a peptide that shares some homology with PTH at the amino terminal and binds to the PTH receptor. The tumors that most commonly are associated with PTHrP are listed in Table 1, but PTHrP production has been described in many tumor types. Tumor production of PTH itself is exceedingly rare. Production of 1,25-$(OH)_2$ vitamin D is the etiology of hypercalcemia in most patients with Hodgkin's disease and has been implicated in non-Hodgkin's lymphoma as well *(20)*.

Hypercalcemia Caused by Lytic Bone Lesions. Hypercalcemia, caused by destruction of the bone and calcium release into the general circulation, is common in patients with multiple myeloma and breast cancer. In multiple myeloma, the mechanism appears to be related to the tumor cells secretion of cytokines (interleukin [IL]-1, IL-6, tumor necrosis factor [TNF]-β, which then either directly or indirectly activate osteoclasts *(2,21)*. While many patients with multiple myeloma develop lytic bone lesions, less than 40% become hypercalcemic. The likelihood of such patients developing hypercalcemia may be due to the varying degrees of renal insufficiency seen in patients with multiple myeloma *(22)*.

In breast cancer, the production of local factors by bone metastases also stimulates osteoclastic bone resorption and thus contributes to the hypercalcemia commonly seen in these patients. These factors include the local production of PTHrP. In fact, neutralizing antibodies to PTHrP reduce the development of destructive bone lesions after inoculation with breast cancer cells in mice. This suggests that PTHrP may actually have a pathogenetic role in the establishment of these lytic bone lesions *(23)*. Finally, it is important to note that patients with breast cancer and skeletal metastases, who do not previously have hypercalcemia, may have their first episode of hypercalcemia after the initiation of hormonal therapy with a selective estrogen receptor modifier *(24)*.

Vitamin D Toxicity and Granulomatous Disease

Vitamin D-mediated hypercalcemia occurs in many granulomatous diseases, such as sarcoidosis, tuberculosis, various fungal infections, Crohn's disease, as well as in some lymphomas (Table 1). In these patients, the hypercalcemia is due to conversion of 25-OH vitamin D to 1,25-$(OH)_2$ vitamin D either by activated macrophages within granulomatous tissue or by lymphoid cells within lymphomatous tissue. This extrarenal conversion bypasses the normally tightly regulated production of 1,25-$(OH)_2$ vitamin D. The ensuing derangement in 1,25-$(OH)_2$ vitamin D levels increases intestinal absorption of calcium and bone resorption. This new milieu, if sufficient 1,25-$(OH)_2$ vitamin D is present, leads to hypercalciuria, hypercalcemia, hyperphosphatemia, and suppression of PTH. Vitamin D intoxication, due to the ingestion of vitamin D or its metabolites, similarly increases intestinal calcium absorption and bone resorption. In fact, it is the increased bone resorption that appears to be primarily responsible for the hypercalcemia in these patients *(25)*. The degree, duration, and severity of the hypercalcemia depend on the potency and half-life of the vitamin D preparation ingested.

Familial Hypocalciuric Hypercalcemia

Familial hypocalciuric hypercalcemia (FHH) is an autosomal dominantly inherited disorder caused by inactivating mutations in the gene for the calcium sensor (CaR) *(26)*. Though there was initially some controversy, most now believe that FHH is an asymptomatic disorder. Blood calcium levels are generally mildly elevated (usually <12 mg/dL), blood phosphate levels are low or low-normal, serum PTH levels are mildly elevated or inappropriately normal, and urinary calcium excretion is usually low. Patients with FHH exhibit varying degrees of loss of function of the calcium sensor and thus, a higher set point for inhibition of PTH secretion by calcium. Additionally, there is renal resistance to calcium and, thus, a lack of compensatory urinary calcium excretion expected for the degree of hypercalcemia and normal parathyroid levels. Because of this abnormality in calcium excretion, parathyroidectomy does not cure the hypercalcemia in these patients.

Milk-Alkali Syndrome

The milk-alkali syndrome was first described in the 1930s when the popular regimen for treatment of peptic ulcer disease included frequent ingestion of bicarbonate and milk. Reports of this condition, which is characterized by hypercalcemia, metabolic alkalosis, and renal failure, became less frequent as this method of treatment became less popular. By the 1990s however, the syndrome was again becoming more common due to the increased consumption of calcium carbonate for the prevention and treatment of osteoporosis. The incidence among inpatients with hypercalcemia was reported to be as high as 12% between 1990–1993 *(27)*. Most cases occur in patients taking over 3 g of calcium daily. The mechanisms involved in the development of the milk-alkali syndrome are not entirely clear, but are thought to involve a vicious cycle, in which the alkalosis causes a decrease in calcium excretion and, hence, an elevation in blood calcium. This elevation in blood calcium suppresses PTH secretion, which increases proximal tubular bicarbonate resorption, thus worsening the alkalosis. Volume depletion, which commonly accompanies the hypercalcemia, is a further stimulus to bicarbonate reabsorption and may further fuel this cycle.

Drug Related Hypercalcemia

While vitamin D preparations are the most common cause of drug-related hypercalcemia, thiazide diuretics and lithium are also associated with hypercalcemia. Thiazides act at the level of the distal tubule to increase calcium reabsorption. In most patients, the transient increase in blood calcium suppresses PTH, and thus, serum calcium levels remain normal. In a small subset of patients, however, PTH levels are not suppressed, and hypercalcemia ensues. It appears that these patients have an underlying abnormality in their parathyroid glands, which is unmasked by thiazide therapy. Indeed in some patients, discontinuing thiazide therapy does not cure the hypercalcemia, and many of these patients are subsequently found to have underlying primary hyperparathyroidism.

Lithium often increases blood calcium levels mildly, and serum calcium levels exceed the normal range in 10–20% of patients. The mechanisms involved are not entirely clear, but may involve effects of lithium on the calcium sensor in the parathyroid gland. The blood calcium levels usually return to normal upon discontinuation of the drug although hyperparathyroidism persists (caused by either hyperplasia or adenoma) in some patients.

Miscellaneous Causes

Thyrotoxicosis can cause mild hypercalcemia due to thyroid hormone-induced bone resorption. Vitamin A intoxication can also cause hypercalcemia by increasing bone resorption. Immobilization can lead to hypercalcemia due to accelerated bone resorption in patients with underlying high bone turnover states (e.g., childhood, adolescence, Paget's disease). Primary adrenal insufficiency has also been associated with hypercalcemia, but the mechanism is unclear. Finally, hypercalcemia is occasionally seen in patients recovering from severe rhabdomyolysis, as the calcium that was deposited in the injured muscle is remobilized. Hypercalcemia in these patients can be quite prolonged.

Differential Diagnosis and Laboratory Evaluation

The evaluation of hypercalcemia is usually initiated when serum calcium levels are found to be elevated upon routine screening. Nonetheless, it is important to think of hypercalcemia when a patient presents with any of the nonspecific symptoms discussed above, and no explanation is obvious. Similarly, some experts recommend that a serum calcium level be measured in patients presenting with calcium stones. When an elevated serum calcium level is found, simultaneous albumin and globulin levels, or preferably an ionized calcium, should be measured to exclude pseudohypercalcemia. Once true hypercalcemia is confirmed, a great deal of information can be obtained from the clinical history, with the initial goal being to try to distinguish primary hyperparathyroidism from malignancy. The absence of symptoms (except perhaps for those of mild depression or fatigue) makes the diagnosis of primary hyperparathyroidism much more likely than hypercalcemia of malignancy. Documentation of a previously elevated calcium level in the remote past (>1 yr) also strongly favors the diagnosis of hyperparathyroidism, as occult malignancy is rarely seen in patients with chronically elevated calcium levels. A possible history of childhood radiation to the head or neck should be assessed, as these patients are predisposed to hyperparathyroidism. Additionally, a careful dietary history should be taken to determine if the hypercalcemia is due to vitamin D toxicity, milk-alkali syndrome, or other nutrition etiologies. A careful family history is useful to assess whether the hypercalcemia is due to an inherited syndrome. Finally, in some patients with malignancy and hypercalcemia, the hypercalcemia is not caused by the malignancy. Indeed, primary hyperparathyroidism is not infrequently seen in patients with coexisting malignancy *(28)*.

The laboratory evaluation of a patient with documented hypercalcemia begins with the measurement of PTH. While serum phosphate levels help suggest certain etiologies (high in vitamin D toxicity, low in primary hyperparathyroidism and humoral hypercalcemia of malignancy), they are not reliable enough to exclude any etiology, especially among patients with some degree of renal failure. The current double antibody, two-site assays for PTH have greatly facilitated the step-wise assessment of hypercalcemic patients. Both two-site immunoradiometric (IRMA) and two-site immunochemiluminometric (ICMA) assays are highly specific and sensitive for primary hyperparathyroidism and separate patients with primary hyperparathyroidism and malignancy reliably (Fig. 2) *(29,30)*. The finding of simultaneously elevated serum calcium and PTH levels is virtually diagnostic of primary hyperparathyroidism, though these findings would be consistent with FHH, lithium administration, or an ectopic PTH-secreting tumor as well. In some patients, serum PTH levels will be in the upper end of the normal range rather than frankly elevated, and this finding is also highly specific for primary hyperparathyroidism. Measuring 24-h urinary calcium excretion is useful in ruling out FHH if it is suspected by the clinical history. In patients with primary hyperparathyroidism, urinary calcium excretion tends to be elevated, whereas it is generally low in FHH.

A PTH level in the low range or the low-normal range (<20–25 pg/mL depending on the assay) is consistent with all other etiologies, including hypercalcemia of malignancy. Serum vitamin D metabolites, including serum 25-OH vitamin D and 1,25-$(OH)_2$ vitamin D levels, should be measured to rule out vitamin D intoxication and those etiologies dependent on 1,25-$(OH)_2$ vitamin D production (e.g., granulomatous disease or lymphoma). If the serum 1,25-$(OH)_2$ vitamin D

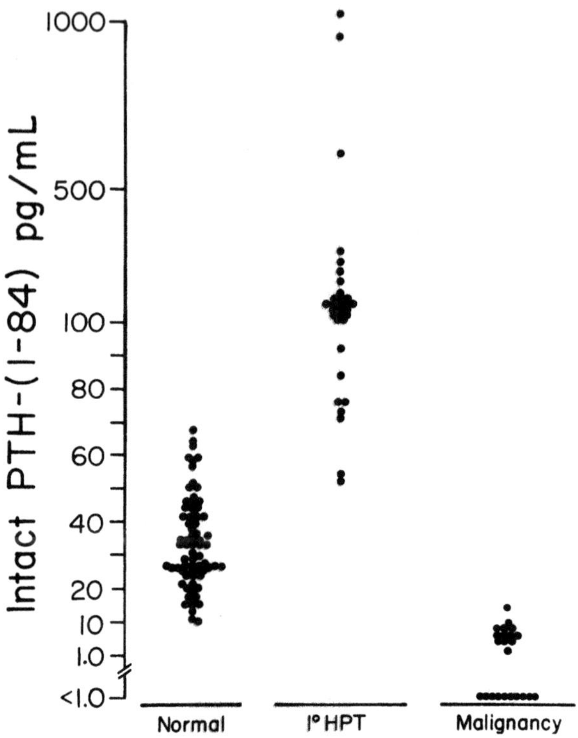

Fig. 2. Intact PTH measured by IRMA in normal individuals, patients with surgically proven hyperparathyroidism, and patients with hypercalcemia of malignancy. From Nussbaum et al. Clin Chem 1987;33:1364–1367, with permission.

level is elevated, and the 25-OH vitamin D level is not, a search for lymphoma or granulomatous disease is warranted. An elevated 1,25-$(OH)_2$ vitamin D level without a documented low or normal PTH is not by itself diagnostic of a vitamin D-dependent mechanism. Indeed, patients with primary hyperparathyroidism often have elevated 1,25-$(OH)_2$ vitamin D levels (though patients with PTHrP-induced hypercalcemia rarely do).

If the cause of hypercalcemia is not apparent, a search for an occult malignancy may be warranted. Initial tests should include a chest X-ray, serum and urine protein electrophoresis, and, in female patients, a mammogram. A chest computed tomography (CT), abdominal CT, and/or bone scan may also be useful. Assays for PTHrP are now available and may be helpful in some patients *(28)*. If this evaluation is not fruitful, one must reconsider one of the rarer causes of hypercalcemia listed, with special attention to the milk-alkali syndrome and other iatrogenic disorders.

The definitive diagnosis of many of these conditions, especially in the case of primary hyperparathyroidism, often comes only after a surgical cure and examination of the pathology specimen. In other instances, response to specific medical treatment helps provide a definitive diagnosis (e.g., response to steroids in granulomatous disease or lymphoma).

HYPOCALCEMIA

Hypocalcemia is an abnormal reduction in the serum ionized calcium concentration. Just as pseudohypercalcemia can be caused by elevations in serum proteins, a reduction in the total blood calcium may occur in patients with hypoalbuminemia and does not necessarily reflect the true ionized calcium concentration. Hypocalcemia is usually caused by abnormalities in the production, secretion, or action of PTH or 1,25-$(OH)_2$ vitamin D. Symptoms of hypocalcemia reflect the importance of calcium in diverse body functions. Although there is considerable individual variability, the extent of symptoms reflects both the degree of hypocalcemia and the rate at which the calcium has fallen (the more acute the drop in calcium, the more severe the symptoms). Exposure of nerves to a low calcium concentration reduces their excitation threshold. Thus, as calcium levels drop, the first symptoms are usually neuromuscular irritability manifested by parasthesias in the hands, feet, and perioral region. Chvostek's sign (contraction of facial muscles elicited by palpation of the facial nerve) and Trousseau's sign (carpal spasm induced by inflation of a blood pressure cuff above systolic pressure for 3 min) are often present even with mild hypocalcemia. As serum calcium levels drop further, blepharospasm, bronchospasm, laryngospasm, and tetany can develop. Central nervous system manifestations include seizures and increased intracranial pressure. Chronic hypocalcemia can cause extrapyramidal disturbances and Parkinsonism *(31)*. These symptoms can occur with or without calcification of the basal ganglia and the dentate nucleus. If calcification is present, these disturbances can persist even after correction of the underlying hypocalcemia *(32)*. As calcium is essential for contraction in cardiac muscle, numerous cardiovascular abnormalities have been associated with hypocalcemia, including a prolonged Q-T interval on electocardiogram (EKG), arrhythmias, and congestive heart failure *(33)*. Ophthalmologic symptoms include mineral deposits in the lens leading to cataracts.

Causes of hypocalcemia can be stratified by underlying mechanism (Table 2). Common causes of hypocalcemia are discussed below.

Hypoparathyroidism

Hypoparathyroidism can be caused by many distinct underlying etiologies. Regardless of the underlying etiology, hypoparathyroidism causes hypocalcemia by inhibiting the mobilization of calcium from bone, inhibiting the renal reabsorption of calcium in the kidney, and inhibiting the absorption of calcium in the gut via down-regulation of renal 1α-hydroxylase activity.

The most common cause of hypoparathyroidism in adults is complete removal of the glands after thyroid or neck surgery or surgical disruption of the blood supply to the glands. In the latter circumstance, the hypoparathyroidism can be temporary. Autoimmune destruction of the glands is often associated with the polyglandular autoimmune syndrome type I (which is also characterized by chronic mucocutaneous candidiasis and adrenal insufficiency) but sometimes occurs sporadically *(34)*. On rare occasions, hypoparathyroidism is caused by destruction of or temporary damage to the parathyroid glands after radioiodine ablation of the thyroid. Severe hypomagnesemia (values <1.0 mg/dL) can cause reversible hypoparathyroidism, both by inhibiting PTH secretion and by causing end organ resistance to PTH *(35,36)*. Rarely, hypoparathyroidism is caused by infiltration of the parathyroid gland in patients with granulomatous diseases, hemochromatosis, and metastases. Finally, hypocalcemia can be caused by heterozygous activating mutations of the calcium sensor gene. These activating mutations cause the gland to sense a greater calcium concentration than actually exists. Thus, patients have low or normal PTH levels despite mild to moderately low calcium levels. They tend to have hypercalciuria, which can be dramatic during treatment with vitamin D analogs. This disorder occurs both in an autosomal dominantly inherited *(37)* and a sporadic form *(38)*.

Pseudohypoparathyroidism

Pseudohypoparathyroidism (PHP) refers to conditions of PTH resistance. In many cases, this resistance is confined only to the kidney, so that hypocalcemia is caused by decreased calcium reabsorption and decreased 1α-hydroxylation of 25-OH vitamin D. The syndrome was first described by Fuller Albright and coworkers who reported three patients exhibiting hypocalcemia and hyperphosphatemia *(39)*. These patients also demonstrated congenital abnormalities including short stature, round face, subcutaneous ossifications, short metacarpals and metatarsals, obesity, and basal ganglia calcification. This phenotype is referred to as Albright's hereditary osteodystrophy (AHO). Patients with PHP have elevated PTH levels and diminished renal response to PTH administration, as determined by measuring the urinary cyclic AMP and phosphate response to PTH infusion (Ellsworth-Howard test).

Since Albright's original description, PHP has been classified into various subtypes. PHP type Ia is an autosomal dominantly inherited disorder characterized by a reduced activity in the α-stimulatory subunit of the guanine nucleotide-binding protein that couples PTH to adenyl cyclase ($G_s\alpha$) *(40)*. Specific mutations in the $G_s\alpha$ have now been reported in some kindreds *(41)*. Of note, patients with PHP type Ia can have resistance to other peptide hormones as well, including

Table 2
Causes of Hypocalcemia

Parathyroid-related	*Vitamin D-related*	*Phosphate-related*	*Other causes*
Hypoparathyroidism: postsurgical (thyroid, parathyroid, neck), autoimmune, infiltrative diseases, metastases, following radioactive iodine ablation, DiGeorge's syndrome	Dietary and environmental vitamin D deficiency	Renal failure	Osteoblastic metastatic disease
	Malabsorption	Tumor lysis	Hungry bone syndrome
	Anticonvolusants	Rhabdomyolysis	Chelation: citrated blood products, foscarnet, EDTA-containing contrast dyes
Impaired PTH secretion: hypomagnesemia, calcium sensor mutations	Impaired 25-hydroxylation: liver disease	Phosphate administration	Biphosphonates
PTH resistance: hypomagnesemia, PHP	Impaired 1α-hydroxylation: renal failure, vitamin D-dependent rickets type 1		Pancreatitis
	Vitamin D resistance: vitamin D-dependent rickets type II		Critical Illness: sepsis, toxic shock syndrome

gonadotropins and thyroid-stimulating hormone. Interestingly, patients who inherit the defective gene from their mothers have the AHO phenotype and PTH resistance, whereas patients who inherit the defective gene from their father may have AHO without PTH resistance (also called pseudo-PHP) *(2)*. Patients with PHP type Ib have inherited resistance to PTH, but normal $G_s\alpha$ activity. They do not exhibit the AHO phenotype. Although it was initially hypothesized that the defect in these patients would be in the PTH receptor gene itself, no such abnormalities have been found. PHP type II is a nonfamilial syndrome characterized by a specific defect only in the phosphaturic response to PTH, without complete PTH resistance.

Vitamin D Deficiency and Resistance

Hypocalcemia may result from vitamin D deficiency, because of decreased intestinal absorption of calcium. While 25-OH vitamin D levels in the low-normal range (15 ng/mL) are associated with a compensatory rise in PTH, more severe deficiency is usually required to cause true hypocalcemia. Vitamin D deficiency can be caused by defects of any of the steps in the pathway of vitamin D synthesis and action. These include dietary insufficiency, lack of sunlight exposure, or intestinal malabsorption. Anticonvulsant use may cause vitamin D deficiency by increasing its metabolism. In patients with severe liver disease, 25-hydroxylation can be impaired, so that serum 25-OH vitamin D levels are reduced. In chronic renal failure, decreased 1α-hydroxylation of 25-OH vitamin D leads to 1,25-$(OH)_2$ vitamin D deficiency.

Vitamin D-dependent rickets type I is an autosomal recessively inherited syndrome characterized by a defect in the 1α-hydroxylation of 25-OH vitamin D. These patients are hypocalcemic, have the pathologic features of childhood rickets, normal 25-OH vitamin D levels, but low 1,25-$(OH)_2$ vitamin D levels. The hypocalcemia in these patients responds to therapy with 1,25-$(OH)_2$ vitamin D. Vitamin D-dependent rickets type II is also an autosomal recessive disorder and is caused by mutations in the vitamin D receptor gene. Such patients are hypocalcemic and hypophosphatemic despite elevated 1,25-$(OH)_2$ vitamin D and PTH levels. The skeletal abnormalities in these patients do not respond well to pharmacological doses of vitamin D metabolites, but can be ameliorated by infusing calcium and phosphate. Such observations suggest that vitamin D itself is not needed for bone mineralization.

Chronic Renal Insufficiency

Chronic renal insufficiency is the most common cause of true hypocalcemia. The mechanisms by which patients with renal failure become hypocalcemic are compound. As renal function deteriorates, phosphate excretion decreases, and 1α-hydroxylase activity is compromised. The resultant hyperphosphatemia, coupled with the reduced 1,25-$(OH)_2$ vitamin D production by the kidney, combine to contribute to the hypocalcemia. PTH secretion increases in an attempt to normalize the serum calcium (secondary hyperparathyroidism). With chronic secondary hyperparathyroidism, autonomous parathyroid function and hypercalcemia can develop (tertiary hyperparathyroidism).

Miscellaneous Causes

Hyperphosphatemia from any cause (rhabdomyolysis, malignant hyperthermia, tumor-lysis) can cause hypocalcemia. Acute pancreatitis, possibly due to chelation of calcium by free fatty acids, is occasionally associated with hypocalcemia. Osteoblastic metastases (most commonly in prostate cancer) can cause hypocalcemia, as calcium is taken out of circulation in the formation of the new bone. Patients receiving blood transfusions often have temporary drops in calcium due to the chelation by citrate in the blood products. Patients with sepsis, toxic shock, and other overwhelming illness can be hypocalcemic, presumably from multiple factors. Bisphosphonate administration can cause hypocalcemia though this reduction is rarely associated with any symptoms in the absence of vitamin D deficiency. Finally, "hungry bone syndrome" (prolonged hypocalcemia due to a rapid shift of calcium and phosphate into bone) occurs both after successful parathyroid tumor resection and occasionally after cure of hyperthyroidism.

Differential Diagnosis and Laboratory Evaluation

The differential diagnosis of hypocalcemia can generally be derived by considering the three major regulators of serum calcium: PTH, vitamin D, and phosphate. Thus, the laboratory evaluation of hypocalcemia can be somewhat more straightforward than that of hypercalcemia. Table 3 shows the laboratory findings in the more common causes of hypocalcemia. As in hypercalcemia, the first step is to confirm the low calcium serum measurement to distinguish true hypocalcemia from low albumin states. Measuring the serum albumin and using a correction equation (add 0.8 mg/dL to the total serum calcium for every 1.0 g/dL fall in serum albumin), while sometimes useful, is not as reliable as measuring the ionized calcium level. Renal failure and hypomagnesemia can be ruled out easily with simple laboratory tests. If these tests are normal, or if the hypocalcemia does not resolve after the magnesium level has been corrected, measuring the serum phosphate level can help in the differential diagnosis. In the absence of renal failure or a condition of tissue breakdown (usually obvious from the clinical presentation), elevated phosphate strongly suggests hypoparathyroidism or PTH resistance (PHP). A low serum phosphate level suggests, but is not diagnostic of, vitamin D deficiency, vitamin D resistance, or an abnormality in vitamin D metabolism.

Simultaneous measurement of the serum PTH concentration, along with the levels of 25-OH vitamin D and 1,25-$(OH)_2$ vitamin D, while the calcium level is low, can distinguish most causes of hypocalcemia. A low serum PTH level, in the absence of hypomagnesemia, is diagnostic of hypoparathyroidism. PTH levels are elevated in other patients with hypocalcemia. In patients with vitamin D deficiency, PTH levels are elevated, 25-OH vitamin D levels are low, and 1,25-$(OH)_2$ vitamin D levels are variable. Indeed, in many patients with severe vitamin D deficiency, serum 1,25-$(OH)_2$ vitamin D levels are frankly elevated. In PHP and vitamin D-dependent rickets type I, 25-OH vitamin D levels are normal, but 1,25-$(OH)_2$ vitamin D levels are low. If not obvious on clinical grounds, the serum phosphate level can help differentiate the two conditions (phosphate is elevated in PHP and low in vitamin D-dependent rickets type I). In vitamin D-dependent rickets type II, PTH levels and 1,25-$(OH)_2$ vitamin D are usually elevated.

In patients with vitamin D deficiency, it is important to determine the underlying cause, as vitamin D deficiency may be a clue to an important underlying disorder. For example, in patients with adequate dietary vitamin D intake, vitamin D deficiency may be a clue to intestinal malabsorption. Similarly, in patients with hypocalcemia due to hypomagnesemia, it is important to consider the many potential causes of magnesium deficiency. Finally, in patients with hypocalcemia and increased PTH levels, in whom the cause of the disorder is not apparent, performance of the Ellsworth-Howard test may be useful.

Table 3
Laboratory Findings in Common Causes of Hypocalcemia[a]

Diagnosis	*Phosphate*	*PTH*	*25-OH vitamin D*	*1,25-(OH)$_2$ vitamin D*
Hypoparathyroidism	Elevated	Low	Normal	Low
PHP	Elevated	Elevated	Normal	Low
Vitamin D deficiency	Low	Elevated	Low	Low, normal, or elevated
Renal failure	Elevated	Elevated	Normal	Low
Vitamin D-dependent rickets type I	Low	Elevated	Normal or elevated	Low
Vitamin D-dependent rickets type II	Low	Elevated	Normal or elevated	Elevated

[a]Adapted from Guise TA, Mundy GR. Clinical review 69: evaluation of hypocalcemia in children and adults. J Clin Endocrinol Metab 1995;80:1473–1478, with permission.

REFERENCES

1. Brown EM, Pollak M, Hebert SC. The extracellular calcium-sensing receptor: its role in health and disease. Annu Rev Med 1998;49:15–29.
2. Bringhurst FR, Demay MB, Kronenberg HM. Hormones and disorders of mineral metabolism. In: Wilson JD, Foster DW, Kronenberg HM, Larsen PR, eds. Williams Textbook of Endocrinology. W.B. Saunders Company, Philadelphia, 1998, pp. 1155–1210.
3. Uy HL, Guise TA, De La Mata J, et al. Effects of parathyroid hormone (PTH)-related protein and PTH on osteoclasts and osteoclast precursors in vivo. Endocrinology 1995;136:3207–3212.
4. McSheehy PM, Chambers TJ. Osteoblastic cells mediate osteoclastic responsiveness to parathyroid hormone. Endocrinology 1986;118:824–828.
5. Frolich A. Prevalence of hypercalcaemia in normal and in hospital populations. Dan Med Bull 1998;45:436–439.
6. Walls J, Ratcliffe WA, Howell A, Bundred NJ. Parathyroid hormone and parathyroid hormone-related protein in the investigation of hypercalcaemia in two hospital populations [see comments]. Clin Endocrinol (Oxf) 1994;41:407–413.
7. Wermers RA, Khosla S, Atkinson EJ, et al. The rise and fall of primary hyperparathyroidism: a population-based study in Rochester, Minnesota, 1965-1992. Ann Intern Med 1997;126:433–440.
8. Salti GI, Fedorak I, Yashiro T, et al. Continuing evolution in the operative management of primary hyperparathyroidism. Arch Surg 1992;127:831–836.
9. Thompson NW, Eckhauser FE, Harness JK. The anatomy of primary hyperparathyroidism. Surgery 1982;92, 814–821.
10. Chan FK, Koberle LM, Thys-Jacobs S, Bilezikian JP. Differential diagnosis, causes, and management of hypercalcemia. Curr Probl Surg 1997;34, 445–523.
11. Potts JT Jr. Hyperparathyroidism and other hypercalcemic disorders. Adv Intern Med 1996;41:165–212.
12. Chandrasekharappa SC, Guru SC, Manickam P, et al. Positional cloning of the gene for multiple endocrine neoplasia-type 1. Science 1997;276:404–407.
13. Mulligan LM, Kwok JB, Healey CS, et al. Germ-line mutations of the RET proto-oncogene in multiple endocrine neoplasia type 2A. Nature 1993;363:458–460.

14. Rosenberg CL, Kim HG, Shows TB, Kronenberg HM, Arnold A. Rearrangement and overexpression of D11S287E, a candidate oncogene on chromosome 11q13 in benign parathyroid tumors. Oncogene 1991;6:449–453.
15. Arnold A, Kim HG, Gaz RD, et al. Molecular cloning and chromosomal mapping of DNA rearranged with the parathyroid hormone gene in a parathyroid adenoma. J Clin Invest 1989;83:2034–2040.
16. Farnebo F, Teh BT, Kytola S, et al. Alterations of the MEN1 gene in sporadic parathyroid tumors [see comments]. J Clin Endocrinol Metab 1998;83:2627–2630.
17. Cryns VL, Rubio MP, Thor AD, Louis DN, Arnold A. p53 abnormalities in human parathyroid carcinoma. J Clin Endocrinol Metab 1994;78:1320–1324.
18. Anonymous. Proceedings of the NIH Consensus Development Conference on diagnosis and management of asymptomatic primary hyperparathyroidism. Bethesda, Maryland, October 29-31, 1990. J Bone Miner Res 1991;6(Suppl 2):S1–S166.
19. Broadus AE, Mangin M, Ikeda K, et al. Humoral hypercalcemia of cancer. Identification of a novel parathyroid hormone-like peptide. N Engl J Med 1988;319:556–563.
20. Seymour JF, Gagel RF. Calcitriol: the major humoral mediator of hypercalcemia in Hodgkin's disease and non-Hodgkin's lymphomas. Blood 1993;82:1383–1394.
21. Garrett IR, Durie BG, Nedwin GE, et al. Production of lymphotoxin, a bone-resorbing cytokine, by cultured human myeloma cells. N Engl J Med 1987;317:526–532.
22. Mundy GR. Hyperacalcemia in hematologic malignancies and solid tumors associated with extensive localized bone destruction. In: Favus, M. J., ed. Primer on the Metabolic Bone Diseases and Disorders of Mineral Metabolism. Lippincott—Raven, Philadelphia, 1996, pp. 203–206.
23. Guise TA, Yin JJ, Taylor SD, et al. Evidence for a causal role of parathyroid hormone-related protein in the pathogenesis of human breast cancer-mediated osteolysis. J Clin Invest 1996;98:1544–1549.
24. Legha SS, Powell K, Buzdar AU, Blumenschein GR. Tamoxifen-induced hypercalcemia in breast cancer. Cancer 1981;47:2803–2806.
25. Selby PL, Davies M, Marks JS, Mawer EB. Vitamin D intoxication causes hypercalcaemia by increased bone resorption which responds to pamidronate. Clin Endocrinol (Oxf) 1995;43, 531–536.
26. Pollak MR, Brown EM, Chou YH, et al. Mutations in the human Ca(2+)-sensing receptor gene cause familial hypocalciuric hypercalcemia and neonatal severe hyperparathyroidism [see comments]. Cell 1993;75:1297–1303.
27. Beall DP, Scofield RH. Milk-alkali syndrome associated with calcium carbonate consumption. Report of 7 patients with parathyroid hormone levels and an estimate of prevalence among patients hospitalized with hypercalcemia. Medicine (Baltimore) 1995;74:89–96.
28. Ratcliffe WA, Hutchesson AC, Bundred NJ, Ratcliffe JG. Role of assays for parathyroid-hormone-related protein in investigation of hypercalcaemia [see comments]. Lancet 1992;339:164–167.
29. Endres DB, Villanueva R, Sharp CF Jr, Singer FR. Immunochemiluminometric and immunoradiometric determinations of intact and total immunoreactive parathyrin: performance in the differential diagnosis of hypercalcemia and hypoparathyroidism [see comments]. Clin Chem 1991;37:162–168.
30. Nussbaum SR, Zahradnik RJ, Lavigne JR, et al. Highly sensitive two-site immunoradiometric assay of parathyrin, and its clinical utility in evaluating patients with hypercalcemia. Clin Chem 1987;33:1364–1367.
31. Soffer D, Licht A, Yaar I, Abramsky O. Paroxysmal choreoathetosis as a presenting symptom in idiopathic hypoparathyroidism. J Neurol Neurosurg Psychiatry 1977;40:692–694.
32. Friedman JH, Chiucchini I, Tucci JR. Idiopathic hypoparathyroidism with extensive brain calcification and persistent neurologic dysfunction. Neurology 1987;37:307–309.
33. Lebowitz MR, Moses AM. Hypocalcemia. Semin Nephrol 1992;12:146–158.

34. Leshin M. Polyglandular autoimmune syndromes. Am J Med Sci 1985;290:77–88.
35. Rude RK, Oldham SB, Singer FR. Functional hypoparathyroidism and parathyroid hormone end-organ resistance in human magnesium deficiency. Clin Endocrinol (Oxf) 1976;5:209–224.
36. Suh SM, Tashjian AH Jr, Matsuo N, Parkinson DK, Fraser D. Pathogenesis of hypocalcemia in primary hypomagnesemia: normal end-organ responsiveness to parathyroid hormone, impaired parathyroid gland function. J Clin Invest 1973;52:153–160.
37. Pollak MR, Brown EM, Estep HL, et al. Autosomal dominant hypocalcaemia caused by a Ca(2+)-sensing receptor gene mutation. Nat Genet 1994;8:303–307.
38. Baron J, Winer KK, Yanovski JA, et al. Mutations in the Ca(2+)-sensing receptor gene cause autosomal dominant and sporadic hypoparathyroidism. Hum Mol Genet 1996;5:601–606.
39. Albright F, Burnett CH. Psuedo-hypoparathyroidism: an example of "Seabright-Bantam syndrome". Endocrinology 1942;30:922–932.
40. Carter A, Bardin C, Collins R, et al. Reduced expression of multiple forms of the alpha subunit of the stimulatory GTP-binding protein in pseudohypoparathyroidism type Ia. Proc Natl Acad Sci USA 1987;84:7266–7269.
41. Patten JL, Johns DR, Valle D, et al. Mutation in the gene encoding the stimulatory G protein of adenylate cyclase in Albright's hereditary osteodystrophy [see comments]. N Engl J Med 1990;322:1412–1419.

13 Osteoporosis

Patrick M. Doran, MD
and Sundeep Khosla, MD

CONTENTS

CLINICAL FEATURES

Definition and Epidemiology

Osteoporosis is a metabolic bone disease characterized by low bone mass and microarchitectural deterioration of the skeleton, leading to enhanced bone fragility and a consequent increase in fracture risk. It is the most prevalent bone disorder in industrialized countries and annually accounts for 1.5 million fractures in the U.S., incurring a total cost estimated at $13.8 billion in 1995 alone *(1)*.

Bone density values in the vertebrae, distal radius, and proximal femur are in the osteoporotic range, as defined by the World Health Organization (see below), in 25% of women at age 65 and in 70% of those above age 80 *(2)*. Caucasian women, without intervention, have a lifetime cumulative fracture risk as high as 60% for hip, spine, distal forearm, or a combination thereof *(3)*. The same lifetime risk for hip fracture alone is 17%, an incidence as great as the risk of breast, endometrial, and ovarian cancers combined. Hip fracture is also significant for being the most costly and catastrophic of the osteoporotic complications. These fractures account for two-thirds of total osteoporosis health care costs *(1)*, about 25% of patients have a fatal outcome (65,000 deaths/yr in the U.S.), half of the survivors are unable to walk unassisted, and a quarter become confined to a long-term care institution (21% of nursing home residents are admitted with this diagnosis *[4]*). However, other types of osteoporotic fractures also present a considerable disease burden (approx 5.6

From: *Contemporary Endocrinology: Handbook of Diagnostic Endocrinology*
Edited by: J. E. Hall and L. K. Nieman

million postmenopausal women suffer from vertebral fractures in the U.S. *[5]*), and can cause significant functional impairment *(1,6)*.

Even though osteoporosis is more common in women, men also incur substantial bone loss with aging *(7)*. Osteoporosis occurs in aging men at a frequency of 20–30% that of aging women, and elderly men have age-specific hip and vertebral fracture rates that are at least half those in women *(8)*. Additionally, recent estimates are that, of the $13.8 billion U.S. healthcare cost attributed to osteoporosis each year, at least $2.7 billion are related to male fractures.

Worldwide, the incidence of osteoporotic fractures has been increasing both in men and in women *(9)*, and this trend will only be magnified by aging of the post-war generation. This fact emphasizes the pressing need for effective and widespread treatment and prevention measures, which themselves depend on the accurate diagnosis of osteoporosis at its earliest stages. This chapter discusses present and future osteoporosis diagnostic approaches, after describing its key clinical manifestations.

Disease Spectrum

Bone is limited in the ways it can respond to illness, and bone loss is the common denominator to many disease processes, both intra- and extraskeletal and often acting in concert. Consequently, what we refer to as osteoporosis is actually a heterogeneous syndrome, with many causes and varying clinical forms. This section concentrates on primary osteoporosis in postmenopausal and aging women and in aging men. The numerous secondary contributors to osteoporosis are discussed in the Diagnostic Evaluation portion of this chapter.

Women undergo two phases of involutional bone loss, whereas men undergo a single one *(10)*, as shown schematically in Fig. 1. Peak bone mass is achieved in young adulthood and determined by multiple genetic and environmental factors. Subsequently, bone mineral density remains relatively constant in both genders until middle life. At menopause, women undergo an accelerated, transient phase of bone loss that is most apparent over the subsequent 10–15 yr and accounts for cancellous (or trabecular) bone losses of 20–30% and cortical bone losses of 5–10% *(10)*. During this phase, the drop in endogenous estrogen levels results in loss of the tonic inhibition exerted by estrogen over bone turnover *(11)*. Cancellous bone has a greater surface area than cortical bone, making it more vulnerable to increased osteoclastic activity. The deeper and more numerous osteoclastic resorption cavities lead to trabecular plate perforation and loss of cancellous bone structural integrity. This process translates clinically, in a subset of women, into fractures that occur at sites rich in cancellous bone, such as painful "crush fractures" of the vertebrae, Colles' fracture of the distal forearm, and fractures of the ankle (a syndrome sometimes referred to as type I osteoporosis) *(12,13)*.

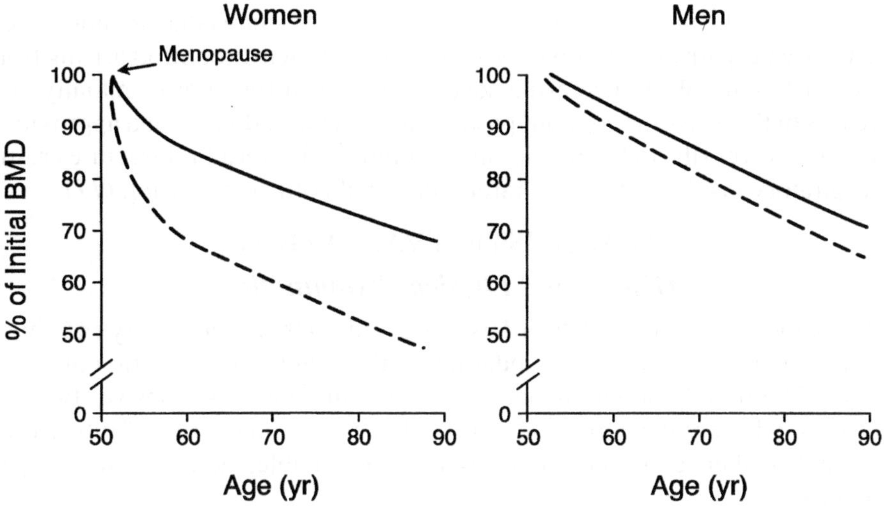

Fig. 1. Schematic representation of changes in bone mass over life in cancellous (broken line) and cortical (solid line) bone in women and men from age 50 yr onward. See text for details. From Riggs BL, Khosla S, Melton LJ III. J Bone Miner Res 1998;13:763–773, with permission.

This accelerated phase is superimposed on and merges asymptotically with an underlying phase of slow bone loss that continues indefinitely. In aging men, the slow continuous phase of bone loss resembles the late slow phase in aging women, and during their lifetimes men undergo two-thirds of the bone loss incurred by women *(14)*. Moreover, after accounting for the lack of a rapid phase in men, the continuous phases of loss in men and women are virtually identical *(15)*. Over life, this slow phase accounts for losses of about 20–30% of cancellous and of cortical bone in both genders *(10)*. The continuous phase of bone loss leads to fractures at sites containing substantial proportions of both types of bone *(12,13)*, namely the hip, proximal humerus, proximal tibia, and pelvis (type II osteoporosis). Vertebral fractures also occur during the slow phase of bone loss and are often of the multiple wedge type, leading to typically painless dorsal kyphosis (sometimes referred to as "dowager's hump").

The spectrum of clinical manifestations of osteoporosis ranges from a silent and progressive risk factor for fractures to a disabling and crippling disease. Osteoporotic fractures may involve any part of the skeleton except the skull *(16)*. The clinical implications of hip fracture have been described above. Most vertebral body fractures result in loss of stature—on average approx 1 cm/fracture—and result in increased thoracic kyphosis and flattening of the lordotic curve, depending on their location. This loss of vertebral height leads to compensatory contraction of the paraspinal muscles, so that even fractures that are not associated with acute pain often ultimately lead to chronic back discomfort arising from muscular fatigue. With increasing severity, vertebral fractures eventually produce loss of the waistline contour, protuberance of the abdomen, and approximation of the lower ribs to the pelvic rim. Uncommonly, vertebral fractures result in respiratory insufficiency and, rarely, in spinal cord compression *(17)*.

DIAGNOSTIC EVALUATION

History and Physical Examination

As for most other medical disorders, a focused yet thorough history and physical examination establish the foundation for the diagnostic evaluation of osteoporosis. The initial patient encounter aims to simultaneously answer two key questions: what are the current severity of bone loss and the risk of future fractures, and are there additional, and potentially reversible, factors contributing to bone loss.

The Current Severity of Bone Loss and Risk of Future Fractures

The question of bone loss severity will ultimately be answered more accurately by densitometry techniques (see below). Nevertheless, one can obtain a wealth of clinical information that is both complementary to the bone mineral density (BMD) measurement and essential in further refining the prediction of future fracture risk, ultimately to determine who is most likely to derive benefit from prevention and treatment. Patient characteristics associated with increased bone loss (Table 1) and/or trauma resulting in fractures, include a history of previous falls, visual impairment, dementia, frailty, and poor overall physical condition. Advanced age, which is associated with both an increase in fall propensity and a reduced capacity to break fall impact, has been recognized as a fracture risk factor independent of BMD *(18)*. Moreover, in the very elderly, a tendency to fall is even more predictive of future hip fracture than is BMD *(19)*.

Previous fragility fractures, which are arbitrarily defined as those occurring from trauma equal or less than a fall from a standing height, doubles the relative risk of future fractures, independently of BMD *(19,20)*. Thus, it is imperative to confirm that such fracture or fractures have indeed occurred and to review pertinent radiographs whenever possible. Diagnostic information can also be obtained from the symptomatology of previous fractures; delayed fracture union is atypical for osteoporosis and would suggest the presence of other skeletal disorders, such as Paget's disease, osteomalacia, hyperparathyroidism, or occult osteogenesis imperfecta (see below). Similarly, vertebral fractures that cause referred pain, long tract symptoms, or for which the acute pain syndrome lasts much beyond 6 wk (after excluding paraspinal muscular pain), should raise one's index of suspicion for an etiology other than simple osteoporosis, such as multiple myeloma or bony metastases *(16)*.

Table 1
Factors That May Contribute to Bone Loss *(16,21,22)*

Genetic	Hypercortisolemia
Caucasian or Asian ethnicity	Hyperparathyroidism
Positive family history of osteoporosis/fragility fracture	Hyperthyroidism
Small body habitus	Type 1 diabetes mellitus
Lifestyle	Addison's disease
Smoking	Hematologic/marrow replacment disorders
Excessive exercise (producting amenorrhea)	Multiple myeloma
Excessive alcohol consumption	Lymphoma/leukemia
Nutritional/gastrointestinal factors	Metastatic disease
Lactose intolerance	Anemias (sicle cell, thalassemia)
Prolonged low dietary calcium intake	Systemic mast cell disease
Vitamin C deficiency	Gaucher's disease
Vitamin D deficiency	Other medical disorders
Prolonged high caffeine intake	Chronic renal failure
Prolonged high protein/phosphorus intake	Hepatic insufficiency
Prolonged parenteral nutrition	Rheumatoid arthritis and other inflammatory arthropathies
Malabsorption (e.g., gastrectomy, celiac disease, Crohn's disease)	Anorexia nervosa
Menstrual status	Osteogenesis imperfecta (occult)
Late menarche	Medications
Oligomenorrhea/amenorrhea	Glucocorticoids
Nulliparity	Heparin
Early menopause	Anticonvulsants (e.g., phenytoin, phenobarbital)
Endocrine disorders	Excessive thyroid hormone
Hypogonadism	Gonadotropin-releasing hormone agonists or antagonists
Hyperprolactinemia	Chemotherapeutics
	Chronic lithium therapy
	Chronic phosphate-binding antacid use

The physical examination should be directed by the information obtained from the history and aim to detect and quantify the stigmata of osteoporosis described above. A baseline, maximally stretched height should be obtained, as well as an arm span, in order to estimate any loss in height. This portion of the clinical evaluation will also serve as a baseline against which the effectiveness of further interventions will be measured.

Additional Factors Contributing to Bone Loss

As already mentioned, osteoporosis is a heterogeneous syndrome that can be caused and exacerbated by a number of factors (Table 1), giving rise to "secondary osteoporosis." It should be emphasized that primary (i.e., postmenopausal/

age-related) and secondary osteoporosis are not mutually exclusive; in fact, one most commonly finds the latter superimposed on the former. For this reason, and given that 20% of women and 40% of men with osteoporosis are found to have at least one major, and potentially reversible, exacerbating factor *(10)*, a search for such factors should be undertaken in all patients with bone loss. Suspicion for a complicating factor should be heightened if the patient has an age-adjusted BMD more than 2 standard deviations (SD) below the mean (see below). As a general rule, the lower the BMD, the younger the patient, or the more atypical the presentation, the more diligent one should be at seeking out exacerbating conditions.

As before, the physical examination should be influenced by the history. In addition, the clinician should actively search for telling stigmata, such as blue sclerae in some types of osteogenesis imperfecta, band keratopathy in hyperparathyroidism, tremor and hyperreflexia in hyperthyroidism, hepatosplenomegaly in some hematologic malignancies, thin skin and ecchymoses in hypercortisolemia, etc.

Screening Laboratory Tests

Because a significant percentage of osteoporotic patients have at least one additional exacerbating condition, it is appropriate to perform simple screening laboratory studies in each patient during the initial evaluation. Among these, a serum biochemistry profile, including calcium, phosphorus, and alkaline phosphatase, may uncover otherwise unsuspected primary hyperparathyroidism, Paget's disease, or osteomalacia. The latter has been shown to be present in an important fraction of the elderly population with fractures *(19)*. Hypovitaminosis D amongst medical inpatients in general appears to be more frequent than originally suspected *(23)*. Given their central roles in bone metabolism, renal and hepatic functions should also be assessed. A complete blood count can provide the first indications of multiple myeloma, other hematological malignancies, hemoglobinopathies, or malnutrition. Also to rule out the presence of myeloma, serum protein electrophoresis should be considered in patients over age 40 yr (a normal result excludes myeloma in 90% of cases). A 24-h urinary calcium <100 mg suggests vitamin D malnutrition or malabsorption. A serum thyrotropin level performed with a sensitive assay should be considered, given that hyperthyroidism can be both readily reversed and difficult to diagnose clinically, particularly in the elderly. For the same reasons, male hypogonadism should also be confirmed or ruled out with serum sex steroid levels, particularly in men with an inordinate degree of bone loss.

Further laboratory tests should be performed as indicated by the information obtained through the history, physical examination, and screening tests (e.g., a serum 25-hydroxyvitamin D in a patient with low serum and urine calcium, a 24-h urinary free cortisol in a patient with Cushingoid features). Once again, the

Table 2
Principal Markers of Bone Remodeling Used Clinically

Formation
Serum:
Total and bone-specific alkaline phosphatase.
Osteocalcin (bone Gla-protein).
Procollagen I C-terminal (PICP) and N-terminal (PINP) extension peptides.
Resorption
Plasma/serum:
Tartrate-resistant acid phosphatase (TRAP).
Free pyridinoline.
Free deoxypyridinoline.
Type I collagen N- and C-telopeptide breakdown products (NTx and CTx).
Urine:
Urinary pyridinoline and deoxypyridinoline (collagen cross-links).
Type I collagen N- and C-telopeptide breakdown products (NTx and CTx).
Urinary hydroxylysine glycosides.

intensity of the search should match the level of one's index of suspicion. Bone biopsies are now rarely required, except in the uncommon patient in whom a diagnosis of osteomalacia or other disorder is clinically suspected and cannot otherwise be confirmed or excluded. Other than for diagnosing fractures that cannot be detected on X-rays, bone scintigraphy is of little use in osteoporosis. The increased uptake of technecium-99m diphosphonate at the site of vertebral fractures is of variable duration and cannot be used to reliably estimate the age of a fracture. Tests that specifically evaluate bone remodeling, mass and structure will be discussed next.

Biochemical Markers of Bone Remodeling

The rate of bone formation or degradation can now be assessed by two approaches. One consists of measuring enzymatic activity of the osteoblastic or osteoclastic cells, such as alkaline phosphatase and acid phosphatase, respectively (Table 2). The other is by measuring components of the bone matrix released into the circulation during its formation or resorption, such as osteocalcin and collagen cross-links, respectively.

It is now generally agreed that fasting urinary calcium and urinary hydroxyproline are too nonspecific and variable to be useful in osteoporosis. Both formation and resorption markers tend to rise with increased bone turnover, given the coupling of these processes at the bone remodeling unit. A thorough discussion of each of the turnover markers is beyond the scope of this chapter, but the interested reader is referred to some excellent reviews *(24–26)*.

As a group, bone turnover markers have shown promise by supplying dynamic information on the rate of bone loss, which is complementary to the static BMD measurement. Furthermore, rapid bone remodeling is a risk factor for fracture, independently of BMD *(27)*. Clinically, turnover markers may be used as an adjunct to decide on whether or not to initiate therapy in a patient with borderline BMD results. However, the most practical use so far has been for monitoring therapy, and patients with high turnover tend to show the best response to antiresorptive agents *(28,29)*.

Nevertheless, remodeling markers still have some limitations. Marker levels can be influenced by factors other than bone turnover, including metabolic clearance, and currently available assays are of variable accuracy. The use of markers still cannot substitute for direct BMD measurements for detecting the presence of osteoporosis, and elevated levels cannot distinguish between the various pathophysiologic mechanisms of bone loss. There are no studies so far to indicate that formation and resorption marker levels can be combined to assess remodeling imbalance. Most relevant to clinical practice, however, is the fact that all data supporting a role for markers in predicting rates of bone loss and response to treatment are based on group data, and it remains to be demonstrated that the changes seen in individual patients are sufficiently great and consistent to provide interpretable information *(26)*. Still, the prospective French Epidémiologie de l'Ostéoporose (EPIDOS) study found that the combination of resorption marker and hip BMD measurements was as sensitive and more specific than hip BMD alone at predicting hip fracture risk in a cohort of postmenopausal women *(30)*. Therefore, the clinical use of bone markers in the assessment of fracture risk in individual postmenopausal women may be envisaged, once thresholds of increased bone resorption become established for each marker and fracture type.

Bone Densitometry

Biomechanical studies have shown that approx 85% of the variance of bone strength is determined by its mineral content *(31)*. Before the advent of bone densitometry, the diagnosis of osteoporosis usually depended on the presence of a fragility fracture. Our current ability to measure BMD before the onset of fractures has been one of the greatest advances in the diagnosis and management of osteoporosis. Several prospective studies have shown that the relative risk of fracture increases exponentially with reductions in bone mass *(18,20,32)*. Estimates consistently show a risk gradient between 1.5 and 3.0 for each SD decrease in BMD with all absorptiometry techniques. Elderly women with hip BMD 1 SD below the mean are 7× more likely to suffer a hip fracture than an age-matched woman with a BMD 1 SD above the mean *(32)*, and BMD predicts fracture risk in men as it does in women, especially when BMD is corrected for bone volume *(33)*. Overall, the relationship between bone density and fracture risk is as strong

Table 3
WHO Criteria for Osteoporosis *(35)*

Normal	BMD within 1 SD of young adult reference mean.
Low bone mass (osteopenia)	BMD between –1 SD and –2.5 SD below young adult reference mean.
Osteoporosis	BMD –2.5 SD or more below young adult reference mean.
Severe (established) osteoporosis	Osteoporosis with one or more fragility fractures.

or stronger than the relationship between serum cholesterol levels and the incidence of coronary disease *(34)*.

In light of the above data, and in an effort to more fully define the prevalence of osteoporosis worldwide, the World Health Organization (WHO) convened an expert panel to define osteoporosis on the basis of bone mass measurements *(35,36)*. This classification is based on T-scores, i.e., the number of SD units a given individual is below the healthy young adult mean BMD, or mean peak bone mass (Table 3).

A cutoff of -2.5 SD below the mean normal peak BMD was chosen, since over 95% of individuals who ultimately fracture have a bone mass below this level. Such a value at a single site suffices for the diagnosis of osteoporosis. The recognition of individuals with osteopenia is also clinically relevant since, if left unidentified, they may unknowingly continue to lose bone and become at increased risk for fractures.

Optimal screening regimens for osteoporosis and osteopenia have yet to be determined, but most authorities have recommended against universal screening *(37)*. With the objective of detecting patients with fracture risk who were likely to benefit from intervention, the National Osteoporosis Foundation (NOF) has presented guidelines recommending BMD testing for the following individuals *(38,39)*:

1. Women 65 yr of age or older, regardless of osteoporosis risk factors.
2. Postmenopausal women less than 65 yr who have at least one additional risk factor for osteoporosis other than menopause.
3. Other individuals at significant risk for bone loss or with fragility fractures.
4. All postmenopausal women who present with fractures.
5. Individuals with roentgenographic findings consistent with osteoporosis.
6. Women who are considering osteoporosis treatment and for whom BMD test results would influence this decision.

The choice of anatomical measurement sites for BMD will depend on instrument availability (see below), patient characteristics, the underlying cause of bone loss, and whether BMD is performed to simply determine bone loss and the overall fracture risk or to also predict the risk of a particular fracture. Within the limitations of accuracy, a diagnosis of generalized osteoporosis and an estimation of the overall risk of fracture can be made from any site *(40)*, and although some have suggested that the diagnostic sensitivity may be increased by measuring at more than one site, the gain is small *(41)*. A notable caveat is found in patients over age 65 and in younger patients with spondylarthropathies, where the lumbar spine BMD may be spuriously elevated with some techniques (see below). In these patients, a second site such as the proximal femur should be considered in order to obtain a more representative reading.

Disorders that preferentially involve cancellous bone loss may be more accurately assessed by measuring BMD at a site rich in cancellous bone, such as the vertebrae or the ultradistal radius, which consists of 70% cancellous bone. Conversely, disorders characterized by greater cortical bone involvement, such as primary hyperparathyroidism, may be better evaluated by measuring a predominantly cortical site, such as the mid radius.

Although osteoporosis is generally a systemic disease, the correlation coefficients (r) between BMD values at different skeletal sites are typically only in the order of 0.7 *(42)*. Considerable evidence also suggests that fracture risk at any particular site is best evaluated by a measurement at that site *(43)*; in the Study of Osteoporotic Fractures, the risk ratio for each 1 SD decrease in BMD for hip fracture was 1.5 for a measurement at the mid-radius, compared to 2.8 for one done at the femur *(43)*. Given that the most clinically serious osteoporotic fractures occur at the hip and spine, most patient evaluations will include BMD measurements performed at both of those sites.

BMD values remain the cornerstone for quantification of bone mass and of the risk of fracture, given that they represent a composite, cumulative index of multiple bone loss contributors, both past and present. However, some of the limitations of BMD measurements in general should be discussed in order to view these techniques from a proper perspective.

1. BMD values do not determine the cause of bone loss or if the patient has sustained fractures (this latter task is best performed by plain X-rays).
2. BMD is only one of several factors determining bone strength. Other factors include trabecular connectivity (as assessed by the novel technique of microscopic computerized tomography), chemical matrix properties, and ability to heal microfractures, all commonly referred to as "bone quality". Readily measurable structural characteristics may also be important.
3. Normal BMD ranges for populations other than women over age 30 yr are not as readily available. Also, the normal ranges provided by BMD instrument manufacturers are not always relevant to the population being studied and in such cases can be misleading.
4. Different instruments may give different results, even when from the same manufacturer, measuring the same site, in the same patient. It is thus preferable

to perform further measurements on the same instrument if results are to be compared.

5. The ability to follow a patient for BMD change also depends on the instrument's precision error (i.e., the inter-result variability due to instrument error alone; in contradistinction to accuracy, which is the ability to obtain a result that is similar to the true value it was intended to measure). As a general rule, a measured change in BMD should be 2.8 × the precision error of the instrument used. For example, at least 12 mo should elapse before repeating a dual-energy X-ray absorptiometry (DXA) scan (precision error 1 to 2%) in most clinical situations. However, in cases where bone loss can be rapid (e.g., following initiation of chronic glucocorticoid therapy), a BMD change can be appreciated by DXA 6 mo after the baseline measurement.
6. BMD values should be considered not as intervention thresholds, but rather as fracture thresholds to be interpreted in the context of the overall patient, in order to determine the remaining lifetime fracture probability (RLFP). For example, a T-score of -2 may not require intervention in an 80-yr-old woman without fractures, but would have drastically different therapeutic implications in a 40-yr-old woman presenting with fragility fractures.

The remainder of this section will describe each of the major bone densitometry techniques currently available or in development. Although an exhaustive discussion of these multiple technologies exceeds the scope of this chapter, the interested reader is referred to some selected reviews *(44–47)*. Densitometers function by measuring bone's absorption of radiation or high-frequency sound waves, and techniques differ in the methods they use in accounting for the energy absorbed by neighboring soft tissue, yielding different levels of accuracy and precision when applied clinically (Table 4).

Most instruments provide patient data expressed in 3 different ways: (*i*) as the actual bone mineral content per surface area (in g/cm^2, clinically referred to as BMD); (*ii*) as a percentile of age- and gender-matched normal individuals; and (*iii*) as T-scores (gender-specific, in SD units) and Z-scores (age-adjusted T-scores).

Conventional Bone Radiography

Plain bone X-rays are mentioned here, partly because they were, for a long time, the only means of detecting bone loss. However, such quantification of osteopenia is inaccurate, since it is influenced by technical factors such as radiographic exposure, film development, and soft tissue thickness. As much as 20–40% of bone mass must be lost before a reduction in density can be appreciated *(48)*. Moreover, radiographic osteopenia in not correlated with vertebral fractures *(49)*.

Bone radiographs are the technique of choice for diagnosing fractures and dystrophic calcifications of the lumbar spine, which can result in spuriously elevated BMD with some techniques. The knowledge of a vertebral fracture is relevant, as it significantly elevates the risk of a second fracture. However, vertebral wedge deformities can be difficult to diagnose with certainty, and there is

Table 4
Comparison of Precision Error, Accuracy Error, and Radiation Dose Among Currently Used Techniques for Bone Mineral Measurement

Technique	*Precision error (%)*	*Accuracy error (%)*	*Effective dose equivalent (μSv)*
Conventional radiography			
Lumbar spine (AP)			approx 550
Lumbar soine (lateral)			approx 450
SPA	1–2	4–6	<1
DPA			
Lumbar spine	2–3	2–11	5
Proximal femur	2–5		3
DXA			
PA lumbar spine	1	1–10	1
Lateral lumbar pine			
Decubitus position	2–6		3
Supine position	1–2		3
Proximal femur	1–2		1
Forearm	approx 1		<1
Whole body	1		3
QCT			
SEQCT	2–4	5–15	50
DEQCT	4–6	3–6	100
pQCT	0.5–1	2–8	<1
Quantitative ultrasound			
SOS	0.3–1.2	?	0
BUA	1.3–3.8	?	0

AP, anteroposterior; SPA, single-photon absorptiometry; DPA, dual-photon absorptiometry; DXA, dual-energy X-ray absorptiometry; PA, posteroanterior; QCT, quantitative computed tomography; SEQCT, single-energy QCT; DEQCT, dual-energy QCT; pQCT, peripheral QCT; SOS, speed of sound; BUA, broadband ultrasound attenuation.

Adapted from Jergas M, Genant HK. Current methods and recent advances in the diagnosis of osteoporosis. Arthritis Rheum 1993;36:1649–1662, with permission.

no unanimous agreement on their definition. For practical purposes, most clinicians agree upon a reduction in vertebral body height of 15–20% as a cutoff for significance *(50)*. Spine radiographs can provide a useful baseline on which to compare future fracture events. Also, radiographs will sometimes give clues as to the etiology of the osteopenia, such as pseudofractures in osteomalacia and brown tumors in hyperparathyroidism.

Single-Photon Absorptiometry and Single-Energy X-Ray Absorptiometry

Single-photon absorptiometry (SPA) was one of the first techniques to gain clinical use over 30 yr ago and uses a γ-ray-emitting source. The more recent single-energy X-ray absorptiometry (SXA) differs mainly by its use of an X-ray source. Both are used to measure bone mass at peripheral sites, most commonly at the radius and calcaneus. These densitometers use the difference in radiation absorption between bone and soft tissue. In order to calculate the fraction absorbed by bone, the thickness of soft tissue (which is assumed to have the density of water) is made constant by submerging the measured site in a known volume of water.

The value of measuring bone mass at the calcaneus has been somewhat controversial, because of the potentially confounding relationship between BMD and body weight or exercise at that site. Nevertheless, several studies have shown favorable results for the value of calcaneal measurements in predicting osteoporotic vertebral and femoral neck fractures *(51,52)*, though they are still not as predictive as BMD measurements at those sites. The advantages of SPA and SXA are their low radiation dose, small size, and relatively wide availability. However, they are limited by the inability to measure central sites. Also, BMD values for measurements at the ultradistal radius vary greatly within a relatively small area, thus making accurate positioning critical.

Dual-Photon Absorptiometry and Dual-Energy X-Ray Absorptiometry

An important development in the diagnostic evaluation of osteoporosis has been the ability to measure BMD at the axial skeleton. Both techniques determine peripheral, central, and whole-body BMD, and both use radiation beams of two different energy levels, which are differentially absorbed by bone and soft tissue. A detection algorithm then defines the bone edges, and the radiation absorption within those edges (the region of interest) is reported as the BMD in g/cm^2. While dual-photon absorptiometry (DPA) uses a gadolinium source, DXA uses an X-ray tube that provides a more intense radiation beam, resulting in shortened scan times, enhanced image definition (approaching that of a roentgenogram), and improved precision. For these reasons, and because it can also be used to assess body composition, DXA rapidly replaced DPA after its introduction, and is currently the most thoroughly studied and widely accepted BMD measurement technology.

Since the region of interest contains the entire vertebra and surrounding tissues, dystrophic osteoarthritic vertebral calcifications, vertebral compression, aortic calcifications, and intra-abdominal surgical clips can all spuriously increase BMD results. Lateral DXA has the advantage of excluding the effect of dystrophic vertebral calcification by restricting the region of interest to the predominantly cancellous vertebral body. Compared to the conventional anteroposterior (AP) approach, lateral DXA has shown a higher correlation with quantitative computerized tomography (QCT) *(53)*, which also measures vertebral trabecular bone in isolation. However, the diagnostic potential of lateral DXA remains controversial, since its capacity to better detect small density changes may be offset by poorer precision due to the positioning variability of having the patient assume a lateral decubitus position *(54)*. Further improvements include supine lateral DXA scans using a source and detector supported on a rotating C-arm, as well as synchronized measurements of the spine in AP and lateral positions for calculation of an estimated volumetric density of the vertebral body, but both these approaches require further evaluation.

Quantitative Computerized Tomography

QCT is generally performed using a routine CT scanner with specialized software and a radiographic standard such as K_2HPO_4. Although it can measure BMD at virtually any skeletal site, QCT has more commonly been applied to vertebral bone mass measurement. On a lateral digital radiograph, a slice selection is made at the vertebral levels of three or four consecutive vertebral bodies (usually L1–L3). The average attenuation (in Hounsfield units) of the scanned region of interest is then determined and compared to the simultaneously scanned standard.

QCT has the advantage of being the only currently available method to provide a true density measurement (g/cm^3). It also has the ability of measuring a region of interest, either including the entire vertebra, or limited to either cortical or cancellous bone, thus avoiding the interfering factors described for AP DXA. QCT can also supply high-resolution cross-sectional images for the calculation of geometric properties. Vertebral QCT has been shown to predict fracture risk *(41)*, and in some cross-sectional studies has generally shown better discrimination than DXA between osteoporotic and healthy individuals *(55)*. Additionally, QCT scanners specially designed for peripheral BMD measurements (usually at the mid- and ultradistal radius) share the above advantages, while being portable and requiring short examination times.

However, QCT's limitations include being more expensive, using a higher radiation dose (50–100 μSv), requiring frequent calibrations (before and after each patient), and being significantly affected by marrow fat content, which can lower results as much as 20% below the actual value. Its precision is closely related to meticulous localization of the region of interest and has an error range of 2–4% under optimal circumstances. Moreover, there have been no prospective studies to determine which measurements best predict subsequent vertebral fractures.

Quantitative Ultrasound

Ultrasound techniques used to assess material properties are well known in industrial testing, but the application of ultrasound technology to the evaluation of bone integrity is only a recent one. The calcaneus is the preferred site, since it is easily accessible, has a high percentage of cancellous bone, and has a narrow range of widths in the adult, facilitating the calculation of measurement parameters. Other measurement sites include the patella, and new hand-held devices for assessment of the axial skeleton are currently in development.

The two main parameters provided by quantitative ultrasound (QUS) are broadband ultrasound attenuation (BUA) and speed of sound (SOS), both of which are reduced in osteoporosis. In vitro studies have demonstrated that both measurements seem to provide structural information, and 3-dimensional bone structure may be an important factor in determining bone strength *(56)*. SOS (m/s) is obtained by dividing the propagation distance (the calcaneal width) by the transit time, and is a function of both bone mass and "bone quality," including elastic modulus, trabecular orientation, and fatigue damage *(57)*. BUA (dB/MHz) rests on the fact that a sound wave passing through a structure will be attenuated proportionately to the complexity of that structure and is thought to reflect bone mass as well as trabecular separation, connectivity, and orientation. A third measurement parameter that is often given is the quantitative ultrasound index (QUI) or stiffness index (SI), which is an artificial quantity derived from BUA and SOS.

Although DXA is currently the more widely accepted procedure *(58)*, there is growing evidence that QUS is an effective predictor of fracture risk; and although a numerical range has yet to be determined, its accuracy compares favorably to that of DXA. In a retrospective study of 50 women who had recently sustained a hip fracture, BUA of the calcaneus had diagnostic sensitivity similar to hip DXA and superior to spine DXA *(59)*. In two other studies *(60,61)*, SOS at the calcaneus had a similar diagnostic sensitivity to femoral and spine DXA for distinguishing patients with vertebral fractures from controls. In the prospective EPIDOS study *(62)*, which followed 5895 women for a mean of 33 ± 8.6 mo, the relative risks of hip fracture was 1.9 (confidence interval [CI] 1.6–2.2)/1 SD reduction in calcaneal BUA, as compared with a relative risk of 2.1 (CI 1.78–2.48)/1 SD reduction in femoral neck BMD by DXA. Moreover, after inclusion of femoral neck BMD into a multivariate model, the ultrasound variables remained predictive of hip fracture, in agreement with QUS measuring properties different from BMD. In another study involving 442 women, BUA was compared to hip, spine, and whole-body DXA. After adjusting for age and weight, the relative risk for vertebral fracture was 1.8 (CI 1.4–2.3) for each SD reduction in BUA; for each SD reduction in BMD, the relative risk was 1.7 at the femoral neck and 2.2 at the spine *(63)*. Adjustment for spine, hip, or whole-body BMD did not significantly alter the association between BUA and vertebral fracture.

QUS is a promising approach that involves no radiation and, thus, does not require the operator to be trained in radiologic techniques. Other advantages include the portability of most units and their relatively lower cost, resulting in potentially greater availability. However, the positioning system of most instruments combined with the variability of calcaneal shape in the general population may yield erroneous results by measuring partly outside bone in some individuals. Most epidemiologic data so far has involved elderly women, and no comparable data is yet available for other groups. Until now, the relatively poor reproducibility of QUS has limited its role in following response to therapy. Also, there exist large differences in measurement scales in different instruments, making comparison difficult. Finally, more prospective data must be accrued in order to determine how each QUS parameter relates to BMD vs architectural factors, how the latter contribute to mechanical competence, and if this data is complementary to what is currently provided by other techniques.

CONCLUSIONS

Osteoporosis is by far the most prevalent metabolic bone disease and is expected to become even more widespread with aging of the population. Its optimal management rests on early diagnosis, as well as on the prompt recognition of exacerbating and potentially reversible contributors. The last 10 yr have seen an unsurpassed burgeoning of new technologies being applied to the characterization of bone integrity. With further improvement in both sophistication and availability, these diagnostic tools should lead the way to more effective and rewarding treatment and prevention strategies.

REFERENCES

1. Ray NF, Chan JK, Thamer M, Melton LJ III. Medical expenditures for the treatment of osteoporotic fractures in the United States in 1995: report from the National Osteoporosis Foundation. J Bone Miner Res 1997;12: 24–35.
2. Melton, LJ III. How many women have osteoporosis now? J Bone Miner Res 1995;10:175–177.
3. Melton LJ III, Atkinson EJ, O'Fallon WM, Wahner HW, Riggs, BL. Long-term fracture risk prediction with bone mineral measurements made at various skeletal sites. J Bone Miner Res 1991;6:S136.
4. Miller PD, Bonnick SL, Rosen CJ. Consensus of an international panel on the clinical utility of bone mass measurements in the detection of low bone mass in the adult population. Calcif Tissue Int 1996;58:207–214.
5. Melton LJ III, Lane AW, Cooper C, Eastell R, O'Fallon WM, Riggs, BL. Prevalence and incidence of vertebral deformities. Osteoporosis Int 1993;3:113–119.
6. Osteoporosis prevention, diagnosis, and therapy. NIH consensus statement online (http://consensus.nih.gov/cons/111/111_statement.htm), March 27-29, 2000 (accessed 2/3/2002);17(1):1–36.
7. Orwoll ES, Klein RF. Osteoporosis in men. Endocr Rev 1995;16:87–116.
8. Melton LJ III. Hip fractures: a worldwide problem today and tomorrow. Bone 1993;14:S1–S8.
9. Melton LJ III. Osteoporosis: a worldwide problem. In: Proceedings of the Third International Symposium on Osteoporosis, Washington, DC, March 2-5, 1994. Washington DC, National Osteoporosis Foundation/National Institutes of Health, p 23.
10. Riggs BL, Melton LJ III. Medical progress series: involutional osteoporosis. N Engl J Med 1986;314:1676–1686.
11. Doran PM, Khosla S. Senile Osteoporosis. In: Goltzman D, Henderson J, eds., Bone Primer. Cambridge University Press, New York, in press.
12. Riggs BL, Melton LJ III. Evidence for two distinct syndromes of involutional osteoporosis. Am J Med 1983;75:899–901.
13. Riggs BL, Melton LJ III. Clinical heterogeneity of involutional osteoporosis: implications for prevention and therapy. J Clin Endocrinol Metab 1990;70:1229–1232.
14. Riggs BL, Wahner HW, Dunn WL, Mazess RB, Offord KP, Melton LJ III. Differential changes in bone mineral density of the appendicular skeleton with aging: relationship to spinal osteoporosis. J Clin Invest 1981;67:328–335.

15. Epstein S, Bryce G, Hinman JW, et al. The influence of age on bone mineral regulating hormones. Bone 1986;7:421–425.
16. Kleerekoper M, Avioli LV. Evaluation and treatment of postmenopausal osteoporosis. In: Favus MJ, ed. Primer on the Metabolic Bone Diseases and Disorders of Mineral Metabolism, 3rd ed. Lippincott-Raven, Philadelphia, 1996, pp. 264–271.
17. Taggart HM, Tweedie DR. Spinal cord compression: remember osteoporosis. BMJ 1987;294:1148–1149.
18. Hui SL, Slemenda CW, Johnston CC Jr. Age and bone mass as predictors of fracture in a prospective study. J Clin Invest 1988;81:1804–1809.
19. Orwoll, ES. The special problem of hip fracture. In: Favus MJ, ed. Primer on the Metabolic Bone Diseases and Disorders of Mineral Metabolism, 3rd ed. Lippincott-Raven, Philadelphia, 1996, pp. 272–275.
20. Ross PD, Davis JW, Eptsein R, Wasnich RD. Pre-existing fractures and bone mass predict vertebral fracture incidence in women. Ann Intern Med 1991;114:919–923.
21. Eastell R, Riggs, BL. Diagnostic evaluation of osteoporosis. Endocrinol Metab Clin North Am 1988;17:547–571.
22. Genant HK. Radiology of osteoporosis and other metabolic bone diseases. In: Favus MJ, ed. Primer on the Metabolic Bone Diseases and Disorders of Mineral Metabolism, 3rd ed. Lippincott-Raven, Philadelphia, 1996, pp. 152–163.
23. Thomas MK, Lloyd-Jones DM, Thadani RI, et al. Hypovitaminosis D in medical inpatients. N Engl J Med 1998;338:777–783.
24. Garnero P, Delmas PD. Biochemical markers of bone turnover: applications for osteoporosis. Endocrinol Metab Clin North Am 1998;27:303–323.
25. Delmas PD, Eastell R, Garnero P, Seibel MJ, Stepan J. The use of biochemical markers of bone turnover in osteoporosis. Committee of Scientific Advisors of the International Osteoporosis Foundation. Osteoporos Int 2000;11(Suppl 6):S2–S17.
26. Garnero P. Markers of bone turnover for the prediction of fracture risk. Osteoporos Int 2000;11(Suppl 6):S55–S65.
27. Riggs BL, Melton LJ III, O'Fallon WM. Drug therapy for vertebral fractures in osteoporosis: evidence that decreases in bone turnover and increases in bone mass both determine antifracture efficacy. Bone 1996;18:197S–201S.
28. Civitelli R, Gonnelli S, Zacchei F, Bigazzi S, Vattimo A, Avioli LV, Gennari C. Bone turnover in postmenopausal osteoporosis: effect of calcitonin treatment. J Clin Invest 1988; 82: 1268–1274.
29. Lufkin EG, Wahner HW, O'Fallon WM, et al. Treatment of postmenopausal osteoporosis with transdermal estrogen. Ann Intern Med 1992;117:109.
30. Garnero P, Dargent-Molina P, Hans D, et al. Do markers of bone resorption add to bone mineral density and ultrasonographic heel measurement for the prediction of hip fracture in elderly women? The EPIDOS prospective study. Osteoporos Int 1998;8:563–569.
31. Melton LJ III, Chao EYS, Lane J. Biomechanical aspects of fractures. In: Riggs BL, Melton LJ III, eds. Osteoporosis: Etiology, Diagnosis, and Management. Raven Press, New York, 1988, pp. 111–131.
32. Cummings SR, Black DM, Nevitt MC, et al. Bone density at various sites for prediction of hip fractures. Lancet 1993;341:72–75
33. Melton LJ III, Atkinson EJ, O'Connor MK, O'Fallon WM, Riggs, BL. Bone density and fracture risk in men. J Bone Miner Res 1998;13:1915–1923.
34. Johnell O. Prevention of fractures in the elderly: a review. Acta Orthop Scand 1995;66:90–98.
35. World Health Organization. Assessment of fracture risk and its application to screening for postmenopausal osteoporosis. Report of a WHO Study Group. World Health Organ Tech Rep Ser 1994;843:1–129.

36. Kanis JA, Melton LJ III, Christiansen C, Johnston CC, Khaltaev N. The diagnosis of osteoporosis. J Bone Miner Res 1994;9:1137–1141.
37. Kanis JA, WHO Study Group. Assessment of fracture risk and its application to screening for postmenopausal osteoporosis: synopsis of a WHO report. Osteoporos Int 1994;4:368–381.
38. National Osteoporosis Foundation. Physician's Guide to Prevention and Treatment of Osteoporosis. Excerpta Medica, Belle Mead, NJ, 1998.
39. Heinemann DF. Osteoporosis. An overview of the National Osteoporosis Foundation clinical practice guide. Geriatrics 2000;55:33–36.
40. Kanis JA. Diagnosis of osteoporosis. Osteoporos Int 1997;7(Suppl 3):108–116.
41. Ross PD, Genant HK, Davis JW, Miller PD, Wasnich RD. Predicting vertebral fracture incidence from prevalent fracture and the bone density among non-black, osteoporotic women. Osteoporos Int 1993;3:120–126.
42. Grampp S, Genant HK, Mathur A, et al. Comparisons of noninvasive bone mineral measurements in assessing age-related loss, fracture discrimination, and diagnostic classification. J Bone Miner Res 1997;12:697–711.
43. Gluer CC, Cummings SB, Pressman A, et al. Prediction of hip fractures from pelvic radiographs: the Study of Osteoporotic Fractures. J Bone Miner Res 1994;9:671–677.
44. Blake GM, Fogelman I. Applications of bone densitometry for osteoporosis. Endocrin Metab Clin North Am 1998;27:267–288.
45. Hans D, Fuerst T, Lang T, et al. How can we measure bone quality? Baillieres Clin Rheumatol 1997;11:495–515.
46. Prins SH, Jorgensen HL, Jorgensen LV, Hassager C. The role of quantitative ultrasound in the assessment of bone: a review. Clin Physiol 1998;18:3–17.
47. Genant HK, Majumdar S. High-resolution magnetic resonance imaging of trabecular bone structure. Osteoporos Int 1997;7(Suppl 3):S135–S139.
48. Virtama P. Uneven distribution of bone mineral and covering effect of non-mineralized tissue as reasons for impaired detectability of bone density from roentgenograms. Ann Med Intern Fenn 1960;49:57–65.
49. Smith RW Jr, Rizek J. Epidemiologic studies of osteoporosis in women of Puerto Rico and southeastern Michigan with special reference to age, race, national origin and to other related or associated findings. Clin Orthop 1966;45:31–48.
50. Lukert M. Vertebral compression fractures: how to manage the pain, avoid disability. Geriatrics 1994;49:22–26.
51. Black D, Cummings SR, Melton LJ III. Appendicular bone mineral and a woman's lifetime risk of hip fracture. J Bone Miner Res 1992;7:639–646.
52. Ross PD, Wasnich RD, Heilbrun LK, Vogel JM. Definition of a spine fracture threshold based upon prospective fracture risk. Bone 1987;8:271–278.
53. Yu W, Gluer CC, Grampp S, et al. Spinal bone mineral assessment in postmenopausal women: a comparison between dual X-ray absorptiometry and quantitative computed tomography. Osteoporos Int 1995;5:433–439.
54. Blake GM, Herd RJM, Fogelman I. A longitudinal study of supine lateral DXA of the lumbar spine: a comparison with posteroanterior spine, hip and total body DXA. Osteoporos Int 1996;6:462–470.
55. Pacifici R, Rupich R, Griffin M, Chines A, Susman A, Avioli LV. Dual energy radiography versus quantitative computer tomography for the diagnosis of osteoporosis. J Clin Endocrinol Metab 1990;70:705–710.
56. Parfitt AM. Trabecular bone architecture in the pathogenesis and prevention of fracture. Am J Med 1987;82(Suppl 1B):68–72.
57. Grampp S, Jergas M, Gluer CC, Land P, Brastow P, Genant HK. Radiologic diagnosis of osteoporosis: current methods and perspectives. Radiol Clin North Am 1993;31:1133–1145.

58. Baran DT, Faulkner KG, Genant HK, Miller PD, Pacifici R. Diagnosis and management of osteoporosis: guidelines for the utilization of bone densitometry. Calcif Tissue Int 1997;61:433–440.
59. Stewart A, Reid DM, Porter RW. Broadband ultrasound attenuation and dual energy X-ray absorptiometry in patients with hip fractures: which technique discriminates fracture risk? Calcif Tissue Int 1994;54:466–469.
60. Turner CH, Peacock M, Timmerman L, Neal JM, Johnston CC Jr. Calcaneal ultrasound measurements discriminate hip fractures independently of bone mass. Osteoporos Int 1995;5:130–135.
61. Wuster C, Paetzold W, Scheidt-Nave C, Brandt K, Ziegler R. Equivalent diagnostic validity of ultrasound and dual x-ray absorptiometry in a clinical case-comparison study of women with vertebral osteoporosis. J Bone Miner Res 1994;9(Suppl 1):S211.
62. Dargent-Molina P, Schott AM, Hans D, et al. Separate and combined value of bone mass and gait speed measurements in screening for hip fracture risk: results from the EPIDOS study. Osteoporos Int 1999;9:188–192.
63. Bauer DC, Gluer CC, Genant HK, Stone K. Quantitative ultrasound and vertebral fracture in postmenopausal women. J Bone Miner Res 1995;10:353–358.

14 Hypogonadism and Erectile Dysfunction

Margaret E. Wierman, MD

CONTENTS

INTRODUCTION

This chapter reviews the approach to the male patient with hypogonadism and/or erectile dysfunction. A discussion of the normal physiology of the hypothalamic-pituitary-testicular axis is important in understanding the underlying mechanisms that result in hypogonadism. Defects can occur at any or multiple levels within the axis and can be congenital or acquired. A review of the normal physiology of erection is helpful to understanding the causes of impotence. A careful history, physical exam, and selected laboratory tests allow the appropriate diagnosis to be made and appropriate treatment to be instituted.

NORMAL PHYSIOLOGY OF THE MALE REPRODUCTIVE AXIS

Gonadotropin-releasing hormone (GnRH) is a hypothalamic hormone that is released in an episodic fashion to control pituitary gonadotropin biosynthesis and release (Fig. 1) *(1,2)*. The pituitary gonadotropins, lutenizing hormone (LH) and follicle-stimulating hormone (FSH) are secreted in a pulsatile manner from the anterior pituitary and act at the level of the testes to control both spermatogenesis and the production of steroid hormones and gonadal peptides. LH is the predominant stimulus for testosterone production *(3)*. FSH and inhibin

From: *Contemporary Endocrinology: Handbook of Diagnostic Endocrinology*
Edited by: J. E. Hall and L. K. Nieman

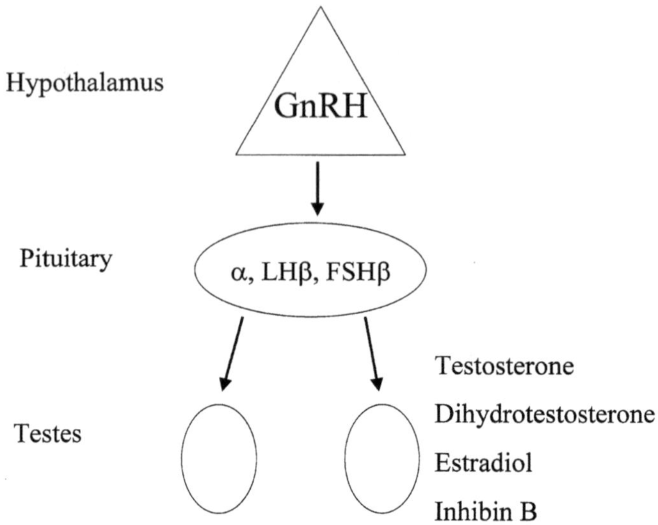

Fig. 1. Diagram of the hypothalamic-pituitary-testicular axis. GnRH from hypothalamic neurons activates the gonadotropin subunit genes (α, LHβ, FSHβ) to release LH and FSH from the pituitary. These in turn stimulate spermatogenesis and production of sex steroids (testosterone, estradiol) and the gonadal peptide, inhibin B.

B together regulate spermatogenesis in the presence of high intratesticular levels of testosterone *(4)*. Testosterone is a prohormone and is converted by 5α-reductase to dihydrotestosterone, a more potent androgen, or by aromatase into estradiol. Although androgens were thought to be the major sex steroid hormone in men, recent studies in animals and humans without an estrogen receptor (ERα) suggest that estradiol plays a critical role in normal spermatogenesis and hormone feedback in the male *(5,6)*. LH levels are controlled primarily by GnRH from the hypothalamus and negative feedback from testosterone and estradiol from the testes *(7–9)*. FSH levels, in contrast, are controlled by GnRH, gonadal steroid hormone feedback and the actions of the gonadal peptides, inhibin B, activin A, and follistatin derived from both the gonad and the pituitary *(10)*. A critical feature of this endocrine system is the negative feedback of steroid hormones on hypothalamic and pituitary hormone production *(2)*. Testosterone levels are secreted in a circadian rhythm with increases at night *(3)*. Another feature is the requirement for an episodic pattern of hormone secretion for normal reproductive function *(1–3)*. Continuous production of GnRH-induced LH secretion turns off the system and is the basis for GnRH analogues used as reversible medical castration in hormone-dependent malignancies such as prostate cancer. This episodic pattern of hormonal signaling is important to remember when obtaining samples for hormone levels.

NORMAL PHYSIOLOGY OF ERECTION

There are two critical events during erection. Dilation of the arterial bed with decreased resistance to allow increased blood flow is coupled with relaxation of the trabecular smooth muscle to compress the venous outflow *(11,12)*. The cavernosal relaxation is mediated by adrenergic receptors activated by norepinephrine released from sympathetic nerves. The autonomic nerves, once thought to be the primary control system, are now thought to act as modulators of the sympathetic activation to maintain flaccidity. Instead, it is the nonadrenergic, noncholinergic system that mediates erection *(13,14)*. Nitric oxide (NO) is released both from the endothelium and the local nerve endings in the corpora cavernosa to trigger smooth muscle relaxation via activation of guanylate cyclase and the generation of cyclic guanine monophosphate (cGMP), resulting in an erection *(15)*. The components of the normal physiology are relevant to the new treatment options for erectile dysfunction and for those under active investigation.

Table 1
Classification of Erectile Dysfunction

Vascular
Neurogenic
Psychogenic
Iatrogenic
Hormonal (hypogonadism)

CLASSIFICATION OF ERECTILE DYSFUNCTION

Erectile dysfunction is defined as the inability to achieve or maintain erection sufficient to permit satisfactory intercourse *(16)*. The prevalence of this disorder increases with age and with associated co-morbidities, such as diabetes, atherosclerosis, hyperlipidemia, or hypertension *(17)*. Impotence can be generally classified into five categories: vascular, neurogenic, psychogenic, iatrogenic (due to a medication the physician prescribes or the patient takes), or hormonal (Table 1). By the time a patient presents for evaluation, he usually, if not always, has multifactorial erectile dysfunction. Table 2 outlines the strategy for evaluation.

Vascular

Associated vascular disease is the most common underlying etiology of patients presenting with impotence and occurs in up to 40% of men *(16,17)*. Arterial insufficiency results in impaired blood flow to the cavernosal muscles. A careful history and physical examination can detect the presence of macro- or microvascular disease. A history of hypertension, hyperlipidemia, or diabetes predicts an underlying vascular component to erectile dysfunction.

Table 2
Approach to the Patient with Impotence

Complete history
Review of medications
Careful physical examination
Laboratory:
LH, FSH, testosterone +/– prolactin, TSH
Glucose
Lipid profile
Liver function tests

Neurogenic

Both trauma, such as spinal cord injury, or systemic diseases, such as diabetes or primary neurologic diseases, impair the normal process of erection *(16–19)*. Disorders that impact on the adrenergic, sympathetic, or nonadrenergic non-cholinergic NO system all result in erectile dysfunction. Additionally, radical prostatectomy, pelvic irradiation, and disorders that cause a peripheral neuropathy, such as toxins and alcohol are associated with impotence *(16–19)*.

Psychogenic

By the time a patient presents to a health care professional for evaluation of erectile dysfunction, there is almost uniformly a psychogenic component to the process *(16–19)*. Performance anxiety can play a role with underlying normal sexual functioning. An acute onset of impotence associated with a major life stressor is a clue for a predominant psychogenic etiology. Patients with underlying primary psychoses or neuroses often have decreased libido and erectile dysfunction when their disease is poorly controlled. In addition, medications given to treat the psychiatric illness are associated with similar symptoms making the underlying trigger often difficult to clarify.

Iatrogenic

Iatrogenic refers to ingestion of compounds or drugs by the patient prescribed by a physician or taken on their own that impair erectile function *(11,12,18,19)*. These include antihypertensive medications such as diuretics, β-blockers, and verapamil. Anti-androgens such as cimetidine, flutamide, and spironolactone can cause gynecomastia and impotence. Most psychiatric medications affect libido, elevate prolactin, and can cause hypogonadism as well as erectile dysfunction. Some over-the-counter medications, including herbal and health food products, cause impotence, although the exact mechanism has not been elucidated. It is important to review all medications, vitamins, or health products with each patient.

Hormonal

Previously, it was argued that hypogonadism is a rare cause of erectile dysfunction, occurring in less than 10% of men *(16,17,19,20)*. However, these studies were conducted in urological practices that included younger men with predominantly psychogenic etiologies. With the renewed interest in erectile dysfunction by primary care physicians, the educational programs available to the patients, and new treatment options, the number of patients presenting with a hormonal component to their erectile dysfunction is increasing. We performed a retrospective review of hormonal measurements in patients presenting to our Impotence Clinic at the Denver VA Medical Center and found that 48% had some endocrine abnormality contributing to their erectile dysfunction *(21)*. Thus, it is our practice to exclude hypogonadism as a contributing factor in all men presenting with impotence. Similarly, Buvat and coworkers suggest screening with a testosterone and prolactin level *(22)*. A discussion of the differential diagnosis of patients presenting with hypogonadism is given below.

CLASSIFICATION OF MALE HYPOGONADISM

There are several ways to classify hypogonadism. Many have used primary and secondary to refer to defects at the level of the testes or central loci. However, this classification is confusing, since congenital and acquired disorders can also be thought of as primary and secondary. A more straightforward approach is to base classification on gonadotropin levels: those associated with low or normal LH and/or FSH (hypogonadotropic hypogonadism) suggests a problem at the level of the brain or pituitary; high LH and/or FSH (hypergonadotropic hypogonadism) suggests a testicular problem. The disorders can then be divided into whether they are inherited or acquired. In addition, one can ask whether the defect is mechanical or hormonal. The approach to disorders of male hypogonadism is presented in Tables 3 and the classifications of such disorders in Tables 4 and 5.

Table 3
Approach to the Patient with Hypogonadism

Complete history
Review of medications
Careful physical examination
Laboratory:
LH, FSH, testosterone
Prolactin, thyroid function panel, free α-subunit,insulin-like growth factor (IGF)-1, cortisol
MRI if hypothalamic or pituitary disorder
Karyotype if suspected Klinefelter's, or genetic screening if familial

Table 4
Causes of Hypogonadotropic Hypogonadism

Hypothalamic disorders:
Congenital GnRH deficiency
Acquired GnRH deficiency
Tumors of the hypothalamus: craniopharyngiomas, dysgerminomas
Pituitary disorders:
Genetic mutations in the GnRH receptor or gonadotropin subunit genes
Pituitary tumors: prolactin, adrenocorticotrophic hormone (ACTH), growth hormone (GH)
Infiltrative diseases of the pituitary: hemachromatosis, sarcoid

Hypogonadotropic Hypogonadism: Low or Normal LH and/or FSH and Low Testosterone (Table 4)

Hypothalamic Disorders

Congenital GnRH Deficiency. GnRH deficiency or idiopathic hypogonadotropic hypogonadism is a disorder of the GnRH pulse generator (3). It occurs in 1/10,000 men and 1/80,000 women (23). The disorder can occur in an X-linked, autosomal dominant, autosomal recessive, and sporadic fashion. The patient presents with a failure to undergo sexual maturation. Patients with associated midline defects and anosmia are said to have Kallmann's syndrome (24). Although one might expect the disorder to be due to a mutation in the GnRH gene, attempts to identify patients with mutations in the gene have been unsuccessful (25). Developmental biologists were the first to provide a clue to the underlying defect. They showed that the GnRH neuronal population is born in the olfactory placode, and the cells must migrate across the cribiform plate into the forebrain and the hypothalamus during development (26). Investigators have shown that the X-linked form of Kallmann's syndrome is due to a mutation in the *KAL* gene whose product has structural features of a neuronal cell adhesion molecule (26–29). An understanding of the exact physiologic role of the KAL protein has been hampered by the fact that the gene is not expressed in rodents (29). Efforts are underway to identify additional molecules that are important in the neuronal migration of the GnRH population that may be miss-expressed in patients with other more common forms of GnRH deficiency syndrome.

Other hypothalamic disorders are associated with hypogonadism. These include Prader-Willi, in which patients have hyperphagia, morbid obesity, and obstructive sleep apnea *(30)*. Similarly, acquired obesity can be associated with hypoventilation and hypogonadism *(31,32)*.

The rare disorder X-linked adrenal hypoplasia, caused by mutations in the *DAX-1* gene is associated with hypogonadotropic hypogonadism as well as adrenal insufficiency *(33,34)*. Studies in a mouse model suggest the primary defect is in the control of secretion of GnRH, since gonadotropin synthesis and secretion was restored with exogenous GnRH administration *(35)*.

Acquired GnRH Deficiency. Acquired GnRH deficiency may occur after radiation or surgery to the hypothalamus *(36,37)*. The hypothalamus is more sensitive to the effects of radiation than the pituitary, and thus, patients we have previously labeled as having panhypopituitarism after radiation, often have their defect at the level of the hypothalamus. The patients have multiple hypothalamic defects resulting in multiple pituitary deficiencies and require lifelong hormone replacement.

Alternatively, men can have acquired defects in the GnRH pulse generator. Although hypothalamic amenorrhea is a well-recognized disorder in women due to the effects of stress, excessive exercise, or eating disorders to inhibit normal reproductive function, it was previously thought to be rare in men. This was based on the fact that GnRH-induced LH pulse frequency of every 2 h is fairly stable in men in contrast to the need for a changing hypothalamic input in the female to maintain normal cyclicity *(3)*. Recent studies however, have documented the acute reversible alteration in GnRH-induced gonadotropin secretion in men with severe stress or with illness *(38,39)*. Additionally, Nachtigall, Crowley and coworkers reported a nonreversible type of acquired GnRH deficiency in men *(40)*. They studied a group of men who had undergone a normal puberty, but then experienced loss of GnRH-induced gonadotropin secretion. Several clinical and biochemical features identified men with this disorder. These included: higher testicular vol (18 vs 3 mL), higher baseline serum testosterone level (78 vs 49 ng/dL), and higher serum inhibin B (119 vs 60 pg/mL) *(40)*.

Tumors of the Hypothalamus. Craniopharyngiomas are tumors that are located at the level of the hypothalamus and pituitary. Patients may present at any age with partial or complete pituitary insufficiency *(41)*. The patients often have associated hyperprolactinemia and, depending on the timing of the development of the tumor, can present with delayed or incomplete puberty or acquired hypogonadism. Patients with dysgerminomas or harmartomas of the hypothalamus or pineal gland may present with either precocious sexual development or acquired hypogonadism *(42)*.

Pituitary Disorders

Defective GnRH Receptor or Gonadotropin Subunit Gene Expression. It has recently been appreciated that there are genetic disorders that cause defects in the reproductive axis, in addition to those associated with GnRH deficiency. A family has been described with mutations in the first and third intracellular loop of the GnRH receptor gene *(43)*. The brother and sister presented with hypogonadotropic hypogonadism and delayed or absent puberty. A homozygous mutation in the LH β-subunit gene has also been reported to cause male hypogonadism *(44)*, and several women with delayed puberty and hypogonadism have been described with mutations in the FSH β-subunit gene *(45,46)*.

Pituitary Tumors. Tumors of the pituitary cause hypogonadism by either mass effect and destruction of gonadotropes or by hormonal production, which inhibits the GnRH pulse generator. The most common type of pituitary tumor is the prolactinoma, which occurs in 40% of patients *(47)*. Although in men, the tumors tend to be macroadenomas (greater than 1 cm in diameter), the mechanism of decreased testosterone levels is not by mass effect. Instead, prolactin acts at all levels of the hypothalamic-pituitary-testicular axis to inhibit function. Studies in hyperprolactinemic men showed that exogenous GnRH administration with a GnRH pump induced normal reproductive function *(48)*. These studies confirm that the major effect of excess prolactin is at the level of the hypothalamus. Recent studies have shown the presence of prolactin receptors on GnRH neuronal cell lines, consistent with the direct effects of prolactin on the GnRH pulse generator. Prolactin has an independent effect on libido that is poorly understood. Thus, men given testosterone replacement for hypogonadism associated with a prolactinoma often will have persistent decreased libido until the prolactin level is normalized.

Other pituitary tumors are often present in men with hypogonadism. Cushing's syndrome, with excess cortisol production from an endogenous or exogenous source, results in inhibition of the reproductive axis. Again, the effects of excess cortisol are to suppress GnRH secretion and induce hypogonadism *(49,50)*. Patients with acromegaly and growth hormone-producing tumors often have decreased testosterone levels. These patients usually have large tumors, so that the effects may be due to mass effect or may due to the fact that the tumors co-secrete prolactin *(51)*. Finally, patients with glycoprotein-secreting pituitary tumors frequently have associated erectile dysfunction and hypogonadism, but with elevated gonadotropins. This will be discussed in further detail below.

Infiltrative Diseases of the Pituitary. There are many uncommon disorders that involve infiltration of the pituitary and gonadotropin deficiency. The most common of these is hemachromatosis, in which excess iron is deposited selectively in gonadotropes *(52,53)*. The carrier frequency is 1/250, and the heterozygote can present with the constellation of clinical features when exposed to excess alcohol. These include severe hypogonadism with prepubertal testosterone levels, loss of body hair, diabetes, bronze discoloration of the skin, cardiomyopathy and arthropathy, in addition to progressive liver disease and cirrhosis. Aggressive phlebotomy is occasionally associated with reversal of the features early in the disease process *(53,54)*. Delayed diagnosis requires life-long androgen replacement.

Other diseases that infiltrate the pituitary and cause hypogonadism include the granulomatous diseases, such as sarcoid *(55)*. These patients more commonly present with hyperprolactinemia and diabetes insipidus, due to the presence of granulomas in the pituitary stalk and hypothalamus. An autoimmune process termed lymphocytic hypophysitis has been associated with acquired hypogonadotropic hypogonadism *(56)*. Infectious agents, such as histoplasmosis, tuberculosis, and rarely, coccidiomycosis or cryptosporosis, can infiltrate the pituitary, often affecting the production of multiple pituitary hormones *(55)*. Additionally, hematopoietic tumors, such as leukemias and lymphomas, have occasionally been reported to involve the pituitary to cause hypofunction *(57)*. Finally, tumors may metastasize to the pituitary *(57)*. These often invade via the posterior pituitary and present with posterior as well as anterior pituitary dysfunction. Tumors with a predilection for the pituitary include: prostate, lung, breast, melanoma, and renal cell cancer.

Table 5
Causes of Hypergonadotropic Hypogonadism

Klinefelter's syndrome
Intrauterine/testicular hypofunction
Genetic defects in gonadotropin action
Mechanical disorders of the testes
Infiltrative diseases of the testes
Glycoprotein-secreting pituitary tumors

Hypergonadotropic Hypogonadism: High LH and/or FSH and Low Testosterone (Table 5)

Klinefelter's Syndrome

Klinefelter's syndrome is a chromosomal disorder (XYY) of nondysjunction that is associated with ultimate hypogonadism *(58,59)*. There is lack of spermatic development and tubules, resulting in small testes at any stage of pubertal development. Initially, the Leydig cells function to produce low levels of gonadal steroids; however, with time, there is progressive tubular fibrosis and decline in androgen production. Men with Klinefelter's present with delayed or halting puberty, eunochoid body habitus, gynecomastia, and small testes. They are infertile and, ultimately, need androgen replacement. Patients with a mosaic karyotype, XXY/XY, have less of the clinical hallmarks, do not have associated gynecomastia, and have less severe and a later onset of their hypogonadism *(58,59)*.

Intrauterine/Testicular Hypofunction

There are several disorders that occur across gestation that result in absent or abnormal testicular function by birth (59,60). Testicular agenesis is associated with absent testes. Vanishing testes syndrome is seen with testicular remnants that disappear soon after birth. Finally, infants with cryptochidism are thought to have had a late insult to the system. With orchiopexy, the reproductive axis in these boys can function normally; although studies have suggested that they have subtle deficiencies in spermatogenesis. With aging, Leydig cell function declines, and patients often require androgen replacement. The underlying insult can be timed by the severity of the defect with the understanding that testicular development occurs prior to ovarian development at 9–11 wk of gestation.

Genetic Defects in Gonadotropin Action

Mutations in the gonadotropin subunit receptor genes have recently been identified that result in abnormal pubertal development. Some mutations of the LH receptor are constitutively active, resulting in gonadotropin-independent precocious puberty or testitoxicosis in boys *(61)*. Inactivating mutations in the LH receptor result in Leydig-cell hypoplasia and under-masculinization in males *(62–64)*. Inactivating FSH receptor mutations are associated with primary gonadal failure in males and hypergonadotropic hypogonadism in females *(65)*.

Mechanical Disorders of the Testes

Torsion of the testes can occur at any age. Normal sexual function can be achieved with only one gonad, so that hypogonadism only occurs when the vascular supply is compromised to both gonads or the remaining gonad is impaired due to another underlying problem.

Infiltrative Disorders of the Testes

Similar to the pituitary, the testes is the locus for a wide variety of disorders (reviewed in ref. *60*). Iron deposition occurs in the testes of patients with hemachromatosis, but the patients usually present with the pituitary rather than the primary testicular defect. Mumps occurring after puberty is associated with risk for subsequent hypogonadism. Additionally, infections, such as tuberculosis, human immunodeficiency virus (HIV), histoplasmosis, and others, have been reported to infiltrate the male gonad. Leukemia and lymphoma infiltration is often seen, but is of unclear clinical relevance.

Glycoprotein-Secreting Pituitary Tumors

Although most patients with elevated gonadotropin and low testosterone levels have a testicular locus of their hypogonadism, some patients with a pituitary disorder present with similar laboratory abnormalities. These are patients with glycoprotein-secreting pituitary tumors, which produce some component of the glycoprotein hormones: α-subunit, LH-β-subunit or FSH-β-subunit or rarely thyroid-stimulating hormone (TSH)-β-subunit *(66–68)*. These tumors, previously called nonfunctional tumors, occur in 30–35% of pituitary tumors. They occur most commonly in older men and present with erectile dysfunction, hypogonadism, and mass effects causing headache or visual disturbance *(66–68)*. Based on the secretory pattern of the glycoprotein tumor, the patient may have elevated FSH with or without elevated LH or α-subunit levels and low, normal, or high testosterone levels. Unfortunately, this is the same pattern of hormonal abnormalities seen in men with early or late testicular failure. Attempts to use other markers, such as elevated prolactin levels, as a signal of stalk compression or gonadotropin response to thyrotropin-releasing hormone (TRH) have been disappointing in discriminating patients with pituitary tumors *(66–68)*. Magnetic resonance imaging (MRI) is the test of choice to exclude a tumor in a patient with hypergonadotropic hypogonadism and symptoms of a mass effect. The tumors are often large at the time of clinical detection and are treated with transphenoidal surgical resection with occasional need for postoperative radiation. After surgery, androgen and other pituitary hormone replacement is often required depending on the status of the residual normal pituitary.

Table 6
Disorders that Present with Variable Patterns of Hypogonadism

Aging
Diabetes
Alcohol
Liver disease

Disorders that Present with Variable Patterns of Hypogonadism (Table 6)

Diabetes

Patients with diabetes often present with a combination of erectile dysfunction with or without hypogonadism *(69)*. Early in the disease process, the lack of metabolic control is associated with a mixed erectile disorder, which is reversed with improved blood glucose control. Later in the disease process, the patient presents with multifactorial erectile dysfunction and hypogonadism, which can be hypogonadotropic or hypergonadotropic, and require androgen replacement.

Aging

Many studies now show a gradual decline in androgen production from the testes with age *(70,71)*. Studies conflict on the timing of the process and the exact number of men that are affected, in contrast to the uniform pattern of ovarian failure seen at menopause in women *(70,71)*. Both hypogonadotropic and hypergonadotropic patterns have been reported. Earlier data was flawed by the inclusion of sick hospitalized men with other disorders that underlie their hypogonadism. Since co-morbid conditions increase with aging, however, the evaluation of all men for androgen deficiency is warranted.

Alcohol and Liver Disease

Excess alcohol has widespread effects on the reproductive axis. It has direct toxic effects on the Leydig cells, decreasing testosterone production *(72–74)*. Additionally, the associated central effects inhibit gonadotropin production *(72)*. Thus, a pattern of high or low gonadotropins with low testosterone can be observed.

TREATMENT ISSUES

Gonadotropin Replacement

In patients with a hypothalamic or pituitary defect, restoration of fertility as well as androgen replacement, are options *(75–77)*. Induction or reinduction of spermatogenesis can be performed using pulsatile GnRH administration or a combination of human menopausal gonadotropins (HMGs) and human chorionic gonadotropins (hCGs). Studies have shown that both are effective, but require parenteral administration and are costly. Successful spermatogenesis is predicted by the size of the testes upon initiation of therapy *(75–77)*, reflecting the severity of the gonadotropin deficiency. When fertility is not desired, androgen replacement options are similar to those with a primary testicular defect (see below).

Androgen Replacement

Androgen replacement should be considered for hypogonadism not only for restoration of sexual function, but for effects on muscle mass, respiratory drive, maintenance of bone mass, and cardioprotection *(78)*. Testosterone historically was available by intramuscular (IM) injection of depotestosterone 200–300 mg IM every (q) 2 to 3 wk. Trough levels just below the normal range, obtained before the 4th dose, help to maintain an optimal level of replacement. Yearly prostatic exams, lipid profiles, and complete blood counts (CBCs) are recommended to avoid side effects of worsening of benign prostatic hypertrophy, increase in low density lipoprotein (LDL) cholesterol levels, or polycythemia. Testosterone therapy is contraindicated in patients with underlying prostatic cancer. The availability of testosterone patches, and, more recently, gel formulations has revolutionized androgen replacement. These products allow a more steady-state replacement strategy without the highs and lows of intramuscular administration. Side effects of contact dermatitis and lack of ability to fine tune the dosing regimen with currently available androgen patches remain problems that should be overcome with future improvements in the drug delivery systems.

Erectile Dysfunction

The currently available treatment options for erectile dysfunction include mechanical devices and local or systemic drugs to modulate penile blood flow. Vacuum devices use suction to induce an erection and constriction rings to maintain the erection. Although cumbersome, they are safe and effective *(79,80)*. Intracavernosal injections of alprostadil are useful in diabetic patients who are comfortable with injections and often have a peripheral neuropathy that diminishes the major side effect of pain after the injection *(81)*. Other side effects include risk of bleeding, infection, and priapism, all which occur only rarely. Compliance with long-term use has been poor with recent studies, suggesting that only 32% of patients continued on the therapy *(82)*. The intraurethral formulation of alprostadil (MUSE) has not been as successful as initial reports suggested *(83,84)*.

The major advancements in the treatment of erectile dysfunction are the oral therapies. Yohimbine hydrochloride is an α-adrenergic antagonist and has been shown to be effective only in psychogenic impotence. The drug was noted to be 20% more effective than placebo when given at 5.4 mg 3×/d *(85)*. In these patients, combination with trazadone, a serotonin agonist, may increase effectiveness *(85)*. The recent availability of sildenafil (Viagra) has popularized the problem of erectile dysfunction. Sildenafil works by inhibiting Type 5 phosphodiesterase, which breaks down cGMP, the downstream target of NO *(86,87)*. Studies have shown the higher effectiveness in those with psychogenic impotence, spinal cord injury, and those men with partial rather than complete erectile dysfunction *(86,87)*. Patients with diabetes or after urological surgery have less response to the drug. Side effects include headache, dyspepsia, blue discoloration of vision, and postural hypotension. Thus, the drug is contraindicated in patients on nitrates. Additionally, the drug half-life can be potentiated by other medications, with aging, or with renal or hepatic disease. Longer clinical experience has suggested that for men with stable coronary artery disease, sildenafil had no deleterious effects on clinical symptoms, exercise capacity, or exercise-induced ischemia assessed by echocardiograpy *(88)*. New agents for erectile dysfunction include oral apomorphine (Ixense, Uprima), an opioid antagonist for psychogenic impotence *(89)*, and phentolamine, which is used to block the norepinephrine-mediated smooth muscle relaxation and vasodilation *(90)*.

SUMMARY

Thus, after a careful history, physical exam, and selected laboratory tests, one can classify patients with erectile dysfunction and/or hypogonadism into specific categories that allow appropriate therapeutic interventions *(91)*. Research is underway to use the new advances in the understanding of the physiology of erection and in disorders of the hypothalamic pituitary gonadal axis to target more specifically the treatment choices.

REFERENCES

1. Belchetz PE, Plant TM, Nakai Y, Keogh EJ, Knobil E. (1978) Hypophysial responses to continuous and intermittent delivery of hypothalamic gonadotropin-releasing hormone. Science 1978;202:631–633.
2. Marshall JC, Kelch RP. Gonadotropin-releasing hormone: role of pulsatile secretion in the regulation of reproduction. N Engl J Med 1986;315:1459–1468.
3. Crowley WF Jr, Whitcomb RW, Jameson JL, Weiss J, Finkelstein JS, O'Dea LS. Neuroendocrine control of human reproduction in the male. [review]. Rec Prog Horm Res 1991;47:27–62.
4. Hayes FJ, Hall JE, Boepple PA, Crowley WF Jr. Clinical review 96: differential control of gonadotropin secretion in the human: endocrine role of inhibin. J Clin Endocrinol Metab 1998;83:1835–1841.
5. Couse JF, Korach KS. Estrogen receptor null mice: what have we learned and where will they lead us? Endocr Rev 1999;20:358–417.
6. Smith EP, Boyd J, Frank GR, et al. Estrogen resistance caused by a mutation in the estrogen-receptor gene in a man. N Engl J Med 1994;331:1056–1061.
7. Finkelstein JS, O'Dea LS, Whitcomb RW, Crowley WF Jr. Sex steroid control of gonadotropin secretion in the human male. II. Effects of estradiol administration in normal and gonadotropin-releasing hormone-deficient men. J Clin Endocrinol Metab 71991;3:621–628.
8. Finkelstein JS, Whitcomb RW, O'Dea LS, Longcope C, Schoenfeld DA, Crowley WF Jr. Sex steroid control of gonadotropin secretion in the human male. I. Effects of testosterone administration in normal and gonadotropin-releasing hormone-deficient men. J Clin Endocrinol Metab 1991;73:609–620.
9. Bagatell CJ, Dahl KD, Bremner WJ. The direct pituitary effect of testosterone to inhibit gonadotropin secretion in men is partially mediated by aromatization to estradiol. J Andrology 1994;15:15–21.
10. Mather JP, Moore A, Li RH. Activins, inhibins, and follistatins: further thoughts on a growing family of regulators. Proc Soc Exp Biol Med 1997;215:209–222.
11. Krane RJ, Goldstein I, Saenz de Tejada I. Medical progress: impotence. N Engl J Med 1989;321:1648–1659.
12. Korenman SG. New insights into erectile dysfunction: a practical approach. Am J Med 1998;105:135–144.
13. Ignarro LJ. Nitric oxide as the physiological mediator of penile erection. J NIH Res 1992;4:59–62.
14. Rajfer J, Aronson WJ, Bush PA, et al. Nitric oxide as a mediator of relaxation of the corpus cavernosum in response to nonadrenergic, noncholinergic neurotransmission. N Engl J Med 1992;326:90–94.
15. Burnett AL, Lowenstein CJ, Bredt DS, et al. Nitric oxide: a physiologic mediator of penile erection. Science 1992;257:401–403.
16. NIH Consensus Conference. Impotence. JAMA 1993;270:83–90.
17. Feldman HA, Goldstein I, Hatzichristal DG, et al. Impotence and its medical and psychosocial correlates: results of the Massachusetts Male Aging Study. J Urol 1994;151:54–61.
18. Saenz de Tejada I, Goldstein I, Azadzoi K, et al. Impaired neurogenic and endothelium-mediated relaxation of penile smooth muscle from diabetic men with impotence. N Engl J Med 1989;320:1025–1030.
19. Wierman ME. Advances in the diagnosis and management of impotence. Adv Intern Med 1999;44:1–17.
20. Korenman SG, Morley JE, Mooradian AD, et al. Secondary hypogonadism in older men: its relation to impotence. J Clin Endocrinol Metab 1990;71:963–969.

21. Mahoney J, Bruder JM, Balanoff A, et al. Effectiveness of laboratory assessment of the pituitary-gonadal axis in patients with impotence [abstract 0038]. Clin Res 1994;42:250.
22. Buvat J, Lemaire A. Endocrine screening in 1,022 men with erectile dysfunction: clinical significance and cost-effective strategy. J Urol 1997;158:1764–1767.
23. Waldstreicher J, Seminara SB, Jameson JL, et al. The genetic and clinical heterogeneity of gonadotropin-releasing hormone deficiency in the human. J Clin Endocrinol Metab 1996;81:4388–4395.
24. Kallmann F, Schoenfeld WA, Barrera SE. The genetic aspects of primary eunuchoidism. Am J Mental Defic 1944;48:203–236.
25. Weiss J, Crowley WF, Jameson JL. Structure of the GnRH gene in patients with idiopathic hypogonadotropic hypogonadism. J Clin Endocrinol Metab 1989;69:299–303.
26. Schwanzel-Fukada M, Bick M, Pfaff DW. Luteinizing hormone-releasing hormone (LHRH)-expressing cells do not migrate normally in an inherited hypogonadal (Kallmann) syndrome. Mol Brain Res 1989;6:311–326.
27. Franco B, Guioli S, Pragliola A, et al. A gene deleted in Kallmann's syndrome shares homology with neural cell adhesion and axonal path-finding molecules. Nature 1991;353:529–536.
28. Legouis R, Hardelin J-P, Levilliers J, et al. The candidate gene for the X-linked Kallmann syndrome encodes a protein related to adhesion molecules. Cell 1991;67:423–435.
29. Rugarli EI, Ballabio A. Kallmann syndrome: from genetics to neurobiology. JAMA 1993;270:2713–2716.
30. Bray GA, Dahms WT, Swerdloff RS, Fiser RH, Atkinson RL, Carrel RE. The Prader-Willi Syndrome: a study of 40 patients and a review of the literature. Medicine 1983;62:59–80.
31. Vermeulen A, Kaufman JM, Deslypere JP, Thomas G. Attenuated luteinizing hormone (LH) pulse amplitude but normal LH pulse frequency, and its relation to plasma androgens in hypogonadism of obese men. J Clin Endocrinol Metab 1993;76:1140–1146.
32. Santamaria JD, Prior JC, Fleetham JA. Reversible reproductive dysfunction in men with obstructive sleep apnoea. Clin Endocrinol 1988;28:461–470.
33. Kruse K, Sippell WG, Schnakenburg KV. Hypogonadism in congenital adrenal hypoplasia: evidence for a hypothalamic origin. J Clin Endocrinol Metab 1984;58:12–17.
34. Muscatelli F, Strom TM, Walker AP, et al. Mutations in the DAX-1 gene give rise to both X-linked adrenal hypoplasia congenita and hypogonadotropic hypogonadism. Nature 1994;372:672–676.
35. Ikeda Y, Luo X, Abbud R, Nilson JH, Parker KL. The nuclear receptor steroidogenic factor 1 is essential for the formation of the ventromedial hypothalamic nucleus. Mol Endocrinol 1995;9:478–486.
36. Samaan NA, Bakdash MM, Caderao JB, Cangir A, Jesse RH Jr, Ballantyne AJ. Hypopituitarism after external irradiation. Ann Intern Med 1975;83:771–777.
37. Constine LS, Woolf PD, Cann D, et al. Hypothalamic-pituitary dysfunction after radiation for brain tumors. N Engl J Med 1993;328:87–94.
38. Woolf PD, Hamill RW, McDonald JV, Lee LA, Kelly M. Transient hypogonadotropic hypogonadism caused by critical illness. J Clin Endocrinol Metab 1985;60:444–450.
39. Spratt DI, Bigos ST, Beitins I, Cox P, Longcope C, Orav J. Both hyper- and hypogonadotropic hypogonadism occur transiently in acute illness: bio- and immunoactive gonadotropins. J Clin Endocrinol Metab 1992;75:1562–1570.
40. Nachtigall LB, Boepple PA, Pralong FP, Crowley WF Jr. Adult-onset idiopathic hypogonadotropic hypogonadism—a treatable form of male infertility. N Engl J Med 1997;336:410–415.
41. Sklar CA. Craniopharyngioma: endocrine abnormalities at presentation. Pediatr Neurosurg 1994;1:18–20.
42. Raisanen JM, Davis RL. Congenital brain tumors. Pathology 1993;2:103–116.
43. de Roux N, Young J, Misrahi M, Genet R, Chanson P, Schaison G, Milgrom E. A family with hypogonadotropic hypogonadism and mutations in the gonadotropin-releasing hormone receptor. N Engl J Med 1997;337:1597–1602.

44. Weiss J, Axelrod L, Whitcomb RW, Harris PE, Crowley WF, Jameson JL. Hypogonadism caused by a single amino acid substitution in the β subunit of Luteinizing hormone. N Engl J Med 1992;326:179–183.
45. Matthews CH, Borgato S, Beck-Peccoz P, et al Primary amenorrhoea and infertility due to a mutation in the beta-subunit of follicle-stimulating hormone. Nat Genet 1993;5:83–86.
46. Layman LC, Lee E-J, Peak DB, et al. Delayed puberty and hypogonadism caused by mutations in the follicle-stimulating hormone beta-subunit gene. N Engl J Med 1997;337:607–611.
47. Carter JN, Tyson JE, Tolis G, et al. Prolactin-secreting tumors and hypogonadism in 22 men. N Engl J Med 1978;299:847–852.
48. Bouchard P, Lagoguey M, Brailly S, Schaison G. Gonadotropin-releasing hormone pulsatile administration restores luteinizing hormone pulsatility and normal testosterone levels in males with hyperprolactinemia. J Clin Endocrinol Metab 1985;60:258–262.
49. Luton J, Thieblot P, Valcke J, Mahoudeau JA, Bricaire H. Reversible gonadotropin deficiency in male Cushing's disease. J Clin Endocrinol Metab 1977;45:488–495.
50. MacAdams MR, White RH, Chipps BE. Reduction of serum testosterone levels during chronic glucocorticoid therapy. Ann Int Med 1986;104:648–651.
51. Molitch ME. Clinical manifestations of acromegaly. Endocrinol. Metab Clin. North Am. 1992;21:597–614.
52. Kelly TM, Edwards CQ, Meikle AW, Kushner JP. Hypogonadism in hemochromatosis: reversal with iron depletion. Ann Int Med 1984;101:629–632.
53. Tavill AS. Clinical implications of the hemochromatosis gene. N Engl J Med 1999;341:755–756.
54. Cundy T, Butler J, Bomford A, Williams R. Reversibility of hypogonadotropic hypogonadism associated with genetic haemochromatosis. Clin Endocrinol 1993;38:617–620.
55. Bell NH. Endocrine complications of sarcoidosis. Endocrinol Metab Clin North Am 1991;20:645–654.
56. Cosman F, Post KD, Holub DA, Wardlaw SL. Lymphocytic hypophysitis: report of 3 new cases and review of the literature. Medicine 1989;68:240–256.
57. McDermott MT. Infiltrative diseases of the pituitary gland. In Wierman ME, ed. Diseases of the Pituitary: Diagnosis and Treatment. Humana, Totowa, NJ, 1997; pp. 305–322.
58. Smyth CM, Bremner WJ. Klinefelter syndrome. Arch Intern Med 1998;158:1309–1314.
59. Diemer T, Desjardins C. Developmental and genetic disorders in spermatogenesis. Hum Reprod 1999;Update 5:120–140.
60. Griffin JE, Wilson JD. Disorders of the testes and the male reproductive tract. In Wilson JD, Foster DW, eds. Williams Textbook of Endocrinology W.B .Saunders, Philadelphia, 1992, pp. 799–852.
61. Kremer H, Martens JW, van Reen M, et al. A limited repertoire of mutations of the luteinizing hormone (LH) receptor gene in familial and sporadic patients with male LH-independent precociouis puberty. J Clin Endocrinol Metab 1999;84:1136–1140.
62. Laue L, Wu SM, Kudo M, et al A nonsense mutation of the human luteinizing hormone receptor gene in Leydig cell hypoplasia. Hum Mol Genet 1995;4:1429–1433.
63. Kremer H, Kraaij R, Toledo SP, et al Male pseudohermaphroditism due to a homozygous missense mutation of the luteinizing hormone receptor gene. Nat Genet 1995;9:160–164.
64. Latronico AC, Anasti J, Arnhold IJP, et al. Testicular and ovarian resistance to luteinizing hormone caused by inactivating mutations of the luteinizing hormone-receptor gene. N Engl J Med.1996;334:507–512.
65. Aittomaki K, Lucena JL, Pakarinen P, et al. Mutation in the follicle-stimulating hormone receptor gene causes hereditary hypergonadotropic ovarian failure. Cell 1995;82:959–968.
66. Snyder PJ. Gonadotroph cell adenomas of the pituitary. Endocr Rev 1985;6:552–563.
67. Jameson JL, Klibanski A, Black PM, et al. Glycoprotein hormone genes are expressed in clinically nonfunctioning pituitary adenomas. J Clin Invest 1987;80:1472–1478.
68. Snyder PJ, Bigdeli H, Gardner DF, et al. Gonadal function in fifty men with untreated pituitary adenomas. J Clin Endocrinol Metab 1979;48:309–314.

69. Dunsmuir WD, Holmes SA. The aetiology and management of erectile, ejaculatory, and fertility problems in men with diabetes mellitus. Diabet Med 1996;13:700–708.
70. Neaves WB, Johnson L, Porter JC, Parker CR, Petty CS. Leydig cell numbers, daily sperm production and serum gonadotropin levels in aging men. J Clin Endocrinol Metab 1984;59:756–763.
71. Swerdloff RS, Hever D. Effects of aging on male reproductive function. In Korenman SG, ed. Endocrine Aspects of Aging. Elsevier Biomedical, New York, 1982, pp. 119–135.
72. Korenman SG, Morley JE, Mooradian AD, et al. Secondary hypogonadism in older men: its relation to impotence. J Clin Endocrinol Metab 1990;71:963–969.
73. Van Thiel DH, Cobb CF, Herman GB, Perez I, Gavaler JS. An examination of various mechanisms for ethanol-induced testicular injury: studies utilizing the isolated perfused rat testes. Endocrinology 1981;109:2009–2015.
74. Iranmanesh A, Velhuis JD, Samojlik E, Rogol AD, Johnson ML, Lizarralde G. Alterations in the pulsatile properties of gonadotropin secretion in alcoholic men. J Androl 1988;9:207–214.
75. Burris AS, Rodbard HW, Winters SJ, Sherins RJ. Gonadotropin therapy in men with isolated hypogonadotropic hypogonadism: the response to human chorionic gonadotropin is predicted by initial testicular size. J Clin Endocrinol Metab 1988;66:1144–1151.
76. Whitcomb RW, Crowley WF. Diagnosis and treatment of isolated gonadotropin-releasing hormone deficiency in men. J Clin Endocrinol Metab 1990;70:3–7.
77. Schopohl J, Mehltretter G, von Zumbusch R, et al. Comparison of gonadotropin-releasing hormone and gonadotropin therapy in male patients with idiopathic hypothalamic hypogonadism. Fertil Steril 1991;56:1143–1145.
78. Bagatell CJ, Bremner WJ. Androgens in men—uses and abuses. N Engl J Med 1996;334:707–714.
79. Baltaci S, Aydos K, Kosa A, et al. Treating erectile dysfunction with a vacuum tumescence device: a retrospective analysis of acceptance and satisfaction. Br J Urol 1995;76:757–760.
80. Vrijhof HJ, Delaere KP. Vacuum constriction devices in erectile dysfunction: acceptance and effectiveness in patients with impotence of organic or mixed aetiology. Br J Urol 1994;74:102–105.
81. Linet OI, Ogring FG. Efficacy and safety of intracavernosal alprostadil in men with erectile dysfunction. N Eng J Med 1996;334:873–877.
82. Sundaram CP, Thomas W, Pryor LE, et al. Long-term follow-up of patients receiving injection therapy for erectile dysfunction. Urology 1997;49:932–935.
83. Padma-Nathan N, Hellstrom WJ, Kaiser FE, et al. Treatment of men with erectile dysfunction with transurethral alprostadil. Medicated Urethral System for Erection (MUSE) Study Group. N Engl J Med 1997;336:1–7.
84. Fulgham PF, Cochran JS, Denman JL, et al. Disappointing initial results with transurethral alprostadil for erectile dysfunction in a urology practice setting. J Urol 1998;160:2041–2046.
85. Montorsi F, Strambi L, Guazzoni G, et al. Effect of yohimbine-trazodone in psychogenic impotence: A randomized double-blind, placebo-controlled study. Urology 1994;44:732–736.
86. Boolell M, Gepi-Attee S, Gingell JC, et al. Sildenafil, a novel effective oral therapy for male erectile dysfunction. Br J Urol 1996;78:257–261.
87. Goldstein I, Lue TF, Padma-Nathan H, et al. Oral sildenafil in the treatment of erectile dysfunction. N Engl J Med 1998;338:1397–1404.
88. Arruda-Olson AM, Mahoney DW, Nehra A et al. Cardiovascular effects of sildenafil during exercise in men with known or probable coronary artery disease: a randomized crossover trial. JAMA 2002;287:766–777.
89. Altwein JE, Keuler FU. Oral treatment of erectile dysfunction with apomorphine SL. Urology International 2001;67:257–263.
90. Wagner, G., Lacy, S., Lewis, R., et al. (1994) Buccal phentolamine: a pilot trial for male erectile dysfunction at three separate clinics. Int J Impot Res 6:D78–D80.
91. Wierman ME, Cassel CK. Erectile dysfunction: a multifaceted disorder. Hosp Pract 1998;33:65–90.

15 Menstrual Dysfunction

Drew V. Tortoriello, MD
and Janet E. Hall, MD

CONTENTS

THE PHYSIOLOGY OF NORMAL MENSTRUAL FUNCTION

A pattern of regular ovulatory menstrual cycles is achieved through the exquisite functional and temporal integration of hormonal secretion from the hypothalamus, the pituitary, and the ovary. This classic endocrine cascade is initiated by pulsatile secretion of gonadotropin-releasing hormone (GnRH) from the hypothalamus into the pituitary portal venous system. The subsequent release of follicle-stimulating hormone (FSH) and luteinizing hormone (LH) from the anterior pituitary stimulates ovarian follicular development, ovulation, and corpus luteum formation. The uterus in turn responds to ovarian steroids by endometrial proliferation, vascularization, and glandular development. In the absence of implantation, ovarian hormonal support wanes, and endometrial shedding ensues. This pattern of events is accompanied by dramatic changes in LH, FSH, estradiol, progesterone, inhibin A, and inhibin B across normal menstrual cycles *(1)* (Fig. 1). In addition, the pulsatile stimulation of pituitary hormone secretion by GnRH results in pulsatile secretion of LH and to a lesser extent FSH, which also varies across the cycle, reflecting changes in the frequency of the GnRH pulse generator *(2)* (Fig. 2).

The median menstrual cycle length of the American woman is 28 d, with a range between 25–35 d considered normal. The 7-yr intervals immediately following menarche and preceding menopause are marked by the greatest amount

From: *Contemporary Endocrinology: Handbook of Diagnostic Endocrinology*
Edited by: J. E. Hall and L. K. Nieman © Humana Press Inc., Totowa, NJ

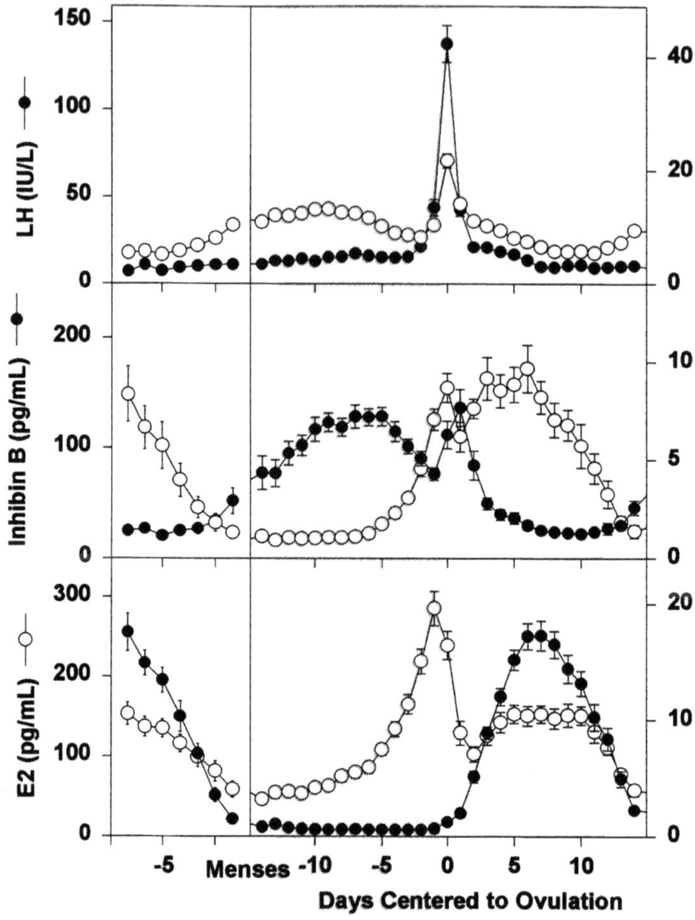

Fig. 1. Dynamic changes in LH, FSH, inhibin B, inhibin A, estradiol (E2), and progesterone (P4) across the menstrual cycle reflect the integration of the hypothalamic-pituitary-ovarian axis. Adapted with permission from ref. *1*.

of cycle variability. The intermenstrual interval is shortest between the ages of 36 and 40 *(3)*. Fluctuations in the length of the follicular phase are primarily responsible for the variations in cycle length noted between women and across the reproductive life span of individual women. The follicular phase begins on the first day of menses and encompasses the period of multiple follicular recruitment, dominant follicle emergence, and endometrial proliferation. The luteal phase of the cycle begins with ovulation and is characterized by the emergence of the progesterone-secreting corpus luteum. Luteal phase duration is more constant, lasting between 10 and 16 d in 95% of cycles. Ovulatory cycles are often, but not always, associated with moliminal symptoms, the term used for the

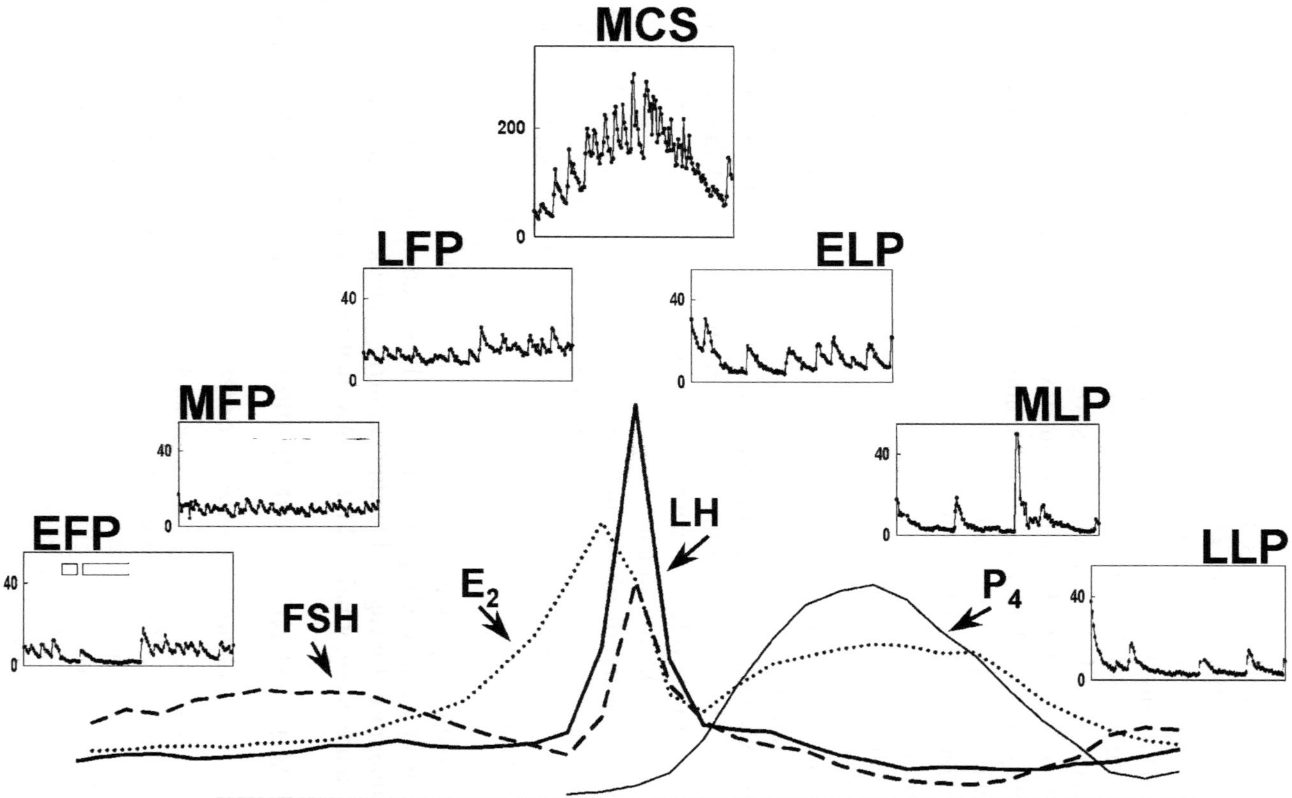

Fig. 2. The pattern of LH secretion across the menstrual cycle is presented in the boxes and in relation to serum levels of LH, FSH, estradiol (E2), and progesterone (P4) during the early, mid, and late follicular phase (EFP, MFP, LFP, respectively), at the midcycle (MCS), and during the early, mid, and late luteal phase (ELP, MLP, LLP, respectively). Pulsatile LH reflects underlying GnRH secretion and indicates the dynamic changes that occur during normal cycles in women. Reproduced with permission from ref. *2*.

combination of bloating, breast tenderness, and food cravings that may occur premenstrually.

This intricate system achieves its precision predominantly through multiple negative feedback pathways. Secretion of estradiol and inhibin B and/or inhibin A from the ovary restrain transcription of gonadotropin subunit genes in the pituitary, thus limiting its responsiveness. Estradiol is also likely to inhibit GnRH pulsatility at the level of the hypothalamus, either directly or through a paracrine neuronal effect *(4–6)*. In the presence of estrogen, progesterone secretion from the ovary diminishes GnRH pulse frequency through interaction with the β-endorphin system *(7)*. In contrast to these inhibitory influences, the initiation of the pre-ovulatory LH surge is uniquely dependent upon the positive feedback that a prolonged elevation of serum estradiol exerts upon the pituitary *(8)*.

Dysfunction at any level of the reproductive system is sufficient to induce menstrual irregularities. Hormonal disorders with seemingly only indirect relationships with the reproductive system, as well as systemic disease, often have a negative impact on reproductive function. Any such disruption may alter the timing of menarche or the frequency and volume of menstrual flow. Menstrual cycle disturbances occur relatively infrequently, with estimates of between 2–8% in large studies. However, both the delayed onset of menstrual function and subsequent menstrual cycle dysfunction serve as sensitive bioassays for general and reproductive health in women.

A framework for the diagnosis and therapy of these disorders can best be constructed by combining functional and anatomic approaches, as will be described below. The first step in determining the etiology of abnormal menstrual function is a thorough history and physical examination (Tables 1 and 2). Based on these findings, appropriate laboratory or imaging studies can be obtained. Although the primary focus of this chapter will be dysfunctional menstrual patterns in women of reproductive age, it is prudent to also review the differential diagnoses for vaginal bleeding occurring outside of this period, which by its very nature is abnormal and frequently anatomic in nature.

MENSTRUAL DYSFUNCTION IN REPRODUCTIVE AGED WOMEN

Amenorrhea/Oligomenorrhea

Amenorrhea refers to the absence of menses. A woman is said to be experiencing primary amenorrhea if she has never menstruated. The first menstrual period or menarche occurs relatively late in the series of developmental milestones that characterize normal pubertal development and the onset of reproductive development. Menarche is generally preceded by pubarche (the onset of pubic hair, which is dependent on both adrenal and gonadal maturation) and thelarche (breast development which is sensitive to very low levels of estrogen secretion). Menarche occurs at 12.7 yr on average in the United States and younger in African-Ameri-

Table 1
History

Developmental history
- Growth, pubertal development.

Previous menstrual history
- Last menstrual period.
- Age and weight at menarche.
- Characteristics of recent cycles (duration, molimina).
- Sexual activity and use of contraception.

Health/lifestyle factors
- Medications, illnesses.
- Pregnancy, uterine instrumentation.
- Stress, diet, weight changes, exercise patterns.

Localizing symptoms
- Presence and pace of androgenic symptoms.
- Nausea, breast tenderness, weight gain.
- Galactorrhea or visual symptoms.
- Significant loss or increase in weight.
- Hot flashes or vaginal dryness.
- Anorectic behavior or perceptions.

Table 2
Physical Examination

General
- Height, weight, arm span.
- Somatic features of Turner's Syndrome.
- Secondary sexual characteristics (Tanner staging).

Skin
- Axillary and pubic hair development.
- Acne, hirsutism (Ferriman-Galwey score), oiliness, acanthosis nigricans.
- Signs of weight loss, hypercarotenemia, lanugo hair, dental caries.
- Centripetal obesity, pigmented striae.

Visual fields

Breasts
- Development.
- Galactorrhea.

Pelvic Examination
- Normal external and internal genitalia.
- Vaginal atrophy.
- Ovarian or uterine enlargement.

can girls. Primary amenorrhea is diagnosed if menarche has not occurred by age 14 in the absence of growth or development of secondary sexual characteristics, or by age 16 regardless of the presence of normal growth and development and the presence of secondary sexual characteristics.

A previously menstruating woman is said to have secondary amenorrhea if menses have ceased for a length of time minimally equivalent to a total of 3 of the usual cycle intervals, generally 3 mo. The relative frequency of presentation of disorders at each level of consideration is influenced by whether amenorrhea is primary or secondary *(9,10)*, with abnormalities originating at the level of the ovary, and outflow tract disorders being relatively more common in primary amenorrhea (Fig. 3). It is important to note that most processes commonly thought to be associated with secondary amenorrhea can also result in primary amenorrhea. In addition, many of the mechanisms underlying the complete absence of menses may also predispose to an abnormal lengthening of the cycle (>36 d) or oligoamenorrhea.

Strict adherence to the criteria for timing of evaluation is at certain times unwarranted and even problematic. Occasionally, physical stigmata on examination readily identify a diagnosis that should be treated immediately. Equally frequent is the patient who presents with such severe anxiety regarding her condition that to delay evaluation until the strict criteria are met would be counterproductive. It is also appropriate to expedite the investigation of amenorrhea in a woman over the age of 35 who wants to conceive, due to decreased success rates in older reproductive aged women.

It is convenient to divide the differential potential diagnoses of amenorrhea/oligoamenorrhea into two categories, those stemming from an abnormality of the reproductive tract, and those that lead to ovulatory dysfunction. Appropriate tests to investigate the cause of amenorrhea are listed in Table 3. Gonadotropin levels are used to help locate the site of the primary abnormality based on the absolute requirement for GnRH stimulation of pituitary gonadotrope secretion and the negative feedback of gonadal steroids and peptides on gonadotropin secretion.

Disorders Associated with Reproductive Tract Abnormalities

Although they comprise a small percentage of cases, it is particularly important to consider disorders involving the uterus or outflow tract in the differential diagnosis of menstrual disorders. This is particularly true with primary amenorrhea, but is also relevant to the diagnosis of secondary amenorrhea. An overt outflow tract anomaly may be immediately diagnosed on pelvic examination. Actual obstruction may occur with an imperforate hymen, cervical stenosis, or a transverse vaginal septum. Such conditions present with moliminal symptoms and severe dysmenorrhea but without vaginal bleeding. A tender mass may be palpated on examination that is consistent with a hematocolpos or hematometra.

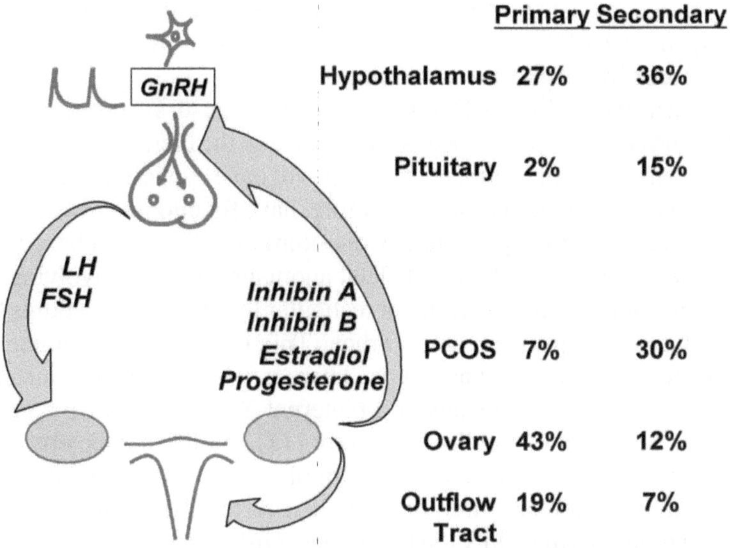

Fig. 3. The reproductive system is tightly integrated, requiring input from the hypothalamic GnRH pulse generator and pituitary and feedback from the ovary, for regular ovulatory function. The uterus acts as an end organ for the effects of ovarian steroids. The incidence of menstrual disorders involving each level of this system differs depending on whether amenorrhea is primary or secondary. Hypothalamic and pituitary disorders will be hypogonadotropic while disorders resulting from ovarian failure will be associated with high levels of FSH and LH.

Table 3
Diagnostic Testing

First-order tests

- β-hCG.
- Prolactin.
- FSH.

Second-order tests

- LH.
- Estradiol or progestin challenge (10 mg medroxyprogesterone for 5 d to induce withdrawal bleed).

Other tests if clinically indicated

- TSH.
- Androgens: Testosterone, dehydroepiandrosterone sulfate (DHEAS), 17-hydroxyprogesterone, urinary 17-ketosteroids.
- Pelvic ultrasound/hysterosalpingogram.
- Cranial MRI.

The retrograde menstrual flow can also create a hematoperitoneum, thereby increasing the risk of severe endometriosis. These conditions are corrected with surgical and/or hysteroscopic resection.

Mullerian agenesis (Mayer-Rokitansky-Kuster-Hauser syndrome) is a congenital anomaly consisting of the absence or hypoplasia of the uterus and/or vagina. Those patients with a normal or rudimentary uterus will have cyclic abdominal pain. These patients are genetically female and, therefore, have functioning ovaries. Radiologic imaging is indicated, as approximately one-third of patients will have urinary tract abnormalities, and 12% will have skeletal anomalies, usually involving the spine.

Complete androgen insensitivity or testicular feminization accounts for approx 10% of all cases of primary amenorrhea. This condition is characterized by a female phenotype but male karyotype. There exists a congenital insensitivity to androgens, transmitted by means of a maternal X-linked recessive gene responsible for the androgen intracellular receptor *(11)*. Wollfian duct structures do not form; however there is no absence of antimullerian hormone, and therefore, these patients usually do not have uteri or tubes. The testes often descend to the level of the internal inguinal ring. Only the lower one-third of the vagina is present, for this portion derives from the urogenital sinus. The diagnosis is likely when a phenotypic female presents with breast development, primary amenorrhea, scanty or absent pubic and axillary hair, a shortened vagina, and an absent uterus and cervix. Patients characteristically have elevated gonadotropins, especially LH, mildly elevated testosterone, and high estradiol. Spermatogenesis does not occur, and hence, these patients are infertile. Testicular malignant transformation is a concern. To allow female secondary sexual characteristics to reasonably develop, gonadectomy is usually not recommended until the mid to late teens, however, the optimal timing of gonadectomy remains controversial. After gonadectomy, hormonal replacement therapy is indicated.

Asherman's syndrome is a complete or partial obliteration of the uterine cavity with the formation of intrauterine adhesions or synechiae. Patients with this disorder present with menstrual irregularities, usually amenorrhea or scanty bleeding and infertility. The vast majority of cases follow instrumentation or surgery of the uterus. It generally is iatrogenically induced by an overzealous postpartum curettage and may be more prevalent with severe hypoestrogenism. It has also been linked to infectious causes, as with puerperal endometritis, genital tuberculosis, schistosomiasis, or from an intra-uterine device. The diagnosis is suspected by failure of withdrawal bleeding after the administration of exogenous estrogen and progesterone, and is diagnosed by visualization of synechiae on hysterosalpingogram (sharp angled filling defects) or hysteroscopy. The preferred treatment involves hysteroscopically directed resection of intrauterine adhesions with high-dose estrogen therapy to foster endometrial overgrowth *(12)*. Repeated attempts may be necessary to restore menses, but eventually about 75% of patients achieve a successful pregnancy.

Disorders Associated with Ovulatory Dysfunction

Pregnancy

Pregnancy is the single most common cause of secondary amenorrhea in the reproductive age female. It is, therefore, essential to rule out pregnancy in all women even remotely likely to possess reproductive capacity who present with as little as a single missed menses.

Hypogonadotropic Hypogonadism: the Hypothalamus

Hypogonadotropic hypogonadism may result from anatomic or functional abnormalities that interfere with the normal pattern of secretion of hypothalamic GnRH or, less commonly, with pituitary responsiveness to GnRH. Thus, hypoestrogenism is associated with low to low-normal levels of LH and FSH.

Neuroanatomic Hypothalamic Disease. While neuroanatomic lesions of the hypothalamus are much less frequent than functional hypothalamic disorders, it is critical that they be considered in the differential diagnosis of hypogonadotropic amenorrhea. This is particularly true when the patient has not gone through puberty, has not progressed through puberty at a normal pace, or has other features suggestive of a more widespread endocrinopathy, such as short stature or diabetes insipidus. Infiltrative diseases or tumors that affect the hypothalamus are often associated with other endocrine abnormalities, including hypothyroidism, hypocortisolemia, and diabetes insipidus.

The most common tumor affecting the hypothalamus is the craniopharyngioma, a suprasellar tumor derived embryologically from Rathke's pouch. Craniopharyngiomas may be completely or partially cystic in nature and be calcified. The tumor often presents with growth retardation or headache, but primary or secondary amenorrhea are frequent clues to its presence. Other less common tumors include germinomas, meningiomas, endodermal sinus tumors, midline dermoid tumors, or metastatic tumors.

Histiocytosis X or Hand-Christian-Schuller Disease, is a rare children's disease in which multifocal eosinophilic granulomas destroy the hypothalamus, precipitating delayed puberty, growth retardation, and diabetes insipidus. Other infiltrating lesions, which may impair hypothalamic function, include sarcoidosis, tuberculosis, and Wegener's granulomatosis.

The hypothalamus is highly sensitive to external irradiation, and menstrual irregularities may be as high as 70% following cranial irradiation for the treatment of malignancies. Cranial trauma is another, rare cause of hypothalamic dysfunction.

Idiopathic Hypogonadotropic Hypogonadism. Isolated GnRH deficiency or idiopathic hypogonadotropic hypogonadism (IHH) is more commonly seen in men, but can also be a cause of primary amenorrhea and failure of pubertal development in women. IHH is termed Kallmann's syndrome when it is associated with anosmia or hyposmia. Other associated findings include color blindness, synkinesia, and congenital midline defects. The disease has an incidence of approx 1/10,000 live male births and is even less common in females. The hallmark clinical feature of this disorder, hypogonadism, implies a failure of both gametogenic function and sex steroid production. Primary amenorrhea occurs with ovarian follicles that never pass the primordial stage in the absence of exogenous stimulation. The diagnosis is made in the hypogonadal patient only after exclusion of a hypothalamic or pituitary mass lesion by magnetic resonance imaging (MRI) in the setting of otherwise normal pituitary function. Normalization of pituitary and gonadal function occurs with pulsatile administration of physiologic doses of GnRH *(13)*. With appropriate stimulation by GnRH or exogenous gonadotropins, the ovaries and uterus, which are generally hypoplastic in appearance at the time of diagnosis, increase in size, and ovulation and pregnancy are easily achievable *(14)*.

Although autosomal modes of inheritance are believed to be the most common predisposing factor, the genetic loci for these disturbances have yet to be revealed *(13)*. Approximately 20% of X-linked cases, however, are attributable to a mutation of the *KAL* gene. The absent gene product is a neural adhesion protein, which guides the embryonic migration of GnRH neurons from the olfactory placode into the hypothalamus. The vast majority of patients do not have evidence of deletion of the GnRH gene, nor have point mutations or frameshifts in the coding sequence been identified in these patients. Another specific human gene defect in association with GnRH deficiency and hypogonadism involves the *DAX* gene, whose mutation results in X-linked congenital adrenal hypoplasia.

Mutations in the GnRH receptor gene have been found in association with hypogonadism *(15,16)*. The phenotype is variable and may be associated with partial rather than complete loss of function and responsiveness to high doses of GnRH.

Secondary Hypogonadotropic Hypogonadism. In addition to the neuroanatomic conditions indicated above, there are a number of conditions in which GnRH secretion is reversibly inhibited, resulting in varying degrees of suppression of the reproductive axis and generally low levels of LH, FSH, and estradiol. Acute and chronic illnesses frequently result in menstrual dysfunction. Both hyperthyroidism and hypothyroidism have been associated with anovulation and infertility. The elevated cortisol levels in Cushing's Syndrome or with exogenous steroid use may also suppress normal GnRH secretion.

Nutritionally Related Amenorrhea. The significant impact of nutritional status upon the female reproductive axis is demonstrated by anorexia nervosa, an eating disorder characterized by restrictive eating behaviors and often excessive exercise. It occurs in young women, often peripubertal, from all socioeconomic classes. One study has demonstrated greater than a 1% incidence in English school girls *(17)*. The psychological theories for its emergence include an inability of the patient to cope with incipient adult sexuality and familial pressure to achieve. An attitude of denial with a grossly distorted body image is common.

Anorexia is defined by a weight loss of 25% (or a weight below the 15th percentile for age and height) accompanied by amenorrhea. The following features are common: bradycardia, constipation (often quite severe), lanugo, hypercarotenemia, and diabetes insipidus. Frequently, the physician who encounters these patients does so for complaints of amenorrhea and not for the associated medical and weight disturbances. Anorexia is important to diagnose and follow closely, as mortality ranges from 5–15%.

The starvation state of anorectics induces severe hypothalamic dysfunction with subsequent aberrations in appetite, endocrine secretion, thirst and water conservation, temperature, sleep, and autonomic balance. Cortisol and growth hormone are typically elevated. Thyroid-stimulating hormone (TSH) and thyroxine are normal, however, T_3 levels are diminished, and reverse T_3 levels are elevated, consistent with the hypothyroid-like symptoms manifested by these patients. There appears to be a compensatory shunting of thyroid hormone constituents towards the increased production of the inactive metabolite, reverse T_3, to help combat the state of severe malnourishment. Leptin levels are appropriately low for the diminished body mass of the anorectic patient. Gonadotropins are low, but prolactin is normal. The underlying inhibitory influence upon GnRH pulsatility is possibly mediated by endogenous opioids, and the administration of naltrexone has been shown to restore menstrual cycles in patients with weight loss-related amenorrhea *(18)*.

With weight gain, the metabolic derangements return to normal. A normal response to GnRH is regained at approx 15% below the ideal body weight, and this precedes the onset of menses. The prepubertal gonadotropin levels of the anorectic return to normal in stages that mirror puberty. As with the onset of puberty in normal women, the first step noted with weight gain in the anorectic patient is a sleep associated episodic secretion of LH. As recovery progresses, the GnRH secretory pattern of the normal adult is achieved.

Approximately 50% of anorectics manifest bulimic tendencies, and 1% of female college students exhibit clinically significant bulimia. Bulimics binge on food and thereafter purge through self-induced vomiting or the use of laxatives or diuretics. One study has demonstrated that greater than 25% of bulimics are amenorrheic, and that they also manifest increased cortisol levels and decreased LH pulsatility *(19)*.

The treatment for these disorders begins with communication. A psychiatric consultation and frequent office visits are indicated. Hospital admission should be considered in severe and refractory states. It is also important to provide estrogen replacement therapy in anorectics, especially those who do not exercise, as they are at very high risk for osteoporosis secondary to both their hypogonadal and hypercortisolemic states *(20,21)*.

Exercise-Associated Hypothalamic Amenorrhea. Women who engage in physically demanding activities such as running, weight training, and ballet are at an increased risk for menstrual irregularities and amenorrhea. Up to 66% of daily runners are anovulatory or have shortened luteal phases *(22)*. Menarche is often delayed by as much as 3 yr in women who begin their physical training before puberty.

Recent data demonstrated that low energy bioavailability diminishes LH pulsatility in exercising women and potentially also in patients suffering from other forms of functional hypothalamic amenorrhea *(23,24)*. The degree of slowing of LH pulsatility in interventional studies is dependent upon the source of energy restriction: low energy availability caused by dietary restriction reduces LH pulsatility by 23%, while an equivalent reduction by increasing exercise energy expenditure slows LH pulse frequency by only 10%.

Acute exercise markedly affects the neuroendocrine regulation of the reproductive axis. Gonadotropins are decreased, but prolactin, growth hormone, testosterone, adrenocorticotrophic hormone (ACTH), adrenal steroids, and endorphins are all elevated. Women athletes also have elevated daytime melatonin levels, and amenorrheic athletes have an exaggerated nocturnal secretion of melatonin. Athletes have a relatively low thyroxine level, but amenorrheic athletes have a universal suppression of all thyroid hormones, including reverse T_3. This is in marked contrast to the thyroid status of undernourished women. The diurnal pattern of leptin secretion is lost in amenorrheic athletes and leptin levels are disproportionately low for body mass *(25)*. Secondary to their amenorrhea, female athletes are often markedly hypoestrogenemic, and as such, are at greatly increased risk for bone disease. Drinkwater et al. noted a significant reduction in vertebral bone density in amenorrheic runners as compared to normally cycling controls *(26)*. In one cohort of ballet dancers, Warren noted a 24% incidence of scoliosis and a 61% incidence of stress fractures *(27)*. If a reduction in the severity of the physical training cannot be accomplished, hormone replacement therapy should be initiated to prevent bone loss.

Hypothalamic Amenorrhea. Hypothalamic amenorrhea is a diagnosis of exclusion of other causes of hypogonadotropic hypogonadism in women. It is responsible for approx 20% of all cases of secondary amenorrhea. It is frequently diagnosed in patients whose lifestyle is characterized by high levels of emotional stress and whose diets are significantly lower in fat (50%) and higher in carbohydrate and fiber *(28)*.

Gonadotropins are usually in the low to low normal range in association with hypoestrogenism. FSH levels are often slightly higher than those of LH. Frequent blood sampling studies have revealed LH pulsatility (a reliable although indirect assessment of GnRH pulsatility) to be variably diminished. In a large group of women with hypothalamic amenorrhea, the pattern of pulsatile LH secretion in women with both primary and secondary hypothalamic amenorrhea was heterogeneous among different patients and in the same patient studied over time *(29)*. The most common pattern (43%) was a decrease in pulse frequency. Only 8% of patients were completely apulsatile.

In a majority of women with hypothalamic amenorrhea, LH pulse frequency increases acutely with administration of naloxone *(29)*. These data suggest that abnormal augmentation of the opioidergic inhibition of hypothalamic GnRH neurons may be etiologic in some patients with hypothalamic amenorrhea. There is also evidence for increased dopaminergic tone in over half of women with hypothalamic amenorrhea as administration of metoclopramide, a dopamine antagonist, has been shown to increase LH pulse frequency *(30)*. This feature, as well as the associated hypoestrogenemia, may contribute to the nearly 40% diminution in the 24-h integrated prolactin value that these patients also demonstrate. In a cohort of 10 women with hypothalamic amenorrhea, integrated 24-h cortisol secretion was 17% higher, while prolactin, T_3, and T_4 levels were all significantly reduced compared to normally cycling controls *(31)*.

A number of studies provide evidence for a subclinical eating disorder in weight-stable nonathletic women with hypothalamic amenorrhea and with severe restriction of dietary fat *(28)*. Leptin levels in women with hypothalamic amenorrhea are significantly lower than weight-matched cycling controls *(31)*.

Although hypothalamic amenorrhea is considered to be a reversible disorder, some women will have long-term hypothalamic dysfunction. A follow-up study of women with hypothalamic amenorrhea revealed that rates of recovery exceeded 80% when precipitating factors, such as stress, +/– exercise, or a subclinical eating disorder, were reversed *(32)*.

Women with prolonged hypothalamic amenorrhea may experience osteopenia secondary to hypoestrogenism. In a cross-sectional prospective study, 83% of hypothalamic amenorrheic women had trabecular bone density below the mean for controls *(33)*. Hormone replacement therapy and calcium supplementation are, therefore, indicated in patients with hypothalamic amenorrhea not interested in pregnancy, whose disorder persists after 6 mo. Measurement of bone density may be required in those patients with prolonged amenorrhea who do not want to take hormone replacement.

Ovulation induction therapy easily restores fertility in patients with hypothalamic amenorrheic. Intravenous pulsatile administration of exogenous GnRH is associated with a near universal restoration of ovulation and an increased rate of unifollicular cycles *(14)*. Exogenous gonadotropin treatment is also highly successful. Due to the central nature of this defect and the resultant hypoestrogenism, clomiphene citrate is often ineffective. Neither these medications nor cyclic hormonal therapy has been shown to restore the normal endogenous GnRH pulsatility.

HYPOGONADOTROPIC HYPOGONADISM: THE PITUITARY

Primary Hypopituitarism. Disease processes directly affecting the pituitary may be severe enough to induce hypopituitarism. Evidence of an empty sella turcica on computed tomography (CT) scanning or MRI may be seen in association with infarction of a pituitary tumor, surgery, or radiation. This radiologic appearance may also result from a primary abnormality, in which elevated intracranial pressure remodels the sellar anatomy through an incompetent sellar diaphragm. Most patients present with headache and have no discernable endocrine abnormality, but hypogonadism may be present in up to 6% of cases. In Sheehan's syndrome, hypopituitarism results from postpartum pituitary infarction. This usually occurs in the setting of hypotension secondary to hemorrhagic hypovolemia. The pituitary is highly susceptible to hypotensive necrosis in the puerperium, as estrogen-induced lactotroph hypertrophy renders the gland enlarged and in need of heightened perfusion. The presenting symptoms include mammary involution, fatigue, and hypotension. Lymphocytic hypophysitis is an infiltrative process of the pituitary believed to be autoimmune in nature, occurring frequently in the puerperium. Gonadotropin deficiency is a relatively late manifestation. In women, hemachromatosis rarely presents with hypogonadotropic hypogonadism due to infiltration of the gonadotropes. Pituitary apoplexy is the acute and potentially universal infarction of the pituitary, often secondary to the sudden hemorrhaging of a previously clinically silent hypothalamic or pituitary tumor. It has also occurred in patients with diabetic vasculitis or sickle cell anemia. Pituitary apoplexy is a life threatening condition whose presence or even suspicion necessitates prompt administration of glucocorticoids.

Pituitary Adenomas. Pituitary tumors may cause gonadotropin deficiency as a result of mass compression or secondary to surgery. With the exception of directed proton beam radiation, radiation is more likely to interfere with reproductive function through damage to the hypothalamus rather than the pituitary. In addition, prolactin- and ACTH-secreting tumors, as well as growth hormone-secreting tumors, are more likely to cause hypothalamic dysfunction. However, nonfunctioning adenomas are associated with hypogonadotropic hypogonadism in the large majority of cases. Rarely, these "nonfunctioning" adenomas secrete biologically active gonadotropins, such as FSH, and present with ovarian stimulation. Thyrotropin releasing hormone (TRH) testing reveals paradoxical increases in LH, FSH, and β-subunits *(34)*.

Prolactinomas. At least 70% of all pituitary adenomas are prolactin-only secreting, and up to one-third of women presenting with secondary amenorrhea can be expected to have a prolactinoma. The frequency of the association of amenorrhea with hyperprolactinemia makes measurement of prolactin a key part of the initial work-up of the amenorrheic patient. Up to 25% of patients with acromegaly, due to growth hormone-secreting adenomas, also have hyperprolactinemia, which is a phenomenon likely due to a common progenitor cell.

The characteristic features of hyperprolactinemia are amenorrhea and galactorrhea. Visual disturbances may be present if the adenoma is large enough to compress the optic chiasm. However, the majority of prolactinomas are microadenomas (<1 cm). Hypogonadism associated with hyperprolactinemia is rarely due to a mass effect, but rather to secondary effects of elevated prolactin levels on GnRH secretion. The presence of persistent hyperprolactinemia requires exclusion of the common causes of hyperprolactinemia, such as renal and liver disease, medications, and severe hypothyroidism. Hyperprolactinemia can also be associated with central nervous system tumors that compress the pituitary stalk and, thereby, prevent dopaminergic inhibition of pituitary lactotropes. Therefore, confirmed prolactin elevations mandate pituitary imaging with MRI or enhanced CT scanning.

Traditional therapy of microprolactinomas involves medical treatment with a dopamine agonist. Approximately 80% of patients treated with a dopamine agonist will resume ovulation and achieve pregnancy. Transphenoidal surgery is rarely indicated, as it is invasive, and recurrences have been demonstrated in 80% of cases within 3 yr *(35)*. Hyperprolactinemic patients manifest bone density decrements, which are not correlated with estradiol levels, and their spine mineral density has been shown to remain low up to 9 yr after the restoration of physiological levels of estrogen *(36,37)*. This suggests a direct demineralizing effect of prolactin upon bone, highlighting the need for expedient lactotrope suppression.

Abnormal Gonadotropin Structure. Isolated FSH deficiency has been described in a very small number of woman with primary amenorrhea and failure to go through puberty *(38)*. Fertility was restored with 2 wk of exogenous administration of FSH. LH deficiency has not been described in women.

Hypergonadotropic Hypogonadism: the Ovary

Females begin life at birth with approx 2 million primary oocytes. However, as a result of a natural process of atresia, only 400,000 oocytes remain at the time of puberty, and despite ovulation of only 400 oocytes during reproductive life, ovarian failure occurs between the ages of 45 and 55 yr. Factors that can advance the time of ovarian failure may be genetic, with a decrease in the initial complement of germ cells, accelerated atresia, or acquired secondary to destruction of oocytes. An elevation of FSH >2 standard deviations (SD) above the normal follicular phase range in the setting of amenorrhea and low levels of estrogen is virtually pathognomic of ovarian failure. LH may also be elevated, but FSH is a more sensitive marker of ovarian failure, because of its greater dependence on the negative feedback of estradiol and the inhibins.

Gonadal Dysgenesis. The most common genetic cause of ovarian failure is Turner's syndrome (45,X gonadal dysgenesis) *(39)*. Disorders of gonadal development can present with either primary amenorrhea or premature ovarian failure. Approximately 40% of all patients who present with primary amenorrhea have gonadal streaks due to abnormal development. The vast majority of these patients (50%) have Turner's syndrome (X monosomy). These patients are phenotypic women with specific physical stigmata, including short stature, broad "shieldlike" chest with widely spaced nipples, cubitus valgus, high arched palate, and webbed neck. They have usually depleted their follicular reserve long before puberty, but about 3% of nonmosaic patients retain sufficient ova to have a very short period of normal gonadal activity. A brief period of normal ovarian function occurs in about 12% of individuals with the X/XX mosaicism. Surprisingly, the majority of patients who present with secondary amenorrhea and gonadal dysgenesis have a normal 46,XX karyotype. This syndrome, which when accompanied by neural deafness is termed Perrault's syndrome, may be secondary to an autosomal recessive defect in meiosis. To a lesser extent one will diagnose 45,X/46,XX mosaics, X chromosome deletions, and 47,XXX. The presence of mosaicism with a Y chromosome requires gonadectomy, as the presence of any testicular component carries a high risk for malignant transformation.

Turner's syndrome is also associated with frequent hearing loss, cardiac and renal abnormalities, and a high incidence of autoimmune diseases, including Hashimoto's thyroiditis and Graves' disease. Intestinal telangiectasias, hemangiomatoses, and a higher incidence of inflammatory bowel disease have been reported. Insulin resistance is common, as is hypercholesterolemia. Therefore, follow-up should include echcardiography approximately every 5 yr, hearing evaluation, stool guaiac testing, and tests of thyroid and liver function, screening for diabetes and hyperlipidemia, and blood pressure monitoring, in addition to assessment of bone density.

Premature Ovarian Failure. Premature ovarian failure is a condition of follicular depletion, in which elevated FSH and LH levels are seen in association with hypoestrogenemia in women younger than 40 yr of age. Patients will frequently present with hot flashes, insomnia, and worsening premenstrual symptoms. A population incidence of approx 1% has been estimated *(40)*. In its earlier stages, ovarian function in premature ovarian failure patients is often waxing and waning. Indeed, Taylor et al. showed that 78% of premature ovarian failure patients studied had ultrasound evidence of a developing follicle, and 46% ovulated as determined by an increase in serum progesterone levels *(41)*. Thus, confirmation of the diagnosis may require measurement of FSH levels on several occasions over time. When the syndrome occurs prior to age 30, a karyotype should be performed to rule out chromosomal abnormalities potentially associated with gonadal dysgenesis.

X chromosome deletions have helped to identify two critical regions on the X chromosome associated with hypergonadotropic hypogonadism—POF1 (Xq21.3-q27 or Xq256.1-q27) and POF2 (Xq133-q21.1). Deletions in these regions are not associated with short stature or phenotypic features of Turner's syndrome *(42)*. Galactosemia resulting from mutations in the enzyme galactose-1P-uridyltransferase is associated with hypergonadotropic hypogonadism.

Carriers of the premutation that results in Fragile X mental retardation have early menopause. The premutation is defined as 54–200 CGG repeats in the 5' untranslated region of the *FMR1* gene (Xq27.3). Premutation carriers account for up to 3.3% of sporadic and 12–16% of familial premature ovarian failure. As premutation carriers have a risk of bearing a child with mental retardation, screening for the mutation is recommended *(43)*.

FSH receptor mutations present with primary or secondary amenorrhea and elevated FSH and LH levels *(38)*. Some breast development and menses can occur. The mutations were described in the Finnish population and are rare in North America. LH receptor mutations are also rare. Follicular growth and maturation is normal, but follicles fail to ovulate, resulting in multiple large ovarian cysts. Puberty can be normal, but menses are irregular. LH and FSH levels are only moderately elevated in these patients.

Luborsky et al. reported that 69% of karyotypically normal premature ovarian failure patients have sera positive for oocyte or ovary antibodies *(44)*. Circulating antibodies against the adrenal enzymes 21 hydroxylase and side chain cleavage enzyme, which cross-react with the steroid-producing cells of the ovary, have been reported. However, it is unclear whether this presence of antibodies is etiologic in this disorder.

Autoimmune disorders commonly coexist with premature ovarian failure, even in the absence of detectable ovarian auto-antibodies. Belvisi et al. *(45)* noted that 40% of patients were positive for at least one organ-specific auto-antibody, the most common being antithyroid antibodies (20%). The polyglandular syndromes associated with ovarian failure include hypoparathyroidism, adrenal insufficiency, thyroiditis, and candidiasis. Other rare autoimmune conditions associated with premature ovarian failure include myasthenia gravis, pernicious anemia, idiopathic thrombocytopenic purpura, rheumatoid arthritis, vitiligo, and hemolytic anemia.

As ovarian failure is associated with autoimmune adrenal failure at frequencies of up to 18%, it is important to at least annually assess adrenal function in premature ovarian failure patients *(46)*. Given the high incidence of concomitant antithyroid antibodies, it is also prudent to assess thyroid function. It is imperative to initiate hormone replacement therapy as soon as possible to avoid hypoestrogenic osteoporosis.

Given the significant association between premature ovarian failure and autoimmunity, it has been postulated that corticosteroid-induced immunosuppression may facilitate ovulation induction. However, a recent placebo-controlled randomized and double-blind study using dexamethasone in conjunction with gonadotropins showed no benefit *(47)*. In addition, a randomized controlled trial showed no salutary effect of estradiol replacement therapy upon ovarian function *(41)*. The advent of oocyte donation and in vitro fertilization has recently afforded premature ovarian failure patients a highly successful means to overcome their infertility. These patients can expect the same pregnancy rate as their nonmenopausal counterparts who undergo transfer of embryos derived from oocyte donation *(48)*. For those choosing no treatment, the spontaneous pregnancy rate approaches 10% *(41,49)*.

Finally, systemic chemotherapy or pelvic irradiation may destroy ovarian follicles. Ovaries are more susceptible in older women with higher doses, longer duration of treatment, and multiple agents, resulting in higher incidences of complete ovarian failure. Amenorrheic women can revert back to spontaneous cycling, particularly if they were young at the time of treatment.

Polycystic Ovarian Syndrome

Polycystic ovary syndrome (PCOS) is a prevalent disorder, affecting 5–10% of women of reproductive age. It is the most common cause of hyperandrogenic anovulatory infertility. Affected patients demonstrate the peripubertal onset of a constellation of hormonal and metabolic abnormalities, none of which are pathognomonic *(50–52)*. The 1990 National Institute of Health Meeting defined PCOS by the presence of chronic oligoamenorrhea or amenorrhea, with either clinical or laboratory evidence of hyperandrogenism in the absence of other known causes of hyperandrogenism or irregular cycles *(53)*. While not required for the diagnosis, serum testosterone, free testosterone, and androstenedione are generally elevated in PCOS.

Other common but not obligatory features of PCOS are an elevated LH/FSH ratio, obesity, and insulin resistance. Although the vast majority of women with PCOS have polycystic appearing ovaries on pelvic ultrasound *(54,55)*, the fact that approx 25% of "normal" women display this finding and that it is also present in congenital adrenal hyperplasia has limited its diagnostic importance *(56)*. However, this sensitive, although not specific, finding is associated with an exuberant response to gonadotropin therapy *(57)*.

McArthur et al. in 1958 first documented elevated urinary LH levels in patients with PCOS *(58)*. Further studies have revealed an increase in the frequency and amplitude of pulsatile LH secretion in PCOS *(55,59)*. Although it has been hypothesized that reduced sensitivity to slowing of the GnRH pulse generator in response to progesterone may be etiologic in the neuroendocrine dysfunction associated with PCOS *(60)*, gonadotropin levels decrease in response to progesterone, and ovulation is associated with a decrease in mean LH *(55)*. Both mean LH levels and LH pulse amplitude are negatively related to body weight, and values in obese women with PCOS approach normal *(55,61)*. While LH levels are elevated, serum FSH concentrations in PCOS are generally at the lower end of the normal range and essentially constant. It has been postulated that these chronically low FSH levels are insufficient to initiate folliculogenesis, a disturbance that is easily remedied by the administration of exogenous gonadotropins. The high frequency of GnRH pulses may play a role in this gonadotropin imbalance, as increasing GnRH frequency has been shown to preferentially stimulate pituitary production of LH β-subunit mRNA over that of FSH. In addition, FSH secretion is more sensitive to estradiol negative feedback than is LH. Higher GnRH frequency also stimulates pituitary follistatin production, thereby diminishing activin's ability to induce pituitary FSH release *(62)*.

Although the granulosa cells of PCOS patients appear to function normally when isolated and challenged with gonadotropins in vitro, recent studies suggest that there may be an intrinsic defect favoring increased androgen production in the ovarian theca cells of PCOS patients. Increased 17α-hydroxylase, 3β-hydroxysteroid dehydrogenase, and 17β-hydroxysteroid dehydrogenase enzyme activity have been documented as an enduring trait of cultured theca cells *(63)*.

Women with PCOS have a unique and as yet poorly defined disorder of insulin action. When combined with obesity, approx 20% of PCOS patients will have impaired glucose tolerance or non-insulin-dependent diabetes in their third decade. Increased insulin receptor β-subunit serine phosphorylation has been found in approx 50% of patients *(52)*. Insulin receptor β-subunit tyrosine kinase activity is decreased, impeding the phosphorylation of in vitro substrates *(52)*. This represents a novel postreceptor aberration potentially responsible for diminished intracellular signal transduction in PCOS patients. The link between hyper-insulinemia and hyperandrogenism has now been demonstrated in a number of different models and experimental paradigms *(64)*.

Because of the significant association of PCOS with insulin resistance, all such patients should be screened *(65)*. American Diabetes Association guidelines stipulate that a fasting plasma glucose 125 mg/dL signifies diabetes. Those patients with values between 110 and 125 mg/dL should undergo a 2-h 75-g oral glucose tolerance test. Values between 140 and 200 mg/dL signify impaired glucose tolerance, while values exceeding 200 mg/dL diagnose diabetes. In patients with PCOS, hyperinsulinemia and glucose intolerance are particularly evident following glucose challenge and in the postprandial state. Although further research is required, recent data suggest that the oral insulin-sensitizing medications may improve both the hyperandrogenism and ovulatory dysfunction common in PCOS patients *(64)*.

MENORRHAGIA/MENOMETRORRHAGIA

When menstrual flow is excessive or prolonged, i.e., more than 80 mL or longer than 7 d in duration, menorrhagia is said to exist. When prolonged uterine bleeding occurs at irregular intervals, it is termed menometrorrhagia. While abnormal bleeding patterns are often associated with anovulatory cycles, the presence of systemic or anatomic disease must also be considered.

Patients with disorders of blood coagulation are at high risk for excessive menstrual flow. In fact, coagulation disorders are found in 20% of adolescent females who require hospitalization for abnormal uterine bleeding. It is, therefore, prudent to measure the prothrombin time, the activated partial thromboplastin time, and the bleeding time in patients with menometrorrhagia who give a personal or family history of increased bleeding tendencies or who present with menarcheal hemorrhage. Hypothyroidism is also an infrequent cause of menorrhagia, and a clinical and laboratory assessment of thyroid function should be performed.

The most common cause of heavy or unexpected vaginal bleeding in the reproductive years is pregnancy related. A serum β-human chorionic gonadatropin (hCG) should be performed to assess pregnancy status, and if positive, an endovaginal ultrasound should be performed in concert with the pelvic examination to help ascertain the location and viability of the pregnancy.

The endometrial cavity must be assessed in nonpregnant patients with persistent abnormal bleeding. Uterine lesions, such as endometrial polyps or leiomyomata with intracavitary or submucous locations, frequently produce menorrhagia or menometrorrhagia. Adenomyosis often induces an enlarged globular uterus prone to excessive and painful menstruation. The mechanisms underlying these abnormal bleeding patterns require further elucidation, but may involve increased endometrial surface area or a diminished ability of the distorted uterine body to contract upon itself.

Intermenstrual or heavy prolonged bleeding in perimenopausal or anovulatory premenopausal women should arouse the suspicion of carcinoma. The diagnosis is frequently delayed unnecessarily, because the bleeding is commonly ascribed to benign hormonal fluctuations. Indeed, the mean age of presentation for cervical carcinoma is 52, the age at which most women are experiencing the menopausal transition. Squamous cell carcinoma of the cervix generally presents with light bleeding or postcoital spotting, while endometrial adenocarcinoma generally presents with heavier and more irregular bleeding. Any factor that increases exposure to unopposed estrogen, such as estrogen replacement therapy, anovulatory cycles, obesity, and estrogen-secreting tumors, increases the risk of endometrial cancer, while those factors which limit estrogen exposure or have progestogenic effects, such as smoking or oral contraceptives, diminish the risk. It is important to recognize however, that 35% of patients with endometrial adenocarcinoma are not obese and do not manifest hyperestrogenism *(66)*.

An office endometrial biopsy and Papanicolaou (PAP) smear are the first step in the assessment of abnormal menstrual patterns. Initial attempts to visualize intrauterine mass lesions are traditionally through endovaginal ultrasound *(67)*. In the event of equivocal findings or persistent bleeding, the uterine cavity requires direct visualization. The gold standard for the diagnosis of organic uterine disease is hysteroscopy *(68)*. Saline infusion ultrasonography, a newer, minimally invasive modality, whose diagnostic sensitivity approaches that of hysteroscopy *(69)*, is achieving great popularity. It is limited however, by its inability to effect treatment at the time of diagnosis, a common occurrence with hysteroscopy. In addition, morphologically abnormal areas that do not cause uterine cavity distortion can potentially be missed by both endometrial biopsy and hydrosonogram, but can be directly seen and sampled for histological examination during hysteroscopy.

Dysfunctional Uterine Bleeding. After organic disease of the reproductive tract has been excluded, the etiology of heavy or irregular uterine bleeding is presumed secondary to an imbalance of estrogenic and progestational influences upon the endometrium. Such out of phase bleeding is loosely termed dysfunctional uterine bleeding (DUB). The condition is usually caused by anovulation and tends to occur at the extremes of reproductive life. Immediately post-menarche, adolescents tend to manifest pituitary refractoriness to estrogen positive feedback, implying an element of pituitary immaturity *(70)*. Early follicular phase estradiol concentrations are elevated in perimenopausal women compared with mid-reproductive aged women *(71)*.The perimenopausal ovary, being less responsive to FSH, requires greater circulating quantities of FSH to initiate folliculogenesis. Once started, the FSH rapidly induces relative hyper-estrogenemia. These shortened follicular phases are often not followed by ovulation. When ovulation does occur however, an increased incidence of luteal phase defects is seen. The combination of hyperestrogenic cycles and diminished progesterone secretion predispose women to menorrhagia, endometrial hyperplasia, dysfunctional uterine bleeding, and even endometrial cancer.

There are several general mechanisms potentially responsible for DUB. Estrogen withdrawal bleeding occurs when an acute decrease in estradiol impacts upon the endometrium. An example would be the bleeding encountered after the hyperestrogenic anovulatory cycle of the perimenopausal patient. Estrogen breakthrough bleeding is an irregular sloughing due to an inability of the available estrogen to support the proliferating endometrium. This bleeding is commonly seen after long bouts of anovulatory amenorrhea in PCOS patients. Progesterone breakthrough bleeding is due to an inappropriately high ratio of progesterone to estrogen. This type of bleeding is associated with long acting progestin-only contraceptives.

Patients with DUB can be treated medically, either with ovulation induction therapy if pregnancy is desired, or with progestin therapy to regulate the bleeding pattern. In the latter instance, the treatment of choice is oral medroxyprogesterone acetate, 10 mg/d for 10 d/mo. Combined oral contraceptive pills can be used if the patient desires contraception or if progestin alone fails to normalize the bleeding pattern. In addition, patients with menorrhagia and no obvious organic lesion may experience a significant reduction in their bleeding with prostaglandin synthetase inhibitors, which are believed to work by increasing the ratio of thromboxane A_2 to prostacyclin, thereby favoring platelet aggregation and vasoconstriction *(72)*.

ABNORMAL BLEEDING IN CHILDHOOD

Vaginal bleeding in early childhood, regardless of the duration or quantity, mandates both gynecologic and endocrinologic investigation. Two groups of conditions should be explored. Local lesions include vulvovaginitis, foreign bodies, trauma, urethral prolapse, vulvar skin disorders, botyroid sarcoma, and adenocarcinoma of the cervix or vagina. A detailed medical history and physical examination, including culture, vaginoscopy, and examination under anesthesia, will usually reveal an organic lesion that can be specifically treated.

Isosexual precocity is the onset of sexual maturation at any stage that is 2.5 SD earlier than the norm. Although definitions can vary, the appearance of secondary sexual characteristics before 8 yr of age in white girls and before age 6 yr in African-American girls is generally considered precocious *(73)*. It is important to distinguish central or true precocious puberty, which is characterized by the premature activation of the hypothalamic GnRH pulse generator, from GnRH-independent sexual precocity. This can be accomplished by measurement of LH at baseline or after administration of GnRH, when a sensitive assay is used. In one study, the mean peak serum LH concentration after stimulation was 3.1, 22, and 1.5 IU/L in 100 normal perpubertal children, 58 children with gonadotropin-dependent precocious puberty, and 10 children with gonadotropin-independent puberty, respectively *(74)*. The values for serum FSH are much less useful diagnostically. As tumors of the central nervous system may present with central precocious puberty, a cranial MRI is warranted. Among the lesions that may present are astrocytomas, ependymomas, gliomas, craniopharyngiomas, and hamartomas of the tuber cinereum. Other diseases of the central nervous system, such as hydrocephalus, encephalitis, brain abscess, and traumatic damage may also induce premature GnRH activation. After central nervous system disease has been excluded in the differential diagnosis for central precocious puberty, treatment with a GnRH analogue to suppress pituitary gonadotropin production may be initiated. Measurement of bone age is important both at the time of initial diagnosis and throughout treatment.

GnRH-independent forms of isosexual precocity stem from a direct increase in circulating sex steroids and are incomplete in their presentation *(73)*. Large autonomous ovarian cysts occasionally occur in young girls. As these follicular cysts often secrete estrogen, signs of sexual precocity and anovulatory vaginal bleeding can occur. Although these cysts often regress spontaneously, medroxyprogesterone and, rarely, laparoscopic drainage have been used in their treatment. Estrogen-secreting juvenile granulosa cell tumors of the ovary are another rare cause of GnRH-independent endometrial shedding. McCune-Albright syndrome is an uncommon form of gonadotropin-independent precocious puberty, in which an activating mutation of the α-subunit of the FSH receptor G-protein occurs. Testolactone, an aromatase inhibitor, and medroxyprogesterone are useful forms of therapy for this disease. Endometrial bleeding may also rarely result from inadvertent hormonal stimulation obtained through medications or diet.

ABNORMAL BLEEDING IN POSTMENOPAUSAL WOMEN

The median age of the menopause has been estimated by the Women's Massachusetts Health Study at approx age 51.3 yr. Only 10% of the women studied however, had an abrupt and permanent cessation of monthly menses, giving an indication of how commonly menstrual irregularity exists during the menopausal tradition *(75)*. The postmenopausal endometrium, in the absence of hormone replacement therapy, is atrophic and very thin. Excluding exogenous hormone administration as a cause, atrophic endometritis underlies 30% of all postmenopausal bleeding.

Relative hyperestrogenemia in the postmenopausal patient may occur secondary to extraglandular conversion of androgen, especially with obese patients. Other causes include residual follicular activity, steroid-producing tumors of the ovary, ovarian stromal hyperthecosis, and liver disease with its concomitant decreased level of sex hormone binding globulin production. Surprisingly, these sporadic elevations of estradiol are infrequently accompanied by endometrial withdrawal bleeding.

As endometrial cancer is responsible for 15% of all cases of postmenopausal bleeding, any such bleeding should be considered cancerous in origin until proven otherwise. A more difficult clinical situation occurs in the postmenopausal patient on hormone replacement therapy who experiences abnormal bleeding. Generally, a predictable bleeding pattern occurs in those patients on cyclic regimens, and small amounts of breakthrough bleeding is expected in those patients on continuous regimens. However, whenever the issue is in doubt, a work-up is mandatory. In postmenopausal patients who refuse cavity sampling, an endovaginal ultrasound provides a relatively noninvasive and expedient means of clinical assessment. The risk of uterine malignancy is reportedly very low when the endometrial thickness is <4 mm *(68)*.

CONCLUSION

The etiologies underlying menstrual dysfunction are diverse. These abnormal bleeding patterns are symptoms of an organic lesion or hormonal disturbance. A concise investigational approach, as well as a thorough understanding of the range of conditions that engender abnormal menstruation, is necessary to provide an expedient diagnosis and treatment plan. The initial evaluation includes a detailed history and physical assessment, including speculum and bimanual examinations, followed by selected laboratory studies.

REFERENCES

1. Welt CK, McNicholl DJ, Taylor AE, Hall JE. Female reproductive aging is marked by decreased secretion of dimeric inhibin. J Clin Endocrinol Metab 1999;84:105–111.
2. Hall JE, Martin KA, Taylor AE. Body weight and gonadotropin secretion in normal women and women with reproductive abnormalities. In: Hansel W, Bray GA, Ryan DH, eds. Pennington Center Nutrition Series: Vol 6 Nutrition and Reproduction. Louisiana State University Press, Baton Rouge, 1998, pp. 378–393.
3. Treloar AE, Boynton RE, Borghild GB, Brown BW. Variation of the human menstrual cycle through reproductive life. Int J Fertil 1967;12:77–126.
4. Gharib SD, Wierman ME, Shupnik MA, Chinn WW. Molecular biology of pituitary gonadotropins. Endocr Rev 1990;11:177–199.
5. Shupnik MA. Gonadal hormone feedback on pituitary gonadotropin genes. Trends Endocrinol. Metab. 1996;7:272–276.
6. Couse JF, Korach KS. Estrogen receptor null mice: what have we learned and where will they lead us? Endocr Rev 2000;20:258–417.
7. Herbison AE. Multimodal influence of estrogen upon gonadotropin-releasing hormone neurons. Endocr Rev 1998;19:302–330.
8. Karsch FJ, Bowen JM, Caraty A, Evans NP, Moenter SM. Gonadotropin-releasing hormone requirements for ovulation. Biol Reprod 1997;56:303–309.
9. Reindollar RH, Byrd JR, McDonough PG. Delayed sexual development: a study of 252 patients. Am J Obstet Gynecol 1981;140:371–380.
10. Reindollar RH, Novak M, Tho SP, McDonough PG. Adult-onset amenorrhea: a study of 262 patients. Am J Obstet Gynecol 1986;155:531–543.
11. McPhaul M. Molecular defects of the androgen receptor. J Steroid Biochem Mol Biol 1999;69:315–322.
12. Broome JD, Vancaillie TG. Fluoroscopically guided hysteroscopic division of adhesions in severe Asherman syndrome. Obstet Gynecol 1999;93:1041–1043.
13. Seminara SB, Hayes FJ, Crowley WF Jr. Gonadotropin-releasing hormone deficiency in the human (idiopathic hypogonadotropic hypogonadism and Kallmann's syndrome): pathophysiological and genetic considerations. Endocr Rev 1998;19:521–539.
14. Martin KA, Hall JE, Adams JM, Crowley WF Jr. Comparison of exogenous gonadotropins and pulsatile gonadotropin-releasing hormone for induction of ovulation in hypogonadotropic amenorrhea. J Clin Endocrinol Metab 1993;77:125–129.
15. deRoux N, Young J, Misrahi M, et al. A family with hypogonadotropic hypogonadism and mutations in the gonadotropin-releasing hormone receptor. N Engl J Med 1997;337:1597–1602.
16. Seminara SB, Beranova M, Oliveira LM, Martin KA, Crowley WF Jr, Hall JE. Successful use of pulsatile gonadotropin-releasing hormone (GnRH) for ovulation induction and pregnancy in a patient with GnRH receptor mutations. J Clin Endocrinol Metab 2000;85:556–562.
17. Szmukler GI. Weight and food preoccupation in a population of English schoolgirls. In: Understanding Anorexia Nervosa and Bulimia: Report of the Fourth Ross Conference on Medical Research. Ross Laboratories, Columbus, OH, 1983, p 21.
18. Genazzani AD, Petraglia F, Gastaldi M, et al. Naltrexone treatment restores menstrual cycles in patients with weight loss-related amenorrhea. Fertil Steril 1995;64:951–956.
19. Schweiger U, Pirke KM, Laessle RG, et al. Gonadotropin secretion in bulimia nervosa. J Clin Endocrinol Metab 1992;74:1122–1127.
20. Rigotti NA, Nussbaum SR, Herzog DB, et al. Osteoporosis in women with anorexia nervosa. N Engl J Med 1984;311:1601–1606.
21. Biller BMK, Saxe V, Herzog DB, et al. Mechanisms of osteoporosis in adult and adolescent women with anorexia nervosa. J Clin Endocrinol Metab 1989;68:548–554.
22. Shangold M, Rebar RW, Wentz AC, Schiff I. Evaluation and management of menstrual dysfunction in athletes. JAMA 1990;263:1665–1669.

23. Loucks AB, Heath EM. Dietary restriction reduces luteinizing hormone (LH) pulse frequency during waking hours and increases LH pulse amplitude during sleep in young women. J Clin Endocrinol Metab 1994;78:910–915.
24. Loucks AB, Verdun M, Heath EM. Low energy bioavailability, not stress of exercise, alters LH pulsatility in exercising women. J Appl Physiol 1998;84:37–46.
25. Laughlin GA, Yen SSC. Hypoleptinemia in women athletes: absence of a diurnal rhythm with amenorrhea. J Clin Endocrinol Metab 1997;82:318–321.
26. Drinkwater BL, Nilson K, Chesnut CH III, Bremner WJ, Shainholtz S, Southworth MB. Bone mineral content of amenorrheic and eumenorrheic athletes. N Engl J Med 1984;311:277–281.
27. Warren MP, Brooks-Gunn J, Hamilton LH, Warren LF, Hamilton WG. Scoliosis and fractures in young ballet dancers (relation to delayed menarche and secondary amenorrhea). N Engl J Med 1986;314:1348–1353.
28. Laughlin GA, Dominguez CE, Yen SSC. Nutritional and endocrine-metabolic aberrations in women with functional hypothalamic amenorrhea. J Clin Endocrinol Metab 1998;83:25–32.
29. Perkins R, Hall JE, Martin KA. Neuroendocrine abnormalities in hypothalamic amenorrhea: spectrum, stability, and response to neurotransmitter modulation. J Clin Endocrinol Metab 1999;84:1905–1911.
30. Berga SL, Loucks AB, Rossmanith WG, Kettel LM, Laughlin GA, Yen SS. Acceleration of luteinizing hormone pulse frequency in functional hypothalamic amenorrhea by dopaminergic blockade. J Clin Endocrinol Metab 1991;72:151–156.
31. Warren MP, Voussoughian F, Geer EB, Hyle EP, Adbeg CL, Ramos RH. Functional hypothalamic amenorrhea: hypoleptinemia and disordered eating. J Clin Endocrinol Metab 1999;84:873–877.
32. Perkins RB, Hall JE, Martin KA. Aetiology, previous menstrual function and patterns of neuroendocrine disturbance as prognostic indicators in hypothalamic amenorrhoea. Hum Reprod 2001;16:2198–2205.
33. Biller BMK, Coughlin JF, Saxe V, et al. Osteopenia in women with hypothalamic amenorrhea: a prospective study. Obstet Gynecol 1991;78:996–1001.
34. Snyder PJ. Gonadtroph adenomas. Curr Ther Endocrinol Metab 1997;6:56–68.
35. Serri O, Rasio E, Beauregard H, Hardy J, Soma M. Recurrence of hyperprolactinemia after selective transsphenoidal adenomectomy in women with prolactinoma. N Engl J Med 1983;309:280–283.
36. Klibanski A, Neer RM, Beitins IZ, Ridgway EC, Zervas NT, McArthur JW. Decreased bone density in hyperprolactinemic women. N Engl J Med 1980;303:1511–1514.
37. Schlecte JA, Sherman B, Martin R. Bone density in amenorrheic women with and without hyperprolactinemia. J Clin Endocrinol Metab 1983;56:11203-#1123.
38. Adashi EY, Hennebold JD. Single-gene mutations resulting in reproductive dysfunction in women. N Engl J Med 1999;340:709–718.
39. Saenger P. Current concepts: Turner's syndrome. N Engl J Med 1996;335:1749–1754.
40. Coulam CB, Adamson SC, Annaegers JF. Incidence of premature ovarian failure. Obstet Gynecol 1986;67:604–606.
41. Taylor AE, Adams JM, Mulder JE, Martin KA, Sluss PM, Crowley WF Jr. A randomized, controlled trial of estradiol replacement therapy in women with hypergonadotropic amenorrhea. J Clin Endocrinol Metab 1996;81:3615–3621.
42. Krauss CM, Turksoy RN, Atkins L, McLaughlin C, Brown LG, Page DC. Familial premature ovarian failure due to an interstitial deletion of the long arm of the X chromosome. N Engl J Med 1987;16:125–131.
43. Taylor AE. Should women with premature menopause be screened for FMR-1 mutations? Menopause 2001;8:81–83.
44. Luborsky JL, Visintin I, Boyers S, Asari T, Caldwell B, DeCherney A. Ovarian antibodies detected by immobilized antigen immunoassay in patients with premature ovarian failure. J Clin Endocrinol Metab 1990;70:69–75.

45. Belvisi L, Bombelli F, Sironi L, Doldi N. Organ-specific autoimmunity in patients with premature ovarian failure. J Endocrinol Invest 1993;16:889–892.
46. Betterle C, Rossi A, Dalla Pria S, et al. Premature ovarian failure: autoimmunity and natural history. Clin Endocrinol (Oxf) 1993;39:35–43.
47. van Kasteren YM, Braat DD, Hemrika DJ. Corticosteroids do not influence ovarian responsiveness to gonadotropins in patients with premature ovarian failure: a randomized, placebo-controlled trial. Fertil Steril 1999;71:90–95.
48. Lydic ML, Liu JH, Rebar RW, Thomas MA, Cedars MI. Success of donor oocyte in *in vitro* fertilization-embryo transfer in recipients with and without premature ovarian failure. Fertil Steril 1996;65:98–102.
49. Rebar RW, Cedars MI. Hypergonadotropic forms of amenorrhea in young women. Endocrinol Metab Clin North Am 1992;21:173–191.
50. Taylor AE. Polycystic ovary syndrome. Endocrinol Metab Clin North Am 1998;27:877–902.
51. Legro RS. Polycystic ovary syndrome: the new millenium. Mol Cell Endocrinol 2001;184:87–93.
52. Dunaif A, Thomas A. Current concepts in the polycystic ovary syndrome. Annu Rev Med 2001;52:401–419.
53. Zawadski JK, Dunaif A. Diagnostic criteria for polycystic ovary syndrome: towards a rational approach. In: Dunaif A, Givens J, Haseltine FP, Merriam GH, eds. Current Issues in Endocrinology and Metabolism: Polycystic Ovary Syndrome. Blackwell Scientific Publications, Boston, 1992, pp. 377–384.
54. Dewailly D, Duhamel A, Robert Y, et al. Interrelationship between ultrasonography and biology in the diagnosis of polycystic ovarian syndrome. Ann NY Acad Sci 1993;687:206.
55. Taylor AE, McCourt B, Martin KA, et al. Determinants of abnormal gonadotropin secretion in clinically defined women with polycystic ovary syndrome. J Clin Endocrinol Metab 1997;82:2248–2256.
56. Polson DW, Adams J, Wadsworth J, et al. Polycystic ovaries—a common finding in normal women. Lancet 1988;1:870–872.
57. Buyalos RP, Lee C. Polycystic ovary syndrome: pathophysiology and outcome with in vitro fertilization. Fertil Steril 1996;65:1–10.
58. McArthur JW, Ingersoll FM, Worcester J. The urinary excretion of interstitial-cell and follicle stimulationg hormone activity by women with diseases of the reproductive system. J Clin Endocrinol Metab 1958;18:1202.
59. Waldstreicher J, Santoro N, Hall JE, Filicori M, Crowley WF Jr. Hyperfunction of the hypothalamic-pituitary axis in women with polycystic ovarian disease: indirect evidence for partial gonadotroph desensitization. J Clin Endocrinol Metab 1988;66:165–172.
60. Marshall JC, Eagleson CA. Neuroendocrine aspects of polycystic ovary syndrome. Endocrinol Metab Clin North Am 1999;28:295–324.
61. Arroyo A, Laughlin GA, Morales AJ, et al. Inappropriate gonadotropin secretion in polycystic ovary syndrome: influence of adiposity. J Clin Endocrinol Metab 1997;82:3728#-33733.
62. Kaiser UB, Sabbagh E, Katzenellenbogen RA, Conn PM, Chin WW. A mechanism for the differential regulation of gonadotropin subunit gene expression by gonadotropin-releasing hormone. Proc Natl Acad Sci USA 1995;92:12280–12284.
63. Nelson VL, Legro RS, Strauss JF III, McAllister JM. Augmented androgen production is a stable steroidogenic phenotype of propagated theca cells from polycystic ovaries. Mol Endocrinol 1999;13:946–957.
64. Nestler JE, Stovall D, Akhter N, Iurno MJ, Jakubowicz DJ. Strategies for the use of insulin-sensitizing drugs to treat infertility in women with polycystic ovary syndrome. Fertil Steril 2002;77:209–215.
65. Erhmann DA. Glucose intolerance in the polycystic ovary syndrome: role of the pancreatic beta-cell. J Pediatr Endocrinol 2000;13(Suppl 5):1299–1301.

66. Bokhman JV. Two pathogenetic types of endometrial carcinoma. Gynecol Oncol 1983;15:10–17.
67. Smith P, Bakos O, Heimer G, Ulmsten U. Transvaginal ultrasound for identifying endometrial abnormality. Acta Obstet Gynecol Scand 1991;70:591–794.
68. Townsend DE, Fields G, McCausland, Kauffman K. Diagnostic and operative hysteroscopy in the management of persistent postmenopausal bleeding. Obstet Gynecol 1993;82:419–421.
69. Widrich T, Bradley LD, Mitchinson AR, Collins RI. Comparison of saline infusion sonography with office hysteroscopy for the evaluation of the endometrium. Am J Obstet Gynecol 1996;174:1327–1334.
70. Fraser IS, Michie EA, Wide L, Baird DT. Pituitary gonadotropins and ovarian function in adolescents with dysfunctional uterine bleeding. J Clin Endocrinol Metab 1973;37:407–414.
71. Santoro N, Rosenberg-Brown J, Adel T, Skrunick JH. Characterization of reproductive hormonal dynamics in the perimenopause. J Clin Endocrinol Metab 1996;81:1495–1501.
72. Bonnar J, Sheppard BL. Treatment of menorrhagia during menstruation: randomized controlled trial of ethamsylate, mefenamic acid, and tranexamic acid. BMJ 1996;313:579–582.
73. Palmert MR, Boepple PA. Variation in the timing of puberty: clinical spectrum and genetic investigation. J Clin Endocrinol Metab 2001;86:2364–2368.
74. Brito VN, Batista MC, Borges MF, et al. Diagnostic value of fluiorimetric assays in the evaluation of precocious puberty. J Clin Endocrinol Metab 1999;84:3539–3544.
75. Noci I, Borri P, Scarselli G, et al. Morphological and functional aspects of the endometrium of asymptomatic post-menopausal women: does the endometrium really age? Hum Reprod 1996;11:2246–2250.

16 Differential Diagnosis and Evaluation of Hyperandrogenism

Ricardo Azziz, MD, MPH, MBA

Contents

INTRODUCTION

Androgen excess or hyperandrogenism is one of the most common reproductive endocrinologic defects in women, affecting 5–10% of the reproductive-aged female population. The most common cause of hyperandrogenism is the polycystic ovary syndrome (PCOS), with nonclassic adrenal hyperplasia (NCAH), androgen-secreting tumors, and androgenic drug intake being much less frequent. Hyperandrogenism, the endocrine disorder, should be distinguished from dermatological disorders such as hirsutism, although there is significant overlap. Hirsutism affects approx 6–7% of reproductive-aged women in the United States, and is a common manifestation of androgen excess (Table 1). Nonetheless, hyperandrogenism may present without obvious peripheral manifestations, as in the PCOS patient of Asian extraction with little or absent hirsutism. Alternatively, not all hirsute patients have evidence of detectable androgen excess or endocrine imbalance, as in patients with "idiopathic hirsutism." Finally, androgen excess can also be suspected in those women with other peripheral hyperandrogenic signs, including acne, excessive oiliness or seborrhea, and alopecia. Here, we briefly review the differential diagnosis of androgen excess and denote the diagnostic scheme used for the evaluation of these patients.

Polycystic Ovarian Syndrome (PCOS)

PCOS affects about 4% of the general population of reproductive-aged women *(1)* and between 65–85% of all hirsute women seen. The ovary usually contains intermediate and atretic follicles measuring 2–8 mm in diameter giving the ovary

From: *Contemporary Endocrinology: Handbook of Diagnostic Endocrinology*
Edited by: J. E. Hall and L. K. Nieman © Humana Press Inc., Totowa, NJ

Table1
Differential Diagnosis of Hirsutism

Etiology	*Approximate % of all hirsute patients seen*
PCOS (including hyperthecosis)	approx 80%
Idiopathic hirsutism	approx 15%
HAIRAN syndrome	2–4%
NCAH (21-OH-deficient)	1–2%
Ovarian tumors	Rare
Others	Very rare

a "polycystic" picture on sonography or pathology. A polycystic picture on ultrasound is not diagnostic of PCOS, as approx 25% of normal women with regular ovulatory cycles also demonstrate this pattern. Forty to sixty percent of patients with pathologically diagnosed PCOS are obese, 60–90% are hirsute, 50–90% are amenorrheic, approx 7–16% have regular menses, and 55–75% complain of infertility *(2)*. The etiology(s) of this disorder is unclear, although it appears to have a strong familial association. PCOS appears to be multifactorial, with abnormalities of ovarian and adrenal steroidogenesis, of hypothalamic-pituitary-adrenal or ovarian control, and of insulin action. In fact, approx 50–60% of these patients, regardless of body weight, demonstrate varying degrees of insulin resistance, although generally to a lesser degree than patients with the hyperandrogenic insulin-resistant acanthosis nigricans (HAIRAN) syndrome *(3)*. The role of obesity in this disorder is unclear, although many obese patients with PCOS demonstrate primarily abdominal/visceral (anthropoid) regional fat distribution. This type of fat deposition is associated with an increased risk of metabolic abnormalities (e.g., insulin resistance, glucose intolerance, dyslipidemia, hypertension, etc.).

PCOS patients generally do not present with symptoms of virilization or masculinization. The diagnosis is usually established by the clinical evidence of hyperandrogenism and/or hyperandrogenemia (i.e., elevated circulating levels of testosterone [T], free T, androstenedione [A4] and/or dehydroepiandrosterone sulfate [DHEAS]); after the exclusion of other androgen excess disorders (i.e., NCAH, HAIRAN syndrome, tumors). Prolactin levels are usually normal or only slightly elevated (generally <40 ng/mL). The luteinizing hormone (LH)/folliculestimulating hormone (FSH) ratio may be 2 to 3:1, although this is observed in only 40–60% of patients.

HAIRAN Syndrome

Between 1–5% of hyperandrogenic women suffer from a syndrome characterized by hyperandrogenism, insulin resistance, and acanthosis nicrians (HAIRAN syndrome). This syndrome forms part of a heterogeneous collection of inherited disorders of insulin action on glucose homeostasis (i.e., Kahn Type A). The insulin resistance is most often due to an insulin postreceptor defect, although a few patients may have an insulin receptor abnormality. Very rarely will these women have circulating anti-insulin antibodies. Patients with the HAIRAN syndrome generally exhibit compensatory hyperinsulinemia, with extremely high circulating levels of insulin (generally >80 μU/mL in the fasting state and/or 500 μU/mL following an oral glucose challenge test) *(4,5)*. In the early stages, their fasting glucose levels will be relatively normal in the face of this massive increase in insulin levels. However, as patients age and/or become obese, pancreatic islet β-cell exhaustion becomes apparent, with the appearance of glucose intolerance and, eventually, type 2 diabetes mellitus.

In spite of the relative resistance to insulin at the level of glycemic control, the resultant hyperinsulinemia affects other organs. For example, in the epidermis of the skin, acanthosis nigricans will develop, with hyperplasia of the basal layers of the epidermis. This results in a velvety hyperpigmented change of the crural areas of the skin, particularly the nape of the neck. Likewise, significant dyslipidemia and hypertension may be present, secondary to as yet undetermined mechanisms. At the ovarian level, insulin acts synergistically with LH to stimulate increased androgen production by the theca-stroma cells, resulting in hyperandrogenemia and clinical hyperandrogenism. These girls can be severely hyperandrogenic and can even be masculinized.

This syndrome should not be confused with the milder degrees of insulin resistance noted among many patients with the PCOS (see above). A fasting insulin and glucose level will serve to select and/or diagnose most patients with the HAIRAN syndrome, while some may need to undergo an oral glucose tolerance test (OGTT), measuring both glucose and insulin responses, or an insulin tolerance test, if significant β-cell damage has already occurred.

Nonclassical Congenital Adrenal Hyperplasia (NCAH)

Between 1% and 10% (depending on ethnicity) of hyperandrogenic women suffer from NCAH *(6)*. The most common cause is a deficiency in the activity of adrenocortical 21-hydroxylase (21-OH), resulting from the activity of the enzyme P450c21. The precursors to 21-OH accumulate in excess, specifically, 17α-hydroxyprogesterone (17-HP) and A4. The excessive adrenal production of progestogens and androgens leads to the symptoms of hirsutism, acne, and oligo-ovulation. Clinically, these patients are very difficult to distinguish from other hyperandrogenic patients *(7)*. Furthermore, the levels of the exclusive adrenal androgen DHEAS are not any higher than in other hyperandro-genic women *(8)*. The measurement of a baseline 17-HP obtained in the morning and in the follicular phase can be used to screen for this disorder. If the screening 17-HP is higher than 2 to 3 ng/mL, then the patient should undergo an acute andrenocorticotrophic hormone (ACTH) stimulation test for diagnosis *(9,10)*. These patients can be easily treated with oral contraceptives, corticosteroid replacement, and/or clomiphene. Other, much more uncommon causes of NCAH include deficiencies of 11α-hydroxylase (11-OH) and 3β-hydroxysteroid dehydrogenase (3β-HSD), although since they are so rare, screening for them is not merited.

Androgen-Secreting Tumors

Androgen-producing tumors are relatively rare. They should be suspected when the onset of androgenic symptoms is sudden (i.e., generally <2 yr) and the pace of symptoms is rapid, and when they lead to virilization and masculinization. They may be associated with other systemic symptoms including weight loss, anorexia, a feeling of abdominal bloating, back pain, etc. These tumors usually originate in the ovary or in the adrenal. It is important to know that suppression and stimulation tests can be misleading and are not encouraged for the diagnosis of these neoplasias. It should always be remembered that the best predictor of an androgen-producing tumor is clinical presentation.

Androgen-producing tumors of the adrenal are relatively rare. Adrenal tumors can be suspected when circulating DHEAS is >7000 ng/mL, although the clinical presentation is the most sensitive indicator (i.e., Cushingoid features and/or virilization). Occasional tumors will primarily secrete testosterone. A computed axial tomography (CT) scan of the adrenal usually establishes the diagnosis. Most neoplasms are adrenal carcinomas, frequently associated with Cushingoid features *(11)*. These tumors are generally large (>6 cm) and can be easily identified on CT scan by their irregular outline. Unfortunately, their prognosis is very poor. Adenomas of the adrenal cortex, which secrete DHEA, DHEAS, A4, or T in the absence of glucocorticoids are extremely rare.

Ovarian tumors are somewhat more frequent, occurring in 1/300 to 1/1000 of hyperandrogenic women *(12)*. They are usually palpable on pelvic exam and/or are associated with unilateral ovarian enlargement on ultrasound or CT scan. These tumors are generally not malignant, and include Sertoli-Leydig and lipoid cell tumors. Ovarian tumors can be suspected when the circulating T is persistently greater than 200 or 300 ng/dL (depending on the upper normal limit of T in the specific laboratory used). However, it is important to understand that 20% of androgen-producing ovarian tumors may have T levels below this *(13)*. Furthermore, the majority of women with T levels over 200 ng/dL have HAIRAN syndrome, hyperthecosis, or PCOS and not an ovarian tumor *(12)*.

Androgenic Medications

It is obvious that the excessive ingestion of androgenic drugs can result in masculinization and hirsutism. The use and abuse of androgens (e.g., testosterone propionate, methyltestosterone, stanazol, etc.) for body building in women is a real risk for the development of hirsutism, in addition to amenorrhea and liver dysfunction. The prolonged use of danazol for the treatment of endometriosis, angioneurotic edema, or thrombocytopenia purpura can also result in excess hair growth. However, the most common cause of iatrogenic hirsutism today relates to the use of androgen supplementation (e.g., methyltestosterone orally or testosterone propionate intramuscularly) during menopause. In general, these drugs cause only mild degrees of acne, oily skin, and/or hirsutism.

Idiopathic Hirsutism

The diagnosis of idiopathic hirsutism is reached when the patient is obviously hirsute, and she has regular ovulation. Furthermore, these patients often have normal circulating androgen levels. Approximately 15–30% of hirsute women will have the diagnosis of idiopathic hirsutism *(14)*. However, it should be understood that many of these patients simply demonstrate degrees of hyperandro-genemia that may not be detectable with routine clinical androgen assays. Approximately 40% of hirsute women who claim to have regular menses demonstrate oligo-ovulation when studied more carefully *(15)*. In many of these women, the 5α-reductase activity in the skin and hair follicle may be overactive leading to hirsutism in the face of normal circulating levels of T. The measurement of 3α-androstanediol glucuronide in serum may help to confirm the hyperfunction of 5α-reductase, since this hormone is a peripheral metabolite of dihydro-testosterone (DHT). However, this hormone is neither helpful nor necessary to make the diagnosis of idiopathic hirsutism, which is usually established when hirsutism is encountered in the face of regular ovulation.

EVALUATION OF ANDROGEN EXCESS

In evaluating the patient with suspected hyperandrogenism, the differential diagnosis reviewed above should be kept in mind. A thorough history will often serve to focus the evaluation. In taking a history, practitioners should attempt to exclude the use or abuse of androgenic/anabolic drugs and skin irritants. A detailed menstrual history should be obtained, with an emphasis at determining whether evidence of ovulatory function (e.g., premenstrual molimina, such as breast tenderness) is present. The onset and progression of hirsutism, acne, or balding and hair loss should be noted. A history of changes in weight, extremity or head size, or facial contour should be elicited. Finally, a detailed family history of endocrine, reproductive, or metabolic disorders should be obtained. Rapid progression of androgenization, particularly appearing some time after puberty, or in the menopause, is most suggestive of an androgen-secreting neoplasm and not PCOS. Likewise, if the degree of androgenization is severe, resulting in clitoromegaly, male pattern balding, masculinization of the body (i.e., decrease in breast size, increase in muscle mass, loss of hip to waist discordance, etc.) an androgenic tumor or syndrome of severe insulin resistance should be considered.

On the physical exam, the type and pattern of excessive hair growth should be noted and preferably scored. A useful graphical scoring method is that published by Hatch and colleagues, scoring nine body areas *(16)*. The presence of galactorrhea, virilization, masculinization, pelvic and abdominal masses, obesity, Cushingoid features, "bluntness" of facial features, thyroid enlargement, and signs of systemic illness should be excluded. Overall, it is most important during the physical exam to determine whether hirsutism or other hyperandrogenic features are truly present, and whether there are signs or symptoms of related disorders. The presence of Cushingoid features (i.e., "yoke-like" centripetal obesity, muscle wasting of the extremities, moon facies, generalized facial rubor, or purple-red abdominal striae) in association with hirsutism is particularly worrisome. These features suggest the possibility of either an adrenocortical carcinoma, or ACTH excess, due to either an ectopic ACTH-producing tumor or to a pituitary tumor (i.e., Cushing's disease).

The laboratory evaluation should not be excessive nor unfocused *(17)*. For diagnostic purposes, at a minimum, the levels of thyroid-stimulating hormone (TSH), prolactin, and 17-HP should be to exclude thyroid dysfunction, hyperprolactinemia, and 21-OH-deficient NCAH, respectively. Screening for 21-OH deficient NCAH can be done by measuring the circulating 17-HP in the follicular phase of the menstrual cycle (if the patient is ovulatory), preferably in the morning *(10)*. If the 17-HP level is over 2 ng/mL (200 ng/dL) ,and it is certain that the sample was obtained in the pre-ovulatory phase, the patient should undergo an acute adrenal stimulation testing. For this test, 250 µg (1 vial) of 1–24 ACTH (Cortrosyn®, Organon, New Orange, NJ) is injected intravenously, and a 17-HP level is checked 30–60 min later. If the 17-HP level following ACTH-(1–24) administration is >10 ng/mL (or 30 nmol/L), the diagnosis of 21-OH-deficient NCAH is highly probable, and if >15 ng/mL (45 nmol/L), it is established. It is unnecessary to screen for 3β-HSD or 11α-OH-deficient NCAH, since these disorders are extremely rare.

Total and free T and DHEAS, and LH/FSH levels may also be measured, although the added diagnostic value of these tests is probably minimal and may actually serve to confuse or distract the practitioner. For example, the total T level may be useful for determining the severity of the androgen excess and to indicate which patients may need further evaluation for a tumor. As indicated above, the specificity and sensitivity (and positive predictive value) of a serum T level for the prediction of androgen-secreting neoplasms is quite poor *(12)*. Furthermore, the accuracy of laboratory assays for this steroid is questionable. The DHEAS measurement may also suggest a tumor or 3β-HSD deficient NCAH, although it is more useful as a marker of adrenal androgen excess. Patients with very high levels of DHEAS and acne may benefit from corticosteroid suppression, as may some clomiphene-treated oligo-ovulatory infertile patients. Nonetheless, the specificity and sensitivity of DHEAS as a marker for adrenal tumors is poor, and it is clearly not a marker of 21-OH-deficient NCAH.

It should be remembered that PCOS is a disorder of exclusion, i.e., where oligo-ovulation and hyperandrogenism are demonstrated, and other related or similar disorders are excluded. Hence, patients with oligomenorrhea (e.g., <6–8 cycles/yr) and hirsutism have PCOS, if they are found not to have other disorders such as hyperprolactinemia, thyroid dysfunction, NCAH, or an androgen-secreting neoplasm. If a patient has hirsutism (or other peripheral sign of hyperdro-genism) and has regular menses, her ovulatory function should be confirmed by obtaining a basal body temperature chart and a progesterone level on d 22–24 (i.e., 22–24 d after the start of the patients menstrual flow). Likewise, the hirsute patient would have PCOS if she is proven to be oligo-ovulatory, even in the absence of elevated androgen levels.

If a diagnosis of PCOS is confirmed, an assessment of the patient's metabolic status should be made. At a minimum, this may include measuring the fasting glucose level. The addition of a fasting insulin level may also be helpful, since recently Legro and colleagues suggested that a glucose to insulin ratio of <4.5 was a good indicator of insulin resistance *(3)*. However, the measurement of glucose and insulin levels 2-h postprandial, or following the administration of 75 g glucose (or dextrose), may be a more sensitive indicator of hyperinsulinemia (and by inference, insulin resistance). Although specific guidelines do not exist, it may be appropriate to also obtain a lipid profile and a glycosylated hemoglobin (i.e., hemoglobin A1C) every 2 to 3 yr in women with PCOS who are over 35 yr, particularly if they have a strong family history of non-insulin-dependent diabetes mellitus (NIDDM) or cardiovascular disease.

REFERENCES

1. Knochenhauer ES, Key TJ, Kasar-Miller M, Waggoner W, Boots LR, Azziz R. Prevalence of the polycystic ovarian syndrome in unselected black and white women of the southeastern United States: a prospective study. J Clin Endocrinol Metab 1998;83:3078–3082.
2. Goldzieher JW, Axelrod LR. Clinical and biochemical features of polycystic ovarian disease. Fertil Steril 1963;14:631–653.
3. Legro RS, Finegood D, Dunaif A. A fasting glucose to insulin ratio is a useful measure of insulin sensitivity in women with polycystic ovary syndrome. J Clin Endocrinol Metab 1998;83:2694–2698.
4. Barbieri RL, Ryan KJ. Hyperandrogenism, insulin resistance, and acanthosis nigricans syndrome: a common endocrinopathy with distinct pathophysiologic features. Am J Obstet Gynecol 1983;147:90–101.
5. Azziz R. The hyperandrogenic-insulin resistant-acanthosis nigricans (HAIRAN) syndrome: therapeutic response. Fertil Steril 1994;61:570–572.
6. Azziz R, Dewailly D, Owerbach D. Non-classic adrenal hyperplasia: current concepts. J Clin Endocrinol Metab 1994;78:810–815.
7. Moran C, Azziz R, Carmina E, et al. 21-Hydroxylase deficient non-classic adrenal hyperplasia is a progressive disorder: a multicenter study. Am J Obstet Gynecol 2000;183:1468–1474.
8. Kuttenn F, Couillin P, Girard F, et al. Late-onset adrenal hyperplasia in hirsutism. N Engl J Med 1985;313:224–231.
9. Azziz R, Zacur HA. 21-Hydroxylase deficiency in female hyperandrogenemia: screening and diagnosis. J Clin Endocrinol Metab 1989;69:577–584

10. Azziz R, Hincapie LA, Knochenhauer ES, Dewailly D, Fox L, Boots LR. Screening for 21-hydroxylase deficient non-classic adrenal hyperplasia among hyperandrogenic women: a prospective study. Fertil Steril 1999; 72:915–925.
11. Derksen J, Nagesser SK, Meinders AE, Haak HR, Van De Velde CJH. Identification of virilizing adrenal tumors in hirsute women. N Engl J Med 1994;331:968–973.
12. Waggoner W, Boots LR, Azziz R. Total testosterone and DHEAS levels as predictors of androgen-secreting neoplasms: a populational study. Gynecol Endocrinol 1999;13:1–7.
13. Meldrum DR, Abraham GE. Peripheral and ovarian venous concentrations of various steroid hormones in virilizing ovarian tumors. Obstet Gynecol 1979;53:36–43.
14. Azziz R, Carmina E, Sawaya ME. Idiopathic hirsutism. Endocrine Reviews 2000;21:347–362.
15. Azziz R, Waggoner WT, Ochoa T, Knochenhauer ES, Boots LR. Idiopathic hirsutism: an uncommon cause of hirsutism in Alabama. Fertil Steril 1998;70:274–278.
16. Hatch R, Rosenfield RL, Kim MH, Tredway D. Hirsutism: Implications, etiology, and management. Am J Abstet Gynecol 1981;140:815–830.
17. Azziz R. The time has come to simplify the evaluation of the hirsute patient. Fertil Steril 2000;74:870–872.

Index

E

W

X

Y

MIX
Papier aus verantwortungsvollen Quellen
Paper from responsible sources
FSC® C105338

If you have any concerns about our products,
you can contact us on
ProductSafety@springernature.com

In case Publisher is established outside the EU,
the EU authorized representative is:
Springer Nature Customer Service Center GmbH
Europaplatz 3, 69115 Heidelberg, Germany

Printed by Libri Plureos GmbH
in Hamburg, Germany